The Oral-Systemic Health Connection

A Guide to Patient Care

S0-BKI-334

The Oral-Systemic Health Connection

A Guide to Patient Care

Edited by

Michael Glick, DMD

Professor, Oral Diagnostic Sciences
Dean, School of Dental Medicine
University at Buffalo
The State University of New York
Buffalo, New York

quintessence books

Quintessence Publishing Co, Inc

Chicago, Berlin, Tokyo, London, Paris, Milan, Barcelona, Beijing, Istanbul,
Moscow, New Delhi, Prague, São Paulo, Seoul, Singapore, and Warsaw

Library of Congress Cataloging-in-Publication Data

The oral-systemic health connection : a guide to patient care / edited by Michael Glick.
    p. ; cm.
 Includes bibliographical references and index.
 ISBN 978-0-86715-650-8 (softcover)
 I. Glick, Michael, editor of compilation.
 [DNLM: 1. Oral Health. 2. Diagnosis, Oral. 3. Preventive Dentistry--methods. 4. Risk Factors.
 WU 113]
 RK61
 617.6--dc23
                                    2013040070

 5 4 3 2 1

quintessence
books
© 2014 Quintessence Publishing Co Inc

Quintessence Publishing Co Inc
4350 Chandler Drive
Hanover Park, IL 60133
www.quintpub.com

All rights reserved. This book or any part thereof may not be reproduced, stored in a retrieval
system, or transmitted in any form or by any means, electronic, mechanical, photocopying,
or otherwise, without prior written permission of the publisher.

Editor: Leah Huffman
Design: Ted Pereda
Production: Sue Robinson

Printed in China

Contents

Preface

The notion that infections in the oral cavity may influence overall health is not a novel idea. More than 2,000 years ago, Hippocrates was credited with curing arthritis by extracting a presumably infected tooth. The concept of an oral focal infection theory—ie, an infection in the mouth can, through various mechanisms, affect distant sites—was originated in the 1890s by an American microbiologist and dentist, Willoughby D. Miller.[1,2] Dr Miller famously wrote:

> During the last few years the conviction has grown continually stronger, among physicians as well as dentists, that the human mouth, as a gathering-place and incubator of diverse pathogenic germs, performs a significant role in the production of varied disorders of the body, and that if many diseases whose origin is enveloped in mystery could be traced to their source, they would be found to have originated in the oral cavity.

For the next 50 years, this theory was promulgated by many prominent scholars, but challenges to this theory started to emerge in the late 1930s and early 1940s. An important article by Cecil and Angevine in 1938 summarized their and others' opinions about focal infection as discussed at the time: "Focal infection is a splendid example of a plausible medical theory which is in danger of being converted by its enthusiastic supporters into the status of an accepted fact."[3] This cautionary tale still rings true.

The final demise of the focal theory, as it was known at that time, can be traced to a paper published in the *Journal of the American Medical Association* in 1940 entitled "Focal infection and systemic disease: A critical appraisal," by Drs Reimann and Havens.[4] These authors failed to find any scientific rigor or proofs of the claims made that "oral sepsis" was the culprit of the multitude of diseases attributed to it.

In the late 1980s, a renewed interest in the effect of oral infection on overall health started to emerge. Thanks to the gradual increased availability of large databases, significant statistical association specifically between periodontal diseases and systemic diseases and conditions could be inferred. During the past 35 years, thousands of articles have been published on this topic.

Information about the association between oral infections and systemic conditions can be found not only in the biomedical literature but also in the popular press, as sensationalized by talk show hosts and found on numerous websites. The oral-systemic connection is not a simple concept, and new data and theories are evolving that try to explain this association. It is essential that oral health care professionals be knowledgeable about the many different aspects of oral-systemic connections and able to communicate accurate and scientifically valid information to patients and other interested parties. This book brings clarity and insight to an important topic that oral health care professionals must be able to communicate to their patients and use to guide treatment decisions.

References

1. Miller WD. The human mouth as a focus of infection. Dent Cosmos 1891;33:689–713.
2. Miller WD. The human mouth as a focus of infection. Lancet 1891;138:340–342.
3. Cecil RL, Angevine DM. Clinical and experimental observations on the focal infection, with an analysis of 200 cases of rheumatoid arthritis. Ann Intern Med 1938;12:577–84.
4. Reimann HA, Havens WP. Focal infection and systemic disease: A critical appraisal—The case against indiscriminate removal of teeth and tonsils. JAMA 1940;114:1–6.

Contributors

Yiorgos A. Bobetsis, DDS, PhD
Lecturer
Department of Periodontology
National and Kapodistrian University of Athens,
    School of Dentistry
Athens, Greece

Wenche S. Borgnakke, DDS, MPH, PhD
Senior Research Associate
Adjunct Clinical Assistant Professor
Department of Periodontics and Oral Medicine
University of Michigan School of Dentistry
Ann Arbor, Michigan

Donald M. Brunette, PhD
Professor
Department of Oral Biological and Medical
    Sciences
Faculty of Dentistry
University of British Columbia
Vancouver, British Columbia
Canada

Ilene Fennoy, MD, MPH
Professor of Pediatrics
Columbia University Medical Center
Columbia University College of Physicians and
    Surgeons
New York, New York

Marcelo O. Freire, DDS, PhD
Postdoctoral Fellow
Department of Applied Oral Sciences
The Forsyth Institute
Cambridge, Massachusetts

Department of Oral Medicine, Infection and
    Immunity
Harvard School of Dental Medicine
Boston, Massachusetts

Robert J. Genco, DDS, PhD
SUNY Distinguished Professor of Oral Biology
    and Microbiology and Immunology
University at Buffalo
The State University of New York
Buffalo, New York

Filippo Graziani, DDS, MClinDent, PhD
Assistant Professor of Periodontology
Unit of Dentistry and Oral Surgery
University of Pisa
Pisa, Italy

Barbara L. Greenberg, MSc, PhD
Chair, Epidemiology and Community Health
School of Health Science and Practice
New York Medical College
Valhalla, New York

Ira B. Lamster, DDS, MMSc
Professor of Health Policy & Management
Mailman School of Public Health
Dean Emeritus
Columbia University College of Dental
    Medicine
New York, New York

Robert E. Marx, DDS
Professor of Surgery and Chief
Division of Oral and Maxillofacial Surgery
University of Miami
Miller School of Medicine
Miami, Florida

Panos N. Papapanou, DDS, PhD
Professor of Dental Medicine
Chair, Section of Oral and Diagnostic Sciences
Director, Division of Periodontics
Columbia University College of Dental Medicine
New York, New York

Douglas E. Peterson, DMD, PhD,
  FDS RCSEd
Professor of Oral Medicine
School of Dental Medicine
Co-Chair, Program in Head and Neck Cancer
  and Oral Oncology
Neag Comprehensive Cancer Center
University of Connecticut Health Center
Farmington, Connecticut

Frank A. Scannapieco, DMD, PhD
Professor and Chair
Department of Oral Biology
School of Dental Medicine
University at Buffalo
The State University of New York
Buffalo, New York

Mary Tavares, DMD, MPH
Senior Clinical Investigator
The Forsyth Institute
Cambridge, Massachusetts

Program Director, Dental Public Health
Harvard School of Dental Medicine
Boston, Massachusetts

Maurizio S. Tonetti, DMD, PhD, MMSc
Executive Director
European Research Group on Periodontology

Private practice
Milan, Italy

Thomas E. Van Dyke, DDS, PhD
Vice President of Clinical and Translational
  Research
Chair, Department of Applied Oral Sciences
Senior Member of the Staff
The Forsyth Institute
Cambridge, Massachusetts

Alessandro Villa, DMD, PhD, MPH
Assistant Professor of Oral Medicine
Department of General Dentistry
Boston University Henry M. Goldman School
  of Dental Medicine
Boston, Massachusetts

David T. W. Wong, DMD, DMSc
Felix and Mildred Yip Endowed Professor in
  Research
Associate Dean of Research
Professor of Oral Biology and Oral Biology &
  Medicine
Director, UCLA Center for Oral/Head & Neck
  Oncology Research
UCLA School of Dentistry
Los Angeles, California

Sook-Bin Woo, DMD, MMSc
Associate Professor of Oral Medicine, Infection,
  and Immunity
Harvard School of Dental Medicine

Chief of Clinical Affairs
Division of Oral Medicine and Dentistry
Brigham and Women's Hospital
Boston, Massachusetts

1 Screening for Heart Disease, Diabetes, and HIV in a Dental Setting

Barbara L. Greenberg, MSc, PhD

Widespread recognition of the need for improved health promotion and an increased emphasis on disease prevention are significant foundations of the 2010 Affordable Care Act[1] and are likely to lead to an increase in screening initiatives. Major titles of the act advance prevention and reflect an underlying strategy to improve access to clinical preventive services among individuals with private and public health insurance. It is likely that screening for health indicators concurrently with disease risk indicators will be a fundamental component of disease prevention and health promotion strategies. Of note is that one of the major titles of the act is Title IV: The Prevention of Chronic Disease and the Improvement of Public Health. Furthermore, new private and public health insurance plans are required to cover preventive services recommended by the US Preventive Services Task Force at no cost to the individual policyholder.

Moving forward, oral health care providers should have a role in preventing and treating noncommunicable and communicable diseases in an effort to reduce their associated morbidity and mortality. The significant burden worldwide of infectious diseases such as human immunodeficiency virus (HIV), tuberculosis, hepatitis C, and cholera is well recognized and has been highlighted in the Millennium Development Goals, eight international development goals es-

tablished and adopted by 189 countries as part of the 2000 United Nations Millennium Summit.[2] In recent years, there has been a growing appreciation of the global burden of chronic conditions such as coronary heart disease (CHD) and diabetes mellitus (DM). In response to this, in 2011 the United Nations convened a high-level meeting on noncommunicable diseases, which for the first time included oral diseases as noncommunicable diseases associated with significant morbidity.[3]

The emerging recognition of the impact of noncommunicable diseases such as heart disease and diabetes and their relationship to oral health was formally recognized by the Fédération Dentaire Internationale with the release in August 2012 of its policy statement on noncommunicable diseases.[4] This calls for a shift to a more horizontal approach to disease and greater integration with other disciplines that are tackling noncommunicable disease. Integrating oral health care providers into strategies to enhance early identification of individuals at risk of developing disease could be an important component of future public health strategies to prevent and control these diseases.

As well-respected health care providers, dentists and dental hygienists can have an impactful role in promoting health and well-being among their patients. According to data from the National Health and Nutrition Examination Survey (NHANES) and the most recent Behavioral Risk Factor Surveillance, 65% to 70% of adults visit the dentist in a given year, but 10% to 20% of these patients have not seen a physician in the preceding year.[5–7] Coupled with these data is the existence of simple, safe, well-validated, and well-accepted chairside screening tools for CHD, diabetes, and HIV, supporting the potential role of oral health care providers in strategies to prevent the onset or control the severity of diseases with public health significance.

Screening tests are a critical component of strategies to prevent and control disease. Screening is conducted primarily to assess the risk of developing disease among individuals who have no clinical signs or symptoms and to assess disease severity and risk factor control among individuals with confirmed disease. Identification of individuals who are unaware of their increased risk can promote early entry into the medical system when medical and behavioral interventions can impact the risk of developing disease. Screening for disease risk is particularly effective for diseases with well-recognized, modifiable risk factors. The diseases of interest for medical screening in a dental setting—heart disease, diabetes, and HIV—have well-recognized and modifiable risk factors, which include high blood pressure, high cholesterol and high-density lipoprotein levels, smoking, obesity, and high-risk sexual behavior.

Abundant epidemiologic data support the feasibility of CHD, DM, and HIV disease prevention, and numerous efficacy and attitudes studies support the value of medical screening in a dental setting for each of these conditions. This chapter presents an overview of the epidemiology, the support for prevention, and the well-recognized chairside screening tools for each condition of interest.

These medical conditions also have implications for oral health care delivery. The relationship between HIV and oral health has been well documented over the years, and there is now a growing body of literature on the relationship between heart disease and oral health and between diabetes and oral health. The oral health considerations related to these conditions are addressed in other chapters.

Feasibility of Medical Screening in a Dental Setting

Attitudes of oral health care providers and patients

Survey data among practicing oral health care providers and patients reveal strong support and willingness to participate in medical screening in a dental setting. In a nationally based random sample of 1,945 general dentists (with a response rate of 28% and a margin of error of less than 3%), 90% of respondents felt it was important to identify patients who may benefit from interventions to prevent or control the onset of medical conditions, and 83% were willing to incorporate into their practice chairside medical screening that yields immediate results. However, only 45% were willing to incorporate screening that required sending samples to an outside laboratory.[8]

The majority of respondents were willing to screen for specified conditions including hypertension (86%), cardiovascular disease (77%), diabetes (77%), hepatitis (72%), and HIV infection (69%). The majority were also willing to discuss the results with the patient during the visit (76%) and refer the patients as appropriate for a medical follow-up (96%). The majority were also willing to collect the necessary specimens or data, such as saliva (88%) and blood pressure measurements (91%), although fewer were inclined to collect fingerstick blood (56%) and height and weight data (67%). Participants were also questioned about their attitudes toward potential issues associated with incorporating medical screening into their practice, including patient willingness, liability, cost, time, and insurance coverage. While all of these concerns were important to the majority of respondents, patient willingness was the most important factor, and insurance coverage was the least important.[8]

Other US-based studies have reported that the majority of dentists believe that it is important and that they are willing to conduct screenings for medical conditions that patients are unaware of or to address medical conditions such as obesity.[9]

Of critical importance to the implementation of medical screening in a dental setting is the attitude of patients. According to survey data obtained among a convenience sample (N = 470) of patients attending an inner-city dental clinic and community-based practices, the majority of respondents felt chairside medical screening in a dental setting is important and were willing to participate in such activity.[10] Confidentiality was the respondents' most important concern and the fact that the screening was not performed by a physician was the least important.

The majority of patients who responded believed it was important for dentists to conduct medical screening (94%). Most were willing to have a dentist conduct chairside screening during their visit for the following conditions: cardiovascular disease (81%), hypertension (90%), diabetes (83%), HIV (80%), and hepatitis C virus (81%). The majority were also willing to have dentists conduct screening that yields immediate results (91%), discuss results during the visit (88%), receive a referral to a physician (89%), provide saliva specimens (88%), provide fingerstick blood (75%), and pay US$10 to US$20 (69%). The data also suggest that patients felt chairside medical screening was valuable, given that most indicated that their opinion of the dentist would improve for the following characteristics: competence (76%), compassion (76%), knowledge (80%), and professionalism (80%).[10]

A community-based survey regarding random blood glucose testing in a dental setting reported that 84% of the 28 dentists and 44 staff members surveyed felt that "patients will benefit from blood glucose testing" and 81% of the 498 patients surveyed felt "blood glucose testing in the dental office was a good idea."[11] There was some concern among the dentists that the screening would be time-consuming, although it was not considered a significant barrier.

Preliminary studies have also shown that patients support HIV screening in particular. Qualitative interviews among 19 patients attending an inner-city dental clinic suggested that 74% would accept HIV screening offered in the clinic.[12] While data suggest support for HIV testing in a dental setting, both providers and patients have also noted concerns. In addition to the general concerns about chairside medical screening noted earlier,[8,10] studies specific to HIV testing report that dental practitioners are concerned about HIV testing being outside the scope of practice, inadequate reimbursement, low patient acceptance, negative impact on practice, and the need for additional training in HIV counseling and testing.[13] For patients, additional concerns around HIV testing in a dental setting relate to logistic issues if the test has a positive result.[12]

Integration of oral health care providers into disease control and prevention strategies can be fully realized only with the cooperation of primary care physicians. A nationally based survey of 1,508 practicing primary care physicians (with a response rate of 22% and a margin of error of less than 3%) found that the majority felt that point-of-care screening was effective and that chairside screening with medical referral was valuable for the specified conditions, which were hypertension (77%), heart disease (61%), diabetes (71%), and HIV infection (64%).[14] The majority would be willing to discuss the results with the dentist (76%) and accept a medical referral from the dentist (89%), and the majority of respondents felt it was unimportant that the referral came from a dentist and not a physician (52%). The majority of physicians reported that the most important consideration was patient willingness, followed by the level of training of the dentist; duplication of roles by the dentist and the physician was the least important consideration.

Studies of efficacy

Studies have demonstrated the efficacy and yield of chairside screening strategies to identify asymptomatic individuals who are at increased risk of developing DM- and CHD-associated events. NHANES data from 1999 to 2002 were used to make theoretical calculations about the potential efficacy of screening for CHD in a dental setting.[5] Elevated risk for CHD was determined using the Framingham Risk Score (FRS), which calculates the individual's risk of developing a severe CHD event within 10 years (the FRS is discussed later in the chapter). Elevated diabetes risk was determined using the hemoglobin A_{1c} (HbA$_{1c}$) level (HbA$_{1c}$ is discussed later in the chapter). Clinical and demographic data, including blood pressure, total and high-density lipoprotein values, age, and smoking status, of eligible adults 40 to 85 years of age were used to calculate the FRS for each study subject. Criteria for eligibility included an age of 40 years or older, no reported risk factors of interest, no history of diabetes or heart disease, no relevant medication use, and no visit to a physician in the prior 12 months but an examination by a dentist in that time period.

Among eligible men, 18% had an increased 10-year global risk of a CHD event (greater than 10% FRS); among those with increased risk, 14% had a moderate, above-average risk score (greater than 10% and less than 20%), and an additional 4% had a high risk (20% or greater).[5] No eligible women had an elevated risk for CHD. The study algorithm results were then extrapolated to the 2000 US census data; among men aged 40 to 85 years without reported risk factors who had not seen a physician but had seen a dentist in the past 12 months, 332,262 had a moderate, above-average 10-year CHD risk, while 72,625 had a severe or high 10-year CHD risk.

A subsequent study using NHANES data estimated an increased probability (27% to 53% depending on the sex and race/ethnicity) of undiagnosed diabetes among individuals with a self-reported family history of diabetes, hypertension, high cholesterol levels, and clinical evidence of periodontal disease.[15]

A study based in an inner-city clinic was conducted as a follow-up to the theoretical calculations to assess the efficacy of chairside screening in a dental setting.[16] Calibrated, trained dentists administered a CHD risk screening questionnaire, measured blood pressure, and tested cholesterol, high-density lipoprotein, and HbA$_{1c}$ using fingerstick blood collected from a convenience sample of adult patients at the New Jersey Dental School. The eligibility criteria for inclusion in the study were an age of 40 years or older; not having been told of any CHD-specific risk factors; no reported history

of heart attack, stroke, angina, or DM; and no visits to a physician in the last 12 months. Fingerstick blood was used to measure total cholesterol, high-density lipoprotein levels, and HbA$_{1c}$ levels chairside with validated machines that yield results within 5 to 7 minutes. Clinical measurements and demographic data were used to calculate the FRS.

Among the participants, 17% had an increased 10-year CHD risk (FRS greater than 10%); of these, 14.0% had moderate, above-average risk (greater than 10% and less than 20%), and 2.2% had high risk (20% or greater).[16] One-third of men and 5% of women had an FRS greater than 10%. Data revealed that 71% of patients presented with one major risk factor of interest, while 31% had two or more risk factors. At the time the study was published (2007), the recommended cutoff point for a normal HbA$_{1c}$ level was 7.0%; at that threshold, only one man was found to have an abnormal A$_{1c}$ level. Under the new HbA$_{1c}$ positive screening threshold set by the American Diabetes Association in April 2010 (HbA$_{1c}$ greater than 5.7%),[17] 21% of participants would have been considered at increased risk for DM (unpublished data, 2010).

Another study conducted in an inner-city dental school clinic among adults 40 years of age or older suggested that using HbA$_{1c}$ in conjunction with two dental criteria, at least four missing teeth and at least 26% of teeth with deep (5-mm or greater) periodontal pockets, can improve the sensitivity of each parameter. The use of HbA$_{1c}$ measurements in conjunction with two dental criteria had a 92% sensitivity for identifying unrecognized diabetes, while either HbA$_{1c}$ alone or the two dental parameters alone had 73% to 75% sensitivity.[18]

The dental setting is an underutilized resource that could be used to enhance early identification of individuals at increased risk of disease and who could benefit from early intervention. A preliminary yield study was conducted in Sweden to assess the outcomes of medical referrals for patients found to be at increased risk of death due to heart disease.[19] The screening tool in this study was the European Heart Score, which identifies individuals who are at an increased risk of dying from a CHD event within 10 years. In this setting of universal health care,

6% were identified as being at increased risk of dying from a CHD event; among those patients, 50% subsequently received a medical intervention after evaluation by a physician.

Screening for Coronary Heart Disease

Burden of disease

Cardiovascular disease (CVD) is the leading cause of death in the United States, and this predominance is expected to increase as life expectancy and obesity rates continue to rise. Using the most recent NHANES data (2007 to 2012), the American Heart Association estimates that 15.4 million people have active symptoms of CHD, the condition responsible for 50% of CVD.[20] This is up from the 2009 estimate of 13 million US adults with CHD. CHD alone caused approximately 1 of every 6 deaths in 2009.

While the mortality rates attributable to CVD have decreased 32.7% between 1999 and 2009, morbidity and health care costs continue to rise with increasing disease prevalence. The well-recognized clinical risk factors associated with heart disease and diabetes include obesity, hypertension, hypercholesterolemia, smoking, and, for heart disease, metabolic syndrome and diabetes. NHANES data indicate that among adults older than 30 years, 30% have hypertension, 13.8% have high cholesterol, 8.3% have diabetes, and 34% have metabolic syndrome.

Compounding these dire statistics is the fact that a significant proportion of individuals remain unaware of their risk factors and their elevated risk of developing heart disease. The prevalence of undiagnosed CVD is estimated to be 29% to 82% (depending on the specific risk factor); the greatest proportion of individuals unaware of their risk factor is among those with hypertension.

The most recent complete economic data (2009) estimate the total direct plus indirect costs associated with CVD to be US$312.6 billion.[20] CVD, which is due to CHD 50% of the time, has the greatest economic impact of any other disease diagnostic group.

Support for screening and prevention

One of the primary goals of Healthy People 2020 states: "Improve cardiovascular health and quality of life through prevention, detection, and treatment of risk factors for heart attack and stroke; early identification and treatment of heart attacks and strokes; and prevention of repeat cardiovascular events."[21] Among the 2020 Strategic Impact Goals released in 2012 by the American Heart Association[20] is an objective to improve cardiovascular health by 20% and decrease deaths due to CVD and stroke by 20% by 2020. In conjunction with this goal, the plan calls for promoting the attainment of ideal levels of seven cardiovascular health factors (smoking, blood pressure, blood glucose, total cholesterol, body mass index, physical activity, and dietary content) to prevent CVD and advance cardiovascular health. Trend data reveal that the proportion of the population with ideal levels of all seven of these cardiovascular health factors has decreased in recent decades, from 2.0% in the period from 1988 to 1994 to 1.2% in the years 2005 to 2010. There was also an impact on mortality: Individuals who presented with a greater number of cardiovascular health factors at an ideal level exhibited lower risk of mortality from CVD and CHD.[22]

Primary and secondary prevention activities aimed at modifying well-recognized risk factors associated with these diseases (eg, high blood pressure, high cholesterol, and obesity) have resulted in substantial reductions in disease-specific incidence, morbidity, and mortality. Dietary modifications and increased physical activity are associated with a 35% to 77% reduction in the incidence of hypertension,[23,24] a 4% to 10% reduction in high cholesterol,[25,26] an 11% to 15% reduction in incidence of CVD,[25] and a 27% reduction in CVD mortality.[26] A recent multicenter European trial found that, among persons with a high cardiovascular risk, a modified Mediterranean diet reduced the incidence of major cardiovascular events by 28% to 30% over a period of 4.8 years.[27]

Screening tool of choice

Among the numerous screening tools for CHD-associated events, the well-validated FRS, which uses demographic and clinical measurements, is among the most widely used in the United States.[28] The FRS estimates the 10-year risk of developing a severe CHD outcome based on a quantitative evaluation of multiple demographic and clinical risk factor data, including sex, age, history of smoking, and measurements of blood pressure, total cholesterol, and high-density lipoprotein cholesterol. The score is based on a risk factor algorithm calculated using data collected from the first 12 years of an ongoing population-based longitudinal study, the Framingham Heart Study, which has observed the development of CHD among 2,489 men and 2,856 women aged 30 to 74 years.[29]

Cox proportional hazards regression models were used to assess the relationship between clinical and demographic characteristics and CHD. The 12-year longitudinal data were used in various proportional hazards prediction models to determine sex-specific 10-year CHD incidence estimates using multiple risk factors. For adults 40 years of age and older, an FRS of greater than 10% and less than 20% is considered a moderate, above-average risk, and an FRS of 20% or greater is considered a high risk of developing a CHD event within the next 10 years, both of which warrant referral to a physician for medical follow-up.[28,29]

To calculate the FRS, the aforementioned clinical measurements and demographic data are entered into a computer-based program. A tool for calculating the FRS can be found at a website provided by the National Heart, Lung and Blood Institute's National Cholesterol Education Program.[30]

For this to be a successful chairside screening strategy in a dental setting, the necessary clinical measurements must be available immediately and ideally obtained with a minimal blood specimen. The CardioChek Analyzer (Polymer Technology Systems), a small handheld, well-validated device[31] is used chairside with a fingerstick blood specimen to assess total cholesterol and high-density lipoprotein levels. The machine uses specific test strips to analyze the clinical values of interest. The machine can be used repeatedly, with one test strip used per blood specimen. Results are accurate to ±2% per manufacturer guidelines and are available within 5 to 7 minutes.

Screening for Diabetes Mellitus

Burden of disease

The incidence of diabetes continues to grow at alarming rates. Estimates show that the number of adults with diabetes in the United States has increased by 45% over the last 20 years, primarily driven by the increase in obesity rates and a sedentary lifestyle.[32] Diabetes is the seventh leading cause of death in the United States, a leading cause of morbidity, and a major cause of heart disease and stroke.[32] Cost estimates (direct and indirect) from the American Diabetes Association put the economic burden of diabetes in the United States at US$245 billion for 2012, an increase of 41% from the cost of US$174 billion in 2007.[33,34]

The increasing cost is due primarily to the increasing disease prevalence. From 1995 to 2012, there was an 82.2% median increase in the age-adjusted prevalence of diabetes in the United States.[35] According to the most recent data (2010) from the Centers for Disease Control and Prevention, diabetes affects 25.8 million adults older than 20 years of age or 11.3% of US adults in this age group; of those individuals, 18.8 million are diagnosed and 7 million are undiagnosed.[36] Based on fasting glucose or HbA_{1c} levels, 35% of US adults aged 20 years or older had prediabetes.[36] The prevalence of undiagnosed diabetes and prediabetes is 27% to 53%.[37] Associated with the increasing disease prevalence are increasing levels of disability and growing health care expenditures, both of which are projected to continue to rise.[35]

Type 2 diabetes is responsible for more than 95% of cases and is strongly associated with a number of modifiable risk factors, the most important being obesity and a sedentary lifestyle.[35] A recent study that used NHANES data to assess the attainment of recommended diabetes care goals in the United States between 1999 and 2010 reported that, although there were improvements in risk factor control for diabetes (ie, smoking, obesity, sedentary lifestyle), 33% to 49% did not meet the recommended goals for glycemic control, blood pressure, or low-density lipoprotein cholesterol.[38]

Support for screening and prevention

One of the primary goals of Healthy People 2020 is to "reduce the disease and economic burden of diabetes mellitus and improve the quality of life for all persons who have, or are at risk for, DM."[39] Three of the 16 related objectives of this goal highlight the need for expanded strategies to prevent disease onset and control disease severity[39]:

- "Reduce the annual number of new cases of diagnosed diabetes in the population"
- "Improve glycemic control among persons with diabetes"
- "Increase the proportion of persons with diagnosed diabetes who have at least an annual dental examination"

In addition, Healthy People 2020 has a specific objective for oral health that highlights the role of oral health care professionals as a component of an integrated approach to disease control: "Increase the proportion of adults who are tested or referred for glycemic control from a dentist or dental hygienist in the past year."[40]

The current strategic plan of the American Diabetes Association[41] augments the focus on evidence-based prevention with newly established goals that call for a doubling in the percentage of Americans with prediabetes who are aware of their condition and a 10% increase in the number of individuals engaged in preventive behaviors. Adding significant support to the documented short-term value of prevention are the demonstrated long-term effects of interventions to delay disease onset. The Finnish Diabetes Prevention Study reported sustained lifestyle changes and a 43% decrease in the incidence of diabetes 13 years postintervention.[42] A long-term study in China, the Da Qing Diabetes Prevention Study, reported a 43% reduction as long as 20 years later.[43] A study of the US-based Diabetes Prevention Program documented a 24% decrease in diabetes incidence 10 years after the baseline.[44] Prevention programs have also been effective at changing the risk profile of high-risk individuals. The Diabetes Prevention Program showed a 16% annual risk reduction for developing diabetes accompanied by a decrease in body weight and an increase in moderate physical activity.[44]

Screening tool of choice

The HbA$_{1c}$ test is a nonfasting measure of the 2- to 3-month average level of circulating glycosylated red blood cells. Specifically, the A$_{1c}$ test measures what percentage of circulating hemoglobin is glycosylated. The higher the HbA$_{1c}$ level, the poorer the blood sugar control and the higher the risk for diabetes. An HbA$_{1c}$ level of 5.7% to 6.4% (inclusive) is considered a positive screening result for prediabetes and an indication of increased risk of developing diabetes; a level of 6.5% or greater is considered diagnostic for diabetes. HbA$_{1c}$ screening results of 5.7% or greater warrant referral to a physician for medical follow-up.

In April 2010, the American Diabetes Association recommended the use of the HbA$_{1c}$ test for screening and diagnosis of DM in routine clinical practice.[45] A recent systematic review concluded that the risk of developing diabetes more than doubles with each 0.5% increase in the HbA$_{1c}$ level.[46] The endorsement of the HbA$_{1c}$ test was a significant step forward in the screening for DM, because prior to this, the accepted screening test for DM was fasting plasma blood glucose level. Data suggest that the HbA$_{1c}$ test (threshold of 5.7%) is more specific, less sensitive, and has higher positive predictive value than fasting plasma glucose (threshold of 100 mg/dL).[47]

A review of the literature on different screening cutoff points for HbA_{1c} risk stratification found that the expected number of diabetes cases prevented or delayed is greater when HbA_{1c} cutoff points are lower; a cutoff point of 5.5% will prevent or delay 17% of cases, while a 6.0% threshold will prevent or delay 4% of cases.[48] However, the number of patients that need to be treated in order to prevent one case increases as the HbA_{1c} screening threshold decreases.[48] In summary, the data clearly support the use of the HbA_{1c} test as a valid diabetes screening and diagnostic tool.

The fingerstick blood sample is used with the test kit, one kit per individual, and has a 99% accuracy. Results are available within 5 to 7 minutes. However, certain circumstances may impact the validity of the HbA_{1c} test and lead to false results. These conditions include iron deficiency anemia, chronic bleeding, hemolytic anemia, or a recent blood transfusion. In addition, some people have an uncommon form of hemoglobin, known as *hemoglobin variant*, which can lead to false A_{1c} results. While rare, the HbA_{1c} variant is most common in black people and people of Mediterranean or Southeast Asian descent. The A1C Now testing system (Bayer) can be used to provide an immediate measure of HbA_{1c}. The Bayer test is cleared by the US Food and Drug Administration for home use.

Screening for HIV

Burden of disease

Approximately 1.1 million Americans are living with HIV, a prevalence rate of 3.5%; about 18% of these individuals are unaware of their infection status.[49] The most recent available statistics (2010) indicate that approximately 47,500 individuals are newly infected annually, and the highest incidence is among 25- to 35-year-olds. Since 2007, the rate of HIV diagnosis has been relatively stable in all risk transmission categories except man-to-man sexual contact, for which there has been a steady but slight increase over that time period. Among newly diagnosed patients, 40% have advanced disease and are considered "late testers."

Data from the NHANES show that 70% of people with self-reported HIV risk see the dentist in a 2-year period. Of those, 60% have never been tested and have received no preventive medical care.[6]

Support for screening and prevention

Public health policy support for HIV testing is clearly articulated in two Healthy People 2020 goals.[50] One goal stipulates an "increase in the proportion of persons living with HIV who know their serostatus," specifically increasing from the baseline of 80.6% to a goal of 90.0%. Another goal calls for an increase in the proportion of adolescents and adults who have been tested for HIV in the last 12 months from 17.2% to 18.9%.

In April 2013, the US Preventive Services Task Force (USPSTF) endorsed routine HIV testing for all adults and adolescents.[51] This recommendation has far-reaching significance because the Affordable Care Act mandates that all public and private insurers cover USPSTF-recommended preventive services without cost to the patient.

From the global perspective, one Millennium Development goal is to "combat HIV/AIDS, malaria and other disease."[6] Among the sub-goals are halting the spread of HIV by 2015 and achieving universal access to HIV treatment for those who need it.

Setting the stage for HIV testing in a dental setting began in 2004 with the US Food and Drug Administration clearance of OraQuick HIV point-of-care test (OraSure Technologies) for use with oral mucosal transudate. The OraQuick test allows for a rapid turnaround time for test results, facilitating use in routine health care settings.

The next significant event came in 2006 with the change in the Centers for Disease Control and Prevention's recommendation for HIV screening and testing.[52] The goal of the revisions was to encourage early testing and to reduce those who had a concurrent AIDS diagnosis within 1 year. The revised recommendations call for routine testing in all 13- to 64-year-olds and broaden the health care settings that could serve as testing sites. Prior to this new recommendation, the testing approach was a targeted approach based on risk assessment, and testing was primarily limited to the presence of clinical manifestations and targeted to regions with a prevalence greater than 1%. Based on data from 2004, the CDC estimated that, of the approximately 1 million people living with HIV/AIDS, one-quarter were unaware of their infection status, and 30% of newly diagnosed patient fell into the category of late testers, those who receive an AIDS diagnosis within 1 year of testing positive for HIV; the targeted screening strategy was deemed unsuccessful for preventing new HIV infections.

Studies suggest the beneficial effect of early HIV identification in terms of reductions in high-risk behavior and HIV transmission rates. Estimates show that persons who are unaware of their infection status account for 55% of new infections and have a 3.5 times greater rate of sexual transmission than do those who are aware of their infection status.[53] The results from the HIV Prevention Trial Network, a multicenter randomized clinical trial of discordant HIV-infected pairs, highlighted further the benefits of early HIV identification. These data showed that early treatment was associated with a 96% reduction in transmission rates and 41% reduction in the number of serious clinical endpoints compared with delayed treatment.[53] The transmission hazard ratio for early therapy was 0.11, and the clinical endpoint hazard ratio was 0.59.[54]

Given the evidence for both reduced transmission with early antiretroviral therapy and protection against HIV infection in uninfected persons who use antiretroviral therapy consistently, the recommendations from the US panel of the International Antiretroviral Society were updated to include offering treatment to all HIV-infected patients regardless of CD4 cell count.[55]

Screening tool of choice

Rapid HIV testing takes advantage of high levels of HIV antibodies in crevicular fluid and is effective for all known serotypes.[56] The test is a saliva-based test to measure the antibody response to HIV-1 antigens for envelope proteins gp41, gp120, or gp160.[57] The OraQuick rapid test has a sensitivity of 98% and a specificity of 99%.[58,59] It is easy to use and produces results in 20 minutes; positive tests should be confirmed with an enzyme-linked immunosorbent assay.

Given the availability of a well-validated, sensitive, safe, effective, and inexpensive HIV test with rapid results and the documented beneficial impact of early identification of HIV infection, testing in a dental setting could have added value toward controlling the spread of disease. In a recent review of HIV diagnosis and testing, the authors concluded that HIV testing is "a public health imperative" and that "healthcare professionals in the dental community occupy a key position in HIV diagnosis because they provide routine care to individuals, many of whom do not otherwise interact with the healthcare system on a regular basis."[57]

However, there are some caveats to keep in mind. Rapid HIV testing has been found to have lower sensitivity for detecting early HIV infection than do traditional laboratory-based tests,[60] although this was not found in subsequent field studies.[61] A systematic review and meta-analysis showed that the rapid test has a decreased sensitivity in settings with a low population prevalence rate (less than 1%) and a consequent decrease in the positive predictive value of the test from 98% to 88%, raising questions about its widespread use in areas of low prevalence.[60]

Laboratory Standards

Chairside screening necessitates the availability of tests that have been approved under the Clinical Laboratory Improvement Amendments (CLIA) and are CLIA-waived. This act was established by the US Congress in 1998 to set quality standards for laboratory testing with human specimens to ensure the accuracy and timeliness of results. This act mandates that all facilities examining human specimens must register with the Centers for Medicare and Medicaid Services (CMS) and obtain CLIA certification. Practitioners operating within a larger CLIA-approved organization or institution are covered under that approval. Applications for CLIA certification can be obtained from the CMS website[62] or through state health departments.

Risks and Benefits of Screening

Questions about the benefits of population-based disease screening have been recently reviewed in terms of the risk-benefit ratio.[63] While negative consequences of screening, such as increased risk for depression and stigma, have been noted, the consensus is that population-based screening for CVD, diabetes, and HIV involves little or no harm and has some benefits, albeit of small magnitude.[63]

The use of cost-benefit analysis has been adopted to demonstrate the bottom-line benefits of population-based screening. In general, these studies show a small benefit, although the wide variation across studies in assumptions applied to the cost-benefit models and the different metrics used to formulate benefit limit the ability to combine disease-specific cost-benefit studies into one definitive quantitative conclusion. In his overview of screening, Harris[63] cautiously concluded, "We should not think of screening as our primary prevention strategy but rather use screening to make a real, but limited contribution to population health for a few conditions." He also suggested that screening be targeted to subgroups with the "highest potential benefit and the lowest potential harm."[63] The strategy proposed for screening for heart disease and diabetes in a dental setting is targeted screening, specifically for patients older than 40 years who have no prior diagnosis, have no related medication use, and are not routinely engaged with a primary care provider (eg, have not seen a physician within the prior 12 months).

Conclusion

Given that there are simple, safe, effective, and relatively inexpensive screening strategies to identify at-risk individuals in a dental setting and documented benefits of primary and secondary prevention, careful consideration should be given to the incorporation of the oral health care setting as a component of a health home. Screening for risk of systemic disease and monitoring of disease control in a dental setting should be embraced from a public health perspective and as a means of gaining additional patient information that could inform the practitioner's delivery of oral health care. However, successful widespread implementation will require further research and development of systems to enhance provider training, maximize referral completion, establish structured referral and follow-up mechanisms, and address reimbursement issues.

References

1. Patient Protection and Affordable Care Act, 42 USC §18001-18121 (2010).
2. United Nations Millennium Development Goals. http://www.un.org/millenniumgoals. Accessed 3 August 2013.
3. United Nations 2011 High Level Meeting on Prevention and Control of Non-communicable Diseases. 19–20 Sept 2011. http://www.un.org/en/ga/ncdmeeting2011/index.shtml. Accessed 3 August 2013.
4. Fédération Dentaire Internationale. Policy statement on non-communicable diseases. 31 Aug 2012. http://www.fdiworldental.org/media/11291/Non-communicable%20diseases-2012.pdf. Accessed 3 August 2013.
5. Glick M, Greenberg BL. The potential role of dentists in identifying patients' risk of experiencing coronary heart disease events. J Am Dent Assoc 2005;136:1541–1546.
6. Pollack HA, Metsch LR, Abel S. Dental examinations as an untapped opportunity to provide HIV testing for high-risk individuals. Am J Public Health 2010;100:88–89.
7. Xu F, Town M, Balluz LS, et al. Surveillance for certain health behaviors among states and selected local areas—United States, 2010. MMWR Surveill Summ 2013;62:1–247.

8. Greenberg B, Glick M, Frantsve-Hawley J, Kantor ML. Dentists' attitudes toward chairside screening for medical conditions. J Am Dent Assoc 2010;141: 52–62.

9. Curran AE, Caplan DJ, Lee JY, et al. Dentists' attitudes about their role in addressing obesity in patients: A national survey. J Am Dent Assoc 2010;14: 1307–1316.

10. Greenberg BL, Kantor ML, Jiang SS, Glick M. Patients' attitudes toward screening for medical conditions in a dental setting. J Public Health Dent 2012;72:28–35.

11. Barasch A, Safford MM, Qvist V, et al. Random blood glucose testing in dental practice: A community-based feasibility study from The Dental Practice-Base Research Network. J Am Dent Assoc 2012;143:262–269.

12. VanDevanter N, Combellick MK, Hutchinson MK, Phelan J, Malamud D, Shelley D. A qualitative study of patients' attitudes toward HIV testing in the dental setting. Nurs Res Pract 2012;2012:803169 doi: 10.1155/2012/803169.

13. Siegel K, Abel SN, Pereyra M, Liguori T, Pollack HA, Metsch LR. Rapid HIV testing in dental practices. Am J Public Health 2012;102:625–632.

14. Greenberg BL, Glick M, Kantor ML. Physicians support medical screening in a dental setting. J Dent Res 2013;92(special issue A):371.

15. Borrell LN, Kunzel C, Lamster IB, Lalla E. Diabetes in the dental office: Using NHANES III to estimate the probability of undiagnosed disease. J Periodontal Res 2007;42:559–565.

16. Greenberg BL, Glick M, Goodchild J, Duda PW, Conte NR, Conte M. Screening for cardiovascular risk factors in a dental setting. J Am Dent Assoc 2007;138:798–804.

17. American Diabetes Association. Standards of medical care in diabetes—2010. Diabetes Care 2010;33 (suppl 1):S11–S61 [erratum 2010;33:692].

18. Lalla E, Kunzel C, Burkett S, Cheng B, Lamster IB. Identification of unrecognized diabetes and prediabetes in a dental setting. J Dent Res 2011;90: 855–860.

19. Jontell M, Glick M. Oral health care professionals' identification of cardiovascular disease risk among patients in private dental offices in Sweden. J Am Dent Assoc 2009;140:1385–1391.

20. Go AS, Mozaffarian D, Roger VL, et al. Heart disease and stroke statistics—2013 update: A report from the American Heart Association. Circulation 2013;127:e6–e245 [erratum 2013;127:e841].

21. Healthy People 2020. Heart disease and stroke. http://healthypeople.gov/2020/topicsobjectives2020/overview.aspx?topicid=21. Accessed 3 August 2013.

22. Yang Q, Cogswell ME, Flanders WD, et al. Trends in cardiovascular health metrics and associations with all-cause CVD mortality among US adults. JAMA 2012;307:1273–1283.

23. He J, Whelton PK, Appel LJ, Charleston J, Klag MJ. Long-term effects of weight loss and dietary sodium reduction on incidence of hypertension. Hypertension 2000;35:544–549.

24. He J, Gu D, Wu X, et al. Effect of soybean protein on blood pressure: A randomized controlled trial. Ann Intern Med 2005;143:1–9.

25. Bazzano LA, He J, Ogden LG, Loria CM, Whelton PK. National Health and Nutrition Examination Survey I Epidemiologic Follow-up Study. Dietary fiber intake and reduced risk of coronary heart disease in US men and women: The National Health and Nutrition Examination Survey I Epidemiologic Follow-up Study. Arch Intern Med 2003;163:1897–1904.

26. Bazzano LA, He J, Ogden LG, et al. Fruit and vegetable intake and risk of cardiovascular disease in US adults: The first National Health and Nutrition Examination Survey Epidemiologic Follow-up Study. Am J Clin Nutr 2002;76:93–99.

27. Estruch R, Ros E, Salas-Salvado J, et al. Primary prevention of cardiovascular disease with a Mediterranean diet. N Engl J Med 2013;368:1279–1290.

28. Grundy SM, Pasternak R, Greenland P, Smith S Jr, Fuster V. Assessment of cardiovascular risk by use of multiple-risk-factor assessment equations: A statement for healthcare professionals from the American Heart Association and the American College of Cardiology. Circulation 1999;100:1481–1492.

29. Wilson PW, D'Agostino RB, Levy D, Belanger AM, Silbershatz H, Kannel WB. Prediction of coronary heart disease using risk factor categories. Circulation 1998;97:1837–1847.

30. National Heart, Lung and Blood Institute. National Cholesterol Education Program. Risk assessment tool for estimating your 10-year risk of having a heart attack. http://cvdrisk.nhlbi.nih.gov/calculator.asp. Accessed 26 August 2013.

31. Panz VR, Raal FJ, Paiker J, Immelman R, Miles H. Performance of the CardioChek PA and Cholestech LDX point-of-care analysers compared to clinical diagnostic laboratory methods for the measurement of lipids. Cardiovascc J S Afr 2005;16:112–117.

32. Cheng YJ, Imperatore G, Geiss LS, et al. Secular changes in the age-specific prevalence of diabetes among U.S. adults: 1988-2010 Diabetes Care 2013;36:1406–1412.

33. American Diabetes Association. Economic costs of diabetes in the U.S. in 2007. Diabetes Care 2008; 31:596–615.

34. American Diabetes Association. Economic costs of diabetes in the U.S. in 2012. Diabetes Care 2013; 36:1033–1046.

35. Centers for Disease Control and Prevention (CDC). Increasing prevalence of diagnosed diabetes—United States and Puerto Rico, 1995–2010. MMWR Morb Mortal Wkly Rep 2012;61:918–921.

36. Centers for Disease Control and Prevention (CDC). National Diabetes Fact Sheet: National estimates and general information on diabetes and prediabetes in the United States, 2011. Atlanta: US Department of Health and Human Services, Centers for Disease Control and Prevention, 2011. http://www.cdc.gov/diabetes/pubs/pdf/ndfs_2011.pdf. Accessed 26 August 2013.

37. Mozumdar A, Liguori G. Persistent increase of prevalence of metabolic syndrome among U.S. adults: NHANES III to NHANES 1999-2006. Diabetes Care 2011;34:216–219.

38. Ali MK, Bullard KM, Saaddine JB, Cowie CC, Imperatore G, Gregg EW. Achievement of goals in U.S. diabetes care, 1999-2010. New Engl J Med 2013;368:1613–1624.

39. Healthy People 2020. Diabetes. http://healthypeople.gov/2020/topicsobjectives2020/overview.aspx?topicid=8. Accessed 3 August 2013.

40. Healthy People 2020. Oral health. http://healthypeople.gov/2020/topicsobjectives2020/overview.aspx?topicid=32. Accessed 3 August 2013.

41. American Diabetes Association. 2012–2015 Strategic plan. http://main.diabetes.org/dorg/PDFs/American_Diabetes_Association-2012-2015-Strategic-Plan.pdf. Accessed 3 August 2013.

42. Lindström J, Paltonen M, Eriksson JG, et al. Improved lifestyle and decreased diabetes risk over 13 years: Long-term follow-up of the randomized Finnish Diabetes Prevention Study (DPS). Diabetologia 2013;56:284–293.

43. Li G, Zhang P, Wang J, et al. The long-term effect of lifestyle interventions to prevent diabetes in the China Da Qing Diabetes Prevention study: A 20-year follow-up study. Lancet 2008;371:1783–1789.

44. Diabetes Prevention Program Research Group, Knowler WC, Fowler SE, et al. 10-year follow-up of diabetes incidence and weight loss in the Diabetes Prevention Program Outcomes Study. Lancet 2009;374:1677–1686.

45. Lu ZX, Walker KZ, O'Dea K, Sikaris KA, Shaw JE. A1C for screening and diagnosis of type 2 diabetes in routine clinical practice. Diabetes Care 2010;33:817–819.

46. Zhang X, Gregg EW, Williamson DF, et al. A1C level and future risk of diabetes: A systematic review. Diabetes Care 2010;33:1665–1673.

47. Soulimane S, Simon D, Shaw J, et al. HbA1c, fasting plasma glucose and the prediction of diabetes: Inter99, AusDiab and D.E.S.I.R. Diabetes Res Clin Pract 2012;96:392–399.

48. Gregg EW, Geiss L, Zhang P, Zhuo X, Williamson DF, Albright AL. Implications of risk stratification for diabetes prevention: The case of hemoglobin A1c. Am J Prev Med 2013;44(4 suppl):S375–S380.

49. Centers for Disease Control and Prevention (CDC). CDC's HIV surveillance report. http://www.cdc.gov/hiv/library/reports/surveillance/index.html. Accessed 12 September 2013.

50. Healthy People 2020. HIV. http://healthypeople.gov/2020/topicsobjectives2020/overview.aspx?topicid=22. Accessed 3 August 2013.

51. Moyer VA. Screening for HIV: U.S. Preventive Services Task Force recommendation statement. http://annals.org/article.aspx?articleid=1700660. Accessed 26 August 2013.

52. Branson BM, Handsfield HH, Lampe MA, et al. Revised recommendations for HIV testing of adults, adolescents, and pregnant women in health-care settings. MMWR Recomm Rep 2006;55(RR-14):1–17.

53. Marks G, Crepaz N, Janssen RS. Estimating sexual transmission of HIV from persons aware and unaware that they are infected with the virus in the USA. AIDS 2006;20:1447–1450.

54. Cohen MS, Chen YQ, McCauley M, et al. Prevention of HIV-1 infection with early antiretroviral therapy. N Engl J Med 2011;365:493–505.

55. Thompson MA, Aberg JA, Hoy JF, et al. Antiretroviral treatment of adult HIV infection: 2012 recommendations of the International Antiviral Society-USA panel. JAMA 2012;308:387–402.

56. Lamey PJ, Nolan A, Follett EA, et al. Anti-HIV antibody in saliva: An assessment of the role of the components of saliva, testing methodologies and collection systems. J Oral Pathol Med 1996;25:104–107.

57. Wilson E, Tanzosh T, Maldarelli F. HIV diagnosis and testing: What every healthcare professional can do (and why they should). Oral Dis 2013;19:431–439.

58. Holguin A, Gutierrez M, Portocarrero N, Rivas P, Baquero M. Performance of OraQuick Advanced Rapid HIV-1/2 antibody test for detection of antibodies in oral fluid and serum/plasma in HIV-1+ subjects carrying different HIV-1 subtypes and recombinant variants. J Clin Virol 2009;45:150–152.

59. Pant Pai N, Balram B, Shivkumar S, et al. Head-to-head comparison of accuracy of a rapid point-of-care HIV test with oral versus whole-blood specimens: A systematic review and meta-analysis. Lancet Infect Dis 2012;12:373–380.

60. Patel P, Mackellar D, Simmons P, et al. Detecting acute human immunodeficiency virus infection using 3 different screening immunoassays and nucleic acid amplification testing for human immunodeficiency virus RNA, 2006-2008. Arch Intern Med 2010;170:66–74.

61. Zachary D, Mwenge L, Muyoyeta M, et al. Field comparison of OraQuick ADVANCE Rapid HIV-1/2 antibody test and two blood-based rapid HIV antibody tests in Zambia. BMC Infect Dis 2012;12:183.

62. Centers for Medicare and Medicaid Services. How to Apply for a CLIA Certificate, Including International Laboratories. http://www.cms.gov/Regulations-and-Guidance/Legislation/CLIA/How_to_Apply_for_a_CLIA_Certificate_International_Laboratories.html. Accessed 3 August 2013.

63. Harris R. Overview of screening: Where we are and where we may be headed. Epidemiol Rev 2011;33:1–6.

Causation, Association, and Oral Health–Systemic Disease Connections

Donald M. Brunette, PhD

Print and electronic media often tout studies that show an association between exposure to a factor and a health effect. "Brush teeth to prevent heart disease," read a headline on the BBC News Health website, but later the article noted that "more work is needed to confirm if poor oral health directly causes heart disease or is a marker of risk."[1] Meanwhile, for those concerned about less lethal lifestyle matters, a syndicated column by Dr Oz and Dr Roizen included a headline that read, "Brushing up boosts sex life," which linked erectile dysfunction with inflammation and cardiovascular problems, including blood flow. Their advice to brush up is justified by an aphorism suggesting a mechanism: "If the flow don't go, guys, you're a no-show."[2] Dr Oz's website, however, has a less sanguine story. Headlined "Breaking news: No link between gum disease and heart disease," the article cites a statement from the American Heart Association[3] and has a section heading that states, "No proof that gum disease causes heart disease or stroke."[4] Many other articles could be cited that show there is considerable confusion about causation (or causality) and association in the relationship between oral health and systemic conditions.

The epidemiology of everyday risks, by necessity, has had to rely largely on observational studies, and chronic diseases such as heart disease can be multistage and multifactorial; for example, at least 10 different factors contribute to the occurrence of heart disease. Moreover, there are difficulties in measuring the actual exposure to risk factors over long periods. Kabat[5] noted that many of the strong relationships have already been identified and studied. Examples of "low-hanging fruit" include the relationships between smoking and lung cancer (current smokers have about a 20 times risk) and between alcohol consumption and oral cancer.[6]

Factors that increase risk of a disease only two- to threefold are much more difficult to identify. Dentists should not be surprised that the relationships between oral health and systemic diseases are not necessarily going to be clarified quickly, despite considerable research on the topic. Indeed the editor of the *Journal of the American Dental Association* has suggested that it may be necessary to rethink the whole concept of causation and recognize that many chronic diseases arise from a maze (another metaphor is a web) of interconnected factors that cannot be viewed separately.[7]

The goal of this chapter is to provide dentists with background information to help them better understand current and future evidence on the associations between oral health and general health. The science of epidemiology is concerned with developing measures to prevent or control disease. The basic question is whether exposure to an agent or condition is linked to disease.

For example, there is much current interest in a link between periodontal disease (PD) and coronary heart disease (CHD). It is an important question. CHD is important both in terms of the number of affected individuals and the severity of its effects. PD is a potentially useful epidemiologic exposure variable because it is measureable, has an impact on health, and differs among individuals and populations. Moreover, enough is known about effective ways to treat PD that it is conceivable that treatment may help to prevent or control an associated systemic disease.

It should be emphasized that traditional epidemiology does not determine the cause of a disease in a given individual; it examines relationships or associations between exposures and frequency of disease in populations. Exposures associated with disease are called *risk factors*. When such associations are firmly established, it becomes possible that the exposure might cause the disease, and there may be calls for action, such as occurred with smoking and lung cancer. This chapter reviews common-sense causality, attributable to the 18th-century philosopher David Hume[8,9] and the 19th-century philosopher John Stuart Mill,[10] and its typical use in everyday problem solving in dentistry.

Principles of Causation

Four criteria for causation have evolved from the philosophic musings of Hume and Mill: *(1)* temporality, *(2)* contiguity, *(3)* history of regularity, and *(4)* elimination of alternatives; these criteria form the organizational basis of this chapter. One of Hume's criteria—history of regularity—has in modern times been investigated by sophisticated statistical measures of association, and some of the most common methods, such as calculation of odds ratios and regression analysis, are described.

Moreover, the concepts of causation in epidemiology have evolved to consider complex relationships between putative causes and effects. However, it turns out that the actual acceptance of cause-effect relationships also entails qualitative arguments that involve concepts of plausibility and persuasion. There can be discrepancies between the findings of different studies and the conflicting opinions of experts, so that people can become habitually skeptical about the so-called menaces of everyday life and ignore good advice at their peril.

How such disagreements can be resolved is illustrated by the history of establishing the relationship of smoking as a cause of cancer. Statistics, philosophy, personality, and rhetoric came together to produce a widely accepted causal relationship, and it is likely, for current controversies, that similar outcomes will evolve through similar processes. In the news stories mentioned earlier, as is typically the case, the question of whether an exposure of some kind causes a disease starts with the observation of some association between them. However, the question of whether the exposure is a cause of the disease comes quickly thereafter.

Importance of understanding causation

Causation is a critically important concept in dentistry and medicine as well as in everyday life. Dentists routinely attempt to determine the factors that have caused the need for prosthodontic treatment, such as malocclusion, traumatic occlusion, missing teeth, or poor oral hygiene. Dentists identify causes in order to render appropriate treatment that will eliminate the negative influence and thereby resolve their patients' problems. Indeed Greene[11] listed incorrect cause-effect correlations as one of his "fallacies of failure" in clinical dentistry, noting that if the cause of a clinical problem is unknown or incorrectly identified, a clinician might expect a treatment designed to manage the condition to fail. Greene[11] contended that clinicians who exhibit a theoretical bias to certain problems can often make incorrect cause-effect assessments. Despite abuses of causal reasoning, sound decision making can entail the development of causal models in which observational and/or experimental data as well as logic are combined so that reliable predictions of the outcome of an intervention can be made.

Causal inference

Causal inference is the process of finding causal relationships. Some causes can be directly and deterministically linked to their effects. For example, troubleshooting guides that accompany appliances list an array of possible conditions that could explain the equipment's malfunction; near the top of the list will be a suggestion to see if the machine is in fact turned on or plugged in. No great philosophic acumen is required to understand the reasoning.

Elucidating cause-effect relationships, however, can also be complex, and philosophers such as David Hume[8,9] and John Stuart Mill[10] have proposed criteria for the demonstration and investigation of causality. Their approaches were developed, however, at a time when large data sets and statistical approaches were not available. Most causal claims today eventually rest on probability, and the web of causation is investigated by sophisticated study designs and statistical techniques. Central to this enterprise is distinguishing causation, which entails a time sequence in which the cause precedes the event and reasons for connecting the two, from mere association, which is a statistically discernible relationship between two or more measured variables or counts.

Common-Sense Causation

Regularity of nature

The common-sense view of causality rests on the faith of the regularity or uniformity of nature. It has two tenets:

1. An identical cause will always produce an identical effect, so observations can be repeated.
2. There is a reason for any change, so searching for causes of changes is not necessarily a fruitless task.

The father of experimental medicine, Claude Bernard,[12] posited that the appearance of disease must by caused by some change in either the internal milieu of the body or the environment: "Proof that a given condition is the immediate cause of that phenomenon does not warrant concluding with certainty that a given cause is the immediate cause of that phenomenon. It must still be established that, when this condition is removed, the phenomenon will no longer appear." While Bernard, like other scientists of his era, believed in specific and deterministic causes, modern conceptions of causation include causes that induce only a probability of producing an effect.

Identifying causes

In his *A Treatise of Human Nature*, Hume[8] denied that there could be any logical validity in our conception of cause and effect. In brief, Hume believed that all inferences from experience are effects of custom and not of rigorous reasoning. People can be misled by experience like a turkey who has been fed every day of his life and confidently expects to be fed forever until he is sadly disillusioned by being slaughtered by the farmer for Thanksgiving dinner. Kenneth Clark summarized this philosophic pessimism as follows: "Hume…succeeded in proving that experience and reason have no necessary connection with one another. There is no such thing as a rational belief." He added that the *Treatise* has "made all philosophers feel uneasy till the present day."[13]

Despite his doubts that absolute certainty can ever be obtained, Hume[8] identified eight principles that people use when they identify causes and even included concepts, such as dose-response relationships, that are employed in clinical epidemiology today. The major features of Hume's principles can be condensed into three rules:

1. Temporality: The cause precedes the effect.
2. Contiguity: A connection exists between the cause and the effect that explains how the cause can produce the effect.
3. Association: There is a history of regularity in the relationship of the cause and the effect.

An additional rule can be traced to John Stuart Mill[10]: the elimination of alternatives. Mill developed a methodology for investigating causal relationships, which he called the *canons of induction*[10]:

1. The method of agreement: "If two or more instances of the phenomenon under investigation have only one circumstance in common, the circumstance in which alone all the instances agree, is the cause (or effect) of the given phenomenon."
2. The method of difference: "If an instance in which the phenomenon under investigation occurs, and an instance in which it does not occur, have every circumstance save one in common…the circumstance in which alone the two instances differ is the effect, or cause…of the phenomenon."
3. The joint method of agreement and difference, which employs both of the first two methods on sets of instances.
4. The method of residue, which is a form of the method of difference.
5. The method of concomitant variations, which can be considered as the philosophic antecedent of dose-response relationships.

Mill formulated both experimental and observational versions of his method.[14] For experimental investigations, Mill's canons boil down to advising causal investigators to vary one factor at a time and observe the result. This is the philosophic basis of the randomized controlled trial (RCT), in which the investigator introduces one factor, that is, a treatment, to one of two groups that are theoretically identical because randomization should distribute confounding factors equally between the groups. The canons are less rigorously applied in analytical studies,

where, for example, the researcher compares mortality between those who have decided to quit smoking and those who did not. There are probably differences between the people who decided to quit smoking and those who did not, and such differences mean that the groups differ in more than just one factor of quitting smoking. Analytical application of the canons, in particular the method of agreement, is intended to eliminate all contending (or perhaps pretending) causes except the actual cause.[14]

These common-sense concepts of Hume and Mill continue to be employed in modern investigations. For example, meeting criterion 1 (temporality) is one of the strengths of longitudinal cohort studies as well as clinical trials in which investigators introduce a putative cause and observe the result; cross-sectional surveys do not meet this criterion. The connections between cause and effect (contiguity) must be investigated to clarify the mechanisms of action linking the cause to the effect, as for example the action of radiation on DNA and the subsequent production of mutations and malignancy. The criterion of history of regularity (association) is documented by the use of statistical measures of association.

As an example of common-sense reasoning in dentistry, consider a dentist attempting to diagnose and treat a patient suffering from oral ulcers, which have many putative causes, such as aphthous stomatitis, infections, trauma, burning, poorly fitting dentures, or allergies. All these conditions could, in theory, meet Hume's second criteria, contiguity—a reason to connect the cause to the effect. Besides closely observing the oral tissues and the dentition, the dentist would typically want to know when the condition developed and how it progressed. For example, if the ulcer arose soon after the placement of new dentures, that *possible* cause might be considered a *likely* cause, because it fulfills Hume's first criteria, temporality: The effect occurred after the putative cause.

Although such clinical reasoning seems simple, it is also powerful. Sackett et al[15] stated that clinical reasoning is far more powerful than laboratory evaluation for most patients in most places. Various strategies are used to optimize this reasoning, such as the mnemonic *VINDI-*

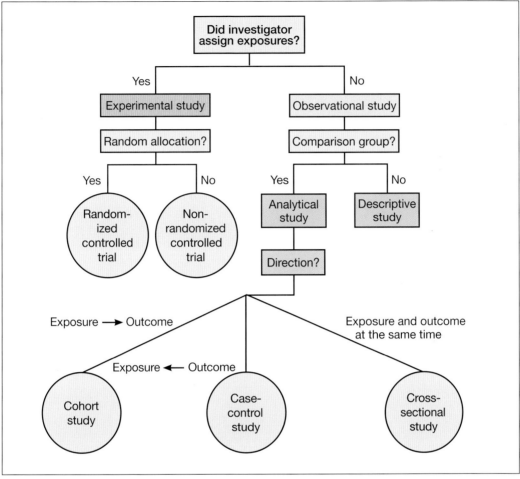

Fig 2-1 Algorithm for classification of study designs. (Reprinted from Grimes and Shulz[16] with permission.)

CATE (vascular, inflammatory, neoplastic, degenerative, idiopathic, congenital, autoimmune/allergic, traumatic, endocrine) for differential diagnoses to systematically cover various possibilities. Sackett et al[15] described the approach adopted in this example as a hypotheticodeductive strategy, which involves "formulation, from the earliest clues about the patient of a short list of potential diagnoses and actions... followed by maneuvers that will best reduce the length of the list." Unlike scientists, who, allegedly, attempt to disprove their hypotheses, clinicians generally seek data that support their working hypothesis. If the dentist in this example

produced a new set of dentures and the ulcer went away, the dentist could use the canons of induction to draw a conclusion: Because only one factor, the dentures, had been changed, the ulcer was caused by the dentures.

However, in real life, situations may be much more complex; the timing between the putative cause and effect may not be clear, a well-established mechanism linking the cause and the effect may not be known, and/or how often the cause is associated with the effect may not be established. Thus, various study designs and measures of association have been developed to clarify these issues (Fig 2-1).[16]

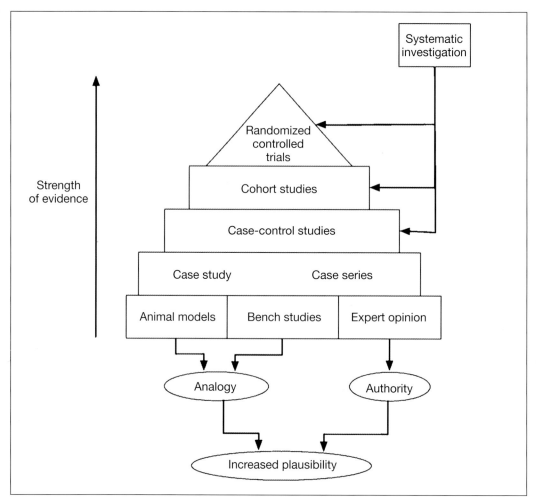

Fig 2-2 Evidence pyramid for investigative approaches and its support by inductive logic through analogy and authority.

Study Designs in Causal Investigation

Most studies linking an exposure with a disease are observational; that is, the people in the study determine their own exposures by their choices and circumstances, for example, by choosing to smoke cigarettes. Compared with clinical trials, such observational studies are inexpensive, particularly when they employ population data collected for other purposes. Moreover, observational studies often have large samples that include a wide range of patients and occur in the real world, with all its variety, rather than the artificial conditions created in RCTs. Ethical issues related to treatment assignment can be avoided because the investigator does not assign subjects to a potentially noxious agent or deny a potentially beneficial therapy. A major problem with observational studies is that there is a risk of selection bias that leads to systematic differences in outcomes because the exposure is chosen rather than randomly assigned.

The strength of study designs is often presented as a pyramid (Fig 2-2), with the strongest type of evidence at the top and the lowest-level evidence at the base. Some versions of the evidence pyramid include filtered information, such as systematic reviews at the top, but this discussion is concerned with primary studies.

There is some debate about aspects of the pyramid; Concato et al[17] have argued against employing such a rigid hierarchy to arbitrarily exclude evidence and found that well-designed observational studies (with either a cohort or a case-control design) do not systematically overestimate the magnitude of the effects of treatment compared with those found in RCTs on the same topic. As of June 2013, the study by Concato et al[17] has been cited some 1,300 times, and there is a vigorous debate on the issue. Nevertheless, it is not just the design of the study that determines the quality of the evidence; the execution and interpretation of the study are major contributors to its usefulness.

Study designs are discussed in order of the causal criterion that is mainly fulfilled by their use.

Criterion 1: Temporality

Case studies or case series

In a case study, patients are treated or exposed to a risk factor, and they or their records are carefully observed; therefore, the investigator does have access to a time sequence. A compilation of case reports can constitute a case series. Inferences are made of the basis of historical controls, that is, the outcome that would have been expected if treatment had not taken place or if a standard treatment had been given. Historical controls are less than ideal, because time and history can mislead as a result of changes such as incremental improvements in equipment, materials, and techniques. The basic flaw is the lack of a control group, and this flaw is not eliminated by considering more cases. Streiner et al[18] noted that case reports involving some 1,500 patients indicated that gastric freezing cured gastric ulcers, but subsequent properly controlled trials showed the treatment to be useless.

Huth[19] argued that only three types of case report merit publication: the unique case, the

case of unexpected association, and the case of unexpected events. Truly dramatic treatment effects or adverse effects can be identified by this method. Venning[20] reported that, of 18 well-recognized, serious adverse drug reactions, 13 were first published as case reports.

Because elaborate equipment need not necessarily be involved, case study or case series is an approach to causal investigation that dentists can perform in their own practices. For example, oral and maxillofacial surgeons first recognized and reported cases of nonhealing exposed bone in the maxillofacial regions in patients treated with bisphosphonates.[21,22]

Finally, the basic case study intervention design "try something and see if it works" is successful in everyday problem solving and probably contributes to the faith people have in this approach.

Cohort studies

In cohort studies, the researcher forms groups on the basis of exposure to the putative causal agent, follows them forward, and measures the incidence of the disease outcome. Incidence rate, that is, the person–time to outcome, is the preferred measure of disease frequency for causal effects. In cohort studies, relative risk (RR) is used to describe the results.

$$RR = \frac{\text{Incidence of outcome with exposure}}{\text{Incidence of outcome without exposure}}$$

The RR expresses how many times more (or less) likely an exposed person is to develop an outcome relative to an unexposed person. A value of RR = 1 indicates that the exposure does not change the risk, while RR > 1 indicates that the person is at increased risk for the disease, and RR < 1 indicates that the person is at less risk. For example, if RR = 0.8, the risk of disease on exposure is decreased by 20%.

The following is a useful formula to calculate the change in risk in percentages:

$$RR \text{ decrease or increase} = |1.0 - RR| \times 100$$

For example, if RR = 0.8 (a decrease), then $|1.0 - 0.8| \times 100 = 0.2 \times 100 = 20\%$ decrease in risk. Similarly, if RR = 1.2 (an increase), then $|1.0 - 1.2| \times 100 = |-0.2| \times 100 = 0.2 \times 100 = 20\%$ increase in risk. The absolute value of $|1.0 - RR|$ is used in the formula, so the same formula is applied for both increases and decreases in risk.

RRs can be used by dentists to advise patients on how to change their risks for certain diseases or conditions. For example, Holm[23] found that the RR of losing one or more teeth was 4.55 among young smokers compared with nonsmokers over a 10-year period. If the baseline rate (BR) for losing one or more teeth over the 10-year period for nonsmoking persons of that age was 10%, the absolute risk for the young smoker would be BR × RR = 10% × 4.55 = 45.5%, an increase of 35.5% over baseline. Such a large change, almost a 50:50 chance of tooth loss at a young age, might give patients pause to consider their behavior. If the BR were very low, as it is for some conditions, say for example BR = 0.01 and RR = 4.5, the absolute risk even in the presence of an exposure would be only 0.045%, which might not provide patients with much incentive to change their behavior.

Additional advantages of cohort studies over the cross-sectional designs (discussed later) are that selection bias in the cohort is rarely problematic and subjects can be matched for possible confounders, although matching can be inefficient.[24] Moreover, unlike in case-control studies, recall of events in the past is not required, and measurement errors of exposure are not expected to differ between the groups.[24] Cohort studies also have several disadvantages: The exposure is not under the investigator's control and may be related to some unknown factor that is correlated with the outcome; they are expensive; and cohort studies take a long time, particularly when rare outcomes are being studied.

Randomized (clinical) controlled trials

Unlike observational designs, RCTs are true experiments in which eligible patients are randomly allocated to groups to receive (experimental group) or not receive (control group) one or more interventions that are being compared.

The investigator controls the timing of the exposure or treatment and subsequently observes the effects, so the criterion of temporality is satisfied. In principle, randomization ensures that the groups are comparable initially and any differences in outcomes can be attributed to the experimental intervention. Trials or experiments in which the groups are formed without randomization can be subject to confounding and bias just like observational studies.

To ensure the validity of the comparison, the RCT normally includes various safeguards against bias. For example, ideally both patients and researchers are "blinded"; that is, they do not know whether the individual patient is receiving a treatment or a sham treatment. The blinding of the recipient of the treatment and its providers and assessors (a double-blind experiment) attempts to remove the expectancy bias that occurs when the observers or the patients expect the treatment to be effective or noxious and this expectation influences their response in the expected direction.

RCTs are generally (but not universally; see Concato et al[17]) agreed to provide the best evidence for determining causation. The results of the treatment are normally reported as the ratio of the risk in the treated group to the risk in the control group.

Limitations on the use of RCTs include situations in which ethics dictate that treatments not be assigned to patients or communities by random assignment. For example, if there is strong suggestive evidence for a beneficial effect, an ethics committee might demand that the treatment be offered to all subjects. In contrast, if there is substantial evidence that a treatment could cause harm, an ethics committee might demand that it not be given by random assignment to any subjects. Another problem with RCTs is that the approach may simply be unfeasible if the outcome of interest is rare.

Criterion 2: Contiguity mechanisms

Animal models and laboratory research are ranked at the lowest level in terms of strength of the evidence of primary sources as applied to investigations involving humans, such as effectiveness of interventions or causation of disease. The ranking of these approaches as low level indicates their contribution when they stand alone. However, they do increase the plausibility of conclusions and thus the overall strength of the evidence. Metaphorically at least, being at the base of the pyramid they raise the strength of all the evidence above them. Animal models and bench research provide support for the role of a risk factor in causing disease through the logic of analogy, a form of inductive argument.

Animal models

In brief, noting that experimental animals and humans share many characteristics, analogy deems it reasonable that they might well respond similarly to various stimuli or treatments. That mice develop tumors in response to components of tobacco smoke painted on their skin supports the contention that such substances may be carcinogenic in humans. Arguments of this type strengthened the case that smoking caused lung cancer.

Laboratory research

Laboratory bench studies can provide a theory or mechanism of how a treatment works, which enables troubleshooting if problems occur. The relationship between clinical evidence and theory is like a bicycle; the optimum stability and predictability occur when there are both strong empirical evidence and a strong underlying theory[18]; having only theory or evidence is like a unicycle, which is inherently unstable.

Criterion 3: History of regularity (association)

Ecologic studies

Ecologic studies compare populations with respect to exposure and outcome, for example, the average sugar consumption per person and the number of decayed, missing, or filled teeth per person in various countries. A serious limitation of these studies is that there is no information about whether the individual's consumption of sugar (exposure) is correlated with the same individual's caries experience (health condition or outcome). The degree of association reported for ecologic studies is often higher than that found when exposures and outcomes for individuals are examined.

Cross-sectional surveys

In cross-sectional (survey) designs, the exposure and health condition are determined simultaneously in individuals; these studies can be used to estimate the prevalence of a disease as well as to explore possible risk factors or causes of disease. They are insufficient for establishing causation because they do not distinguish whether the exposure preceded the disease. Moreover, it is often difficult to determine the direction of causality, that is, if A causes B or B causes A. For example, if poverty and lack of education are correlated, is it because poverty prevents people from affording education or because a lack of education results in low income?

Case-control studies

In case-control designs, the groups are formed by outcome (the "cases" are patients with the disease). The cases are compared with control individuals not known to have the disease of interest. Commonly the controls are selected through some form of matching so that they resemble the cases in all factors save exposure to the risk factor being investigated.

The search for exposure is retrospective, so this design is subject to recall bias, because the cases have generally thought more deeply about their exposure history than the controls have. Another problem is that records from the past may be of dubious quality or omit data that was not considered important at the time. Moreover, investigators generally do not know how confounding variables are distributed among the groups, and there may also be concerns about the suitability of the control group. Another problem can be prevalence-incidence bias (also known as *Neyman bias*)—early deaths or patients in whom evidence of

Table 2-1	Odds ratio: Exposure and disease (2 × 2 table)	
Disease/exposure	Exposure present (+)	Exposure absent (–)
Disease present (+)	a	c
Disease absent (–)	b	d

$$\text{Odds ratio} = \frac{\text{Odds with exposure present}}{\text{Odds with no exposure}} = \frac{a/b}{c/d} = \frac{ad}{bc}$$

exposure has disappeared are not counted appropriately.

Despite these drawbacks, the case-control approach is particularly useful in studying rare diseases or events. In the case-control design, the odds ratio is the usual means of reporting risk levels that have been altered by exposure (Table 2-1).

Calculating association

Association is a statistically discernible relationship between two or more measured variables (or counts). *Correlation* is the term used when the relationship between the variables is linear. Correlation does not imply (in the sense of being sufficient to prove) causation. For example, smoking is associated with oral cancer and with tooth staining. Consequently, through their common cause, smoking, there would likely be a statistical association between tooth staining and oral cancer. However, if the stain were removed from the teeth, the risk of oral cancer would still be increased if the individual, now with pearly white teeth, continued smoking. If the individual stopped smoking, however, his or her risk of oral cancer would be reduced.

According to Edward Tufte,[25] the shortest true statement about correlations and causation is that "Empirically observed covariation is a necessary but not sufficient condition for causality," or, expressed more succinctly, "Correlation is not causation but it sure is a hint."[26] Even so-phisticated methods of exploring relationships, such as multiple regression and multilevel modeling, may be effective for prediction but may still be misinterpreted for causal inference. The method used to calculate association of expo-sure to a risk factor and disease depends on the type of data and the study design.

Categorical data—the 2 × 2 table. The association between exposure and disease is assessed with two general questions:

1. Is there a real effect of the exposure on disease, or could the data be explained adequately by chance?
2. What is the size of the effect?

In the simplest cases, these basic questions can be answered with a 2 × 2 table (see Table 2-1). As an example, Table 2-2 calculates the odds ratio for data in a study by Oğuz et al,[27] who examined the relationship between chronic periodontitis (CP) and erectile dysfunction (ED). In this sample of men aged 30 to 40 years, 42 of 80 men who exhibited ED had chronic periodontitis. Of 82 men who did not have ED, 19 had CP and 63 did not have CP.

The count data in the table are categorical (nominal) scale data that sort variables according to category, such as presence or absence of ED or CP. One test for determining relationships with such categorical data is the chi-square analysis, designated by the Greek letter χ. Chi-square tests whether the actual observed counts differ significantly from what could be expected by chance.

The table itself is called a *contingency table*. The marginal totals of the cells (designated a, b, c, d), which are the characteristics of the whole sample, are used to calculate the expected values in each cell in the contingency table. Then the chi-square statistic is calculated as the sum of the four cells of the table's [(square of the

Table 2-2	Odds ratio of relationship between chronic periodontitis (CP) and erectile dysfunction (ED)		
Disease/exposure	CP +	CP −	Total
ED +	a 42	c 38	80
ED −	b 19	d 63	82

Data from Oğuz et al.[27]

$$\chi^2 = \frac{(ad - bc)^2(a + b + c + d)}{(a + b)(c + d)(b + d)(a + c)}$$

In this case, $\chi^2 = 14.84$; $P < .05$. The critical value of χ^2 for 3 degrees of freedom is 3.84. The null hypothesis (chance alone can explain the variation in the table) is roundly rejected.

$$\text{Odds ratio} = \frac{\text{Odds with exposure present}}{\text{Odds with no exposure}} = \frac{a/b}{c/d} = \frac{ad}{bc} = \frac{42 \cdot 63}{19 \cdot 38} = 3.7.$$

The 95% confidence interval for OR = 1.87–7.19.

observed − expected value) divided by the expected value]:

$$\chi^2 = \Sigma \frac{(O-E)^2}{E}$$

where O is the frequencies observed and E is the frequencies expected. Calculations on the data reported by Oğuz et al[27] reveal that the association of PD with ED is unlikely to be explained by chance (see Table 2-2).

Once it is known that the effect is real, the size of the effect can be determined. A useful approach for analyzing these kinds of data from case-control studies is the odds ratio (OR), calculated as the ratio between the odds of experiencing the disease after exposure to a risk factor and the odds of experiencing the disease with no exposure (see the Glossary at the end of the chapter). If the OR is greater than 1, the odds of experiencing the disease after exposure to the risk factor are increased. If there is no relationship between an exposure and a disease, the proportions of those with exposure would not differ between those with the disease and those without the disease, so the OR would equal 1. That is, if the exposure does not entail any risk, the value of a/b (risk with exposure present [in this example, those with CP]) divided by the value of c/d (risk with no exposure [those without CP]) should equal 1. If the OR is less than 1, the exposure agent indicates an "inverse association" with the disease and may be protective.

The equation $\frac{a/b}{c/d}$ is algebraically equivalent to $\frac{ad}{bc}$, a formula referred to as the *cross-product ratio*. Thus, for the ED/CP data reported by Oğuz et al,[27] the OR is $(42 \times 63)/(19 \times 38) = 3.7$. The data therefore indicate that a person with CP is 3.7 times more likely to suffer from ED, and CP is said to be positively associated with the disease.

When the OR is used, it is necessary to determine the precision of the estimate. Precision is generally reported by providing the 95% confidence interval. The 95% confidence interval indicates that, if the same study were repeated 100 times, 95 of those repetitions would yield a value for the OR lying between the upper and lower bounds of the confidence interval. A somewhat complex formula is available for calculating the confidence interval for the OR (calculators are available on the Internet).

When the formula is applied to the CP and ED data reported by Oğuz et al,[27] the 95% interval is 1.87 to 7.19. This confidence interval does not include the value of 1.0 that would be expected if CP had no influence on ED (ie, the null hypothesis), so this finding also indicates that it is unlikely that the observed association can be explained by chance.

Despite its apparent simplicity and wide use, many people find OR difficult to comprehend and confuse OR with relative risk. When the outcome has a low probability, this confusion is not problematic because the values are similar, but for high-probability outcomes (eg, ≈ 55%) the OR is a poor measure of relative risk.[28]

Finally, the crude estimate of OR based on the 2 × 2 table does not take into account the influence of other risk factors; however, the OR may be adjusted for the presence of risk factors by use of logistic regression to produce an adjusted OR.

The OR can be used in clinical decision making. In a case-control study in which the cases experienced dental implant failure, Yip et al[29] found an adjusted OR of 2.69 (adjustment to be discussed later) for middle-aged women who had been treated with oral bisphosphonates. They concluded that their results supported a recommendation for discontinuation of oral bisphosphonates in long-term users to allow for recovery of bone remodeling.

Correlation coefficient. If the relationship between two variables is such that, when one variable (independent variable) changes, the dependent variable changes linearly, such as can be demonstrated with continuous data, the variables are said to be correlated. Figure 2-3 shows the relationship between the height and the weight of students in a graduate class. In this instance, the height is plotted on the x-axis, where the independent variable is usually plotted. This is the variable selected or controlled by the investigator; the term *independent* in this usage does not connote statistical independence. Weight is plotted on the y-axis, which is where the response (also called *outcome* or *dependent*) variable is typically plotted. The graph reveals a roughly linear relationship.

The main purpose of using correlational data is to make predictions, so it would be desirable to have a mathematic model to describe the relationship. One approach is simple linear regression that represents the relationship as follows: $y = \beta_0 + \beta_1 x + \mathcal{E}$, where y is the predicted value of response variable (weight) and x is the height (predictor or explanatory variable). β_0 (a constant, in particular the intercept: the value where the regression line intersects with the y-axis) and β_1 (slope, change in y per unit change in x) are population parameters. $\mathcal{E}$ is the error term that records the deviation of an observed data point from the value predicted by the regression equation.

For this example, the regression line has parameters $\beta_0 = -144.43$ and $\beta_1 = 1.235$.

One advantage of having a mathematic model of this type is that it makes it possible to predict the expected value of y for any value of x. Such prediction is the bread-and-butter use of regression. In fact, typically regression analysis takes the values of x as stated (as if there were no measurement error) and minimizes the sums of squares on the vertical component (ie, the y-axis).[30]

Also plotted in Fig 2-3 are the residuals for two observations. The residuals can be thought of as the error between the observation and value predicted by the model (ie, the least squares fitted line). The pattern of residual values is used to diagnose the assumptions of the linear regression model, including the normality assumption on the errors.

For continuous data, such as blood pressure, dollars, temperature, height, and weight, the degree to which two variables are related is given by the correlation coefficient (r), which can take values between –1 and 1 . A value of $r = 0$ indicates that there is no relationship; that is, the variables are independent. A value of $r = 1$ indicates a perfect positive relationship, and a value of $r = -1$ represents a perfect negative relationship. Typically, researchers test whether there is a significant relationship between the two variables by demonstrating that the value of r significantly differs from 0.

Regression also can be used to explain the data with regard to the amount of variability in the data that is attributable to the independent variable. An interesting property of r is that r^2 (called the *coefficient of determination*) represents the amount of variation in the outcome variable that is explained by the predictor variable. For the height-weight relationship shown in Fig 2-3, $r^2 = 0.7$, so 30% of the variation is unexplained, and therefore it might be prudent to investigate the data in greater detail.

In the height-weight data, the correlation coefficient differs significantly from 0. In this sample, taller people tend to weigh more. However, the values for women are more likely to fall below the regression line than are those for men. Moreover, when the data are considered sepa-

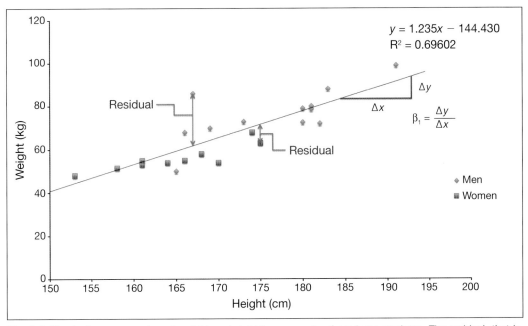

Fig 2-3 Simple linear regression of weight on height for a sample of graduate students. The residual, that is, the deviation of an observed point from the value predicted by the linear equation, is shown for two points. The equation is $y = $ (slope $\times x$) + intercept, where y is the weight (kg) and x is the height (cm). In this case, the slope is 1.235 and the intercept is −144.430. Thus, $y = 1.235x − 144.430$. The points for women tend to be less than those predicted by the model, suggesting that sex might be considered as a predictive variable in a multiple regression model. The coefficient of variation, $R^2 = 0.69602$, indicates that almost 70% of the variation in weight among the sample can be explained by height.

rately for men and women, the regression lines for the two sexes have different slopes. This situation, in which more than one independent (or explanatory) variable has an effect on the dependent (response) variable, is common and can complicate the process of forming conclusions.

Confounding variables. Another problem that can obscure the relationship between a disease and exposure is confounding. A *confounding variable (confounder)* is defined as a risk factor for the disease that is associated with the exposure (the variable of interest in a study) and thereby contributes to the observed association between the exposure and the disease. Smith and Philips[31] concluded that it is likely that many of the associations identified in epidemiologic studies are due to confounding, often by factors that are difficult to measure. Confounding is often offered as an alternative explanation for an association between an exposure and a disease.

There are several criteria for determining a confounding variable: *(1)* There should be an association of the confounder and the disease among the unexposed individuals; *(2)* there is a difference in the distribution of the confounding variable among the different exposure groups; and *(3)* the confounding variable should not lie on the causal pathway between the exposure and the disease. Confounding results from imbalances in risk factors for the outcome (ie, disease) in different exposure groups. Confounding muddies the association of a risk factor with a disease and can either increase or diminish the effect of the exposure variable.

Confounding is often detected by comparing the discrepancy between the crude and adjusted estimates for relative risk. If adjusting for a potential confounder changes the relative risk, the variable is suspected to be a real confounder.

Adjustment. In epidemiologic studies, the possibility that confounding could account for observed associations is managed by demonstrating that the association is independent of the confounding factor.[31] An exposure is said to be independently associated with the outcome if the association remains after the levels of other exposures are held fixed; this process is called *controlling*, *adjusting*, or *conditioning* for other exposures.

Oğuz at al,[27] in their study of ED, avoided the potential problem of the effects of age and smoking on ED simply by restricting the study to nonsmokers in a certain age range. However, that approach (restriction) is often not feasible when there are multiple possible confounders, so that forming well-defined groups with adequate numbers is difficult. Instead, adjustment is often made retrospectively by statistical analysis of the data gathered on the participants in the study.

Two major approaches to adjustment are *multiple linear regression*, which is used when the outcome variable is continuous, such as blood pressure, and *logistic regression*, when the outcome variable is binary, such as presence or absence of disease or an event such as tooth loss, death, or heart attack.

Multiple linear regression is a statistical technique for predicting the value of a continuous and normally distributed dependent variable (also described as *response* or *outcome variables*) from a combination of two or more independent variables (also described as *risk factors* or *explanatory* or *predictor variables*, depending on the purpose of the study). For example, multiple linear regression might be used to examine the relationship of an Oral Health Index value (response variable) to age, race, education, and sex (predictor variables). Similar to simple linear regression, the goodness of fit may be measured by the coefficient of determination, R^2, where R, in this case, is a measure of correlation between the outcome variable and the joint set of independent variables.

Multiple regression can be set up so that the model includes covariates. The *covariates* are variables that the investigator thinks may be important and thus may want to control, such as socioeconomic variables. The reason for including such variables in the analysis may not be to determine their separate effects, which could already have been established, but to enable the investigator to determine the effects of other independent variables by adjusting for the covariates. Multiple regression can also be used to examine interactions among the dependent variables, for example, to determine if the effect of a person's sex on Oral Hygiene Index depends on age.

Logistic regression is the technique used to explore questions involving binary outcomes (yes or no), such as the relationship of CP to heart attack. Like multiple regression, logistic regression can include consideration of multiple dependent variables and yields the regression coefficients for the predictor (explanatory or independent) variables. The results are interpreted as the probability that the outcome variable will occur in response to a variable of interest, after adjustment for the effect of the other (independent) variables. The results are usually presented as an OR.

Logistic regression enables the researcher to compare two conditions, such as presence and absence of PD, adjusted for other explanatory variables, on a binary outcome and to obtain an adjusted OR. In the example of CP and ED discussed earlier,[27] the authors used logistic regression to find an adjusted OR of 3.29 (95% confidence interval of 1.36–9.55), a result that was somewhat different but included in the range of the value estimated from the simple 2 × 2 table analysis (see Table 2-2). The result was different because the more sophisticated logistic regression analysis adjusts for potential confounders, including age, body mass index, household income, and education level.

The focus of logistic regression lies in calculating ORs. When newspaper articles use phrases such as, "When adjusted for socioeconomic variables, people with periodontal disease *are three times as likely* to suffer from erectile dysfunction," odds are that the underlying research used logistic regression.

Limitations of statistical adjustment. Statistical adjustment has limitations. Gilbert[30] stated that if the data are observational rather than experimental, the greatest caution must be used when multiple regression is used in an attempt to identify those independent (explanatory) variables (x's) that determine the response value (y). Indeed, in his view, observational data can never guarantee that any observed relationship is cause and effect. Several problems are connected with statistical adjustment:

1. Errors of measurement of x tend to dilute the true size of the functional relationship (but means of dealing with measurement error, such as regression calibration and simulation and extrapolation, are being developed).[32]
2. All the important independent variables (x's) must be included in the analysis. If a missing but important x is correlated with some of the other independent variables, those independent variables may well appear erroneously as more important than they actually are.
3. The assumption that the effects of the independent variables are linear and additive must hold.

Important problems related to calculation and interpretation of association.

Misclassification and exposure measurement error. In general, it is easier to detect meaningful associations when the measurement of exposures and diagnosis of disease are accurate, but sometimes the methods used to measure the exposure or to classify the disease are unreliable. Misclassification is related to the sensitivity and specificity of the classification method. Janket et al[33] found that there was a significant underestimated relative risk for CHD in studies that used self-reported periodontal status. Dietrich and Garcia[34] suggested that, if a real effect exists, the association between PD and CHD may be stronger than that suggested by currently available cohort studies.

One approach to deciding whether the criteria adopted for classification have unduly influenced the conclusion is to conduct sensitivity analysis, in which the researcher monitors the changes in the estimate of risk if classification criteria are varied.

Bias. As used in epidemiology, *bias* is an error in design or execution of a study that produces results that are consistently distorted in one direction because of nonrandom factors. In contrast, chance (random) distortions tend to cancel each other out. Even when studies are carried out with rigorous methodology, P values and confidence intervals are largely concerned with determination of sampling error, not the problem of bias, which can greatly impact the results and interpretation. The P value is the probability of obtaining a test statistic at least as extreme as the one actually observed, assuming that the null hypothesis (no difference) is true. Values of $P < .05$ indicate that groups are significantly different, that is, any difference present cannot be explained by chance.

Sackett[35] listed 56 biases for clinical studies; however, because biases can arise from subtle sources, the actual number of possible biases to be considered is probably limited only by the imagination of the investigator (Box 2-1). An important skill for epidemiologic investigators is the ability to identify conditions that lead to bias of whatever type in their studies.

A common problem is that those individuals who are available for selection into a sample do not represent the target population (those people for whom the findings of the study are meant to generalize). For example, patients receiving treatment in a clinic set in an undergraduate dental faculty are unlikely to represent the general population.

Some study designs are associated with particular types of bias. For example, study designs that require participants to recall exposure to particular agents are subject to recall bias, because people who have a disease are more likely to have thought more deeply about their past types of exposure than have healthy controls. Bias can also appear as a result of changing conditions over time. As methods of cancer detection improve, patients may be diagnosed at an earlier stage of their disease, when there is greater proportion of slow-growing tumors. Thus, survival time after diagnosis may improve irrespective of changes in methods of treatment because of both the greater lead time resulting from earlier diagnosis and the greater proportion of patients with slow-growing tumors. Finally, bias can also arise because of the complex interrelationships of variables that can occur in causal pathways.

Box 2-1   Biases, as described by Sackett[35]

bias Any factor that produces a systematic error between the observation and the true value or property about which information is desired, as opposed to chance (random) distortions that tend to cancel each other out. An analogy for bias in measurement is the deflection of an arrow from its path to a bullseye by a biasing wind that blows it off course.

Six bias families:
1. *Reading-up the field*, such as the biases of rhetoric, one-sided reference bias, and positive results bias
2. *Specifying and selecting the study sample*, such as volunteer bias, referral filter bias, diagnostic access bias, prevalence-incidence (Neyman) bias, and starting-time bias
3. *Executing the experimental intervention (or exposure)*, such as withdrawal bias, compliance bias, therapeutic personality bias, and recall bias
4. *Measuring exposures and outcomes*, such as insensitive measure bias, expectation bias, recall bias, obsequiousness bias, and family information bias
5. *Data analysis*, such as post hoc significance bias, scale degradation bias, repeated peaks bias, and data dredging bias

6. *Interpretation*, such as magnitude bias, significance bias, correlation bias, and cognitive dissonance bias

Important biases:
- *Measurement bias* A systematic error in the values of a measurement caused by inadequacies in the measurement process, such as an improperly calibrated periodontal probe.
- *Publication bias* Editors of scientific journals prefer not to publish studies with negative results because there are many reasons for studies to fail, including a lack of sensitivity or statistical power. Therefore, for any given intervention that is studied extensively, the studies claiming an effect are published, whereas the ones that found no effect end up in a file drawer.
- *Selection bias* A systematic error in choosing a sample so that some categories of individuals are overrepresented or underrepresented. The favorite example of statisticians is the *Literary Digest* poll that predicted the election of a Republican president based on a biased sample in which wealthy people were overrepresented.
- *Source of support bias* The worry that "The one who pays the piper calls the tune."

Shrier and Platt[36] devised a six-step approach, using directed acyclic graphs, that they believe reduces the degree of bias for the effect estimate in a statistical model.

Suggestions for interpreting OR and RR. There are no hard and fast rules for interpreting the usefulness of the absolute numerical values of OR and RR for clinical decision making. Straus et al[37] suggested that the OR and RR be interpreted in the context of the study design that generated them. Case-control and cohort studies are more susceptible to bias than are RCTs. The general goal is to ensure that the OR or RR is greater than the value that might

be generated by bias and so constitutes a real additional risk. For a case-control study, Straus et al[37] suggested that an OR > 4 be adopted as the cutoff for serious consideration in the case of minor adverse events. They proposed that progressively lower values be deemed sufficient for concern as the severity of the adverse event increases, because it is prudent to be more vigilant in identifying risk of more serious outcomes. There is less potential bias in cohort studies, so they suggested that an OR > 3 can be considered convincing.[37]

A further suggestion, which Straus et al[37] attributed to Prof L. Irwig, is that it is useful to find, if possible, a report that includes some adjustment for confounders. The unadjusted measure of association between a putative causal and outcome variable is then compared with the same measure in which at least one known confounder has been adjusted out. If this adjustment produces a large decline in RR or OR, there is a strong possibility of a spurious association between the putative causal factor and the outcome variable. Conversely, if the adjustment produces little change in the OR or RR or if these ratios rise, confidence in the association becomes greater because the likelihood of a spurious association is smaller.

Criterion 4: Elimination of alternatives

The valid deductive logic used in eliminating alternatives is the disjunctive syllogism: Either A or B; Not A; Therefore B. In theory, this approach can be applied to a series of possible causes, sequentially eliminating all but one. The ghost haunting this logical machine is the possible presence of an unknown potential cause or an unanticipated relationship among variables. This disturbing possibility may be called "Rumsfeld's ghost," as the former US Secretary of Defense once famously remarked, "There are also unknown unknowns. There are things we don't know we don't know."

The elimination of alternatives involves identifying and examining other possible causes and how they are related to the effect. It can entail consideration of more complex causal models.

Expert opinion

Sometimes we leave the consideration of alternatives to experts. When considered as mere opinion, expert opinion is generally ranked as low-level evidence, and there is no shortage of examples where experts got it all wrong. Nevertheless, reasonable people make reasonable decisions, and everyday life often places people in the position of having to take advice from an expert.

Alternatives are often eliminated on the basis of expert opinion when it is used in a legitimate form of argument from authority. This inductive argument is best used when there is objective evidence, the evidence is current and ideally high level, the opinion is representative of experts in the field of study, and the expert has no axe to grind.

Classification of causes

Elimination of alternatives involves the question of determining just what else could have produced the effect. The complex relationships between variables illustrated in the discussion on association imply that the simple conception of direct causation exemplified by simple troubleshooting protocols does not adequately describe the myriad possible causal relationships found in the medical, dental, and social sciences. Indeed there are multiple approaches to defining a cause, the advantages and disadvantages of which have been discussed by Parascandola and Weed,[38] and there are models of varying complexity to describe relationships.

Deterministic production. A cause is something that produces an effect. This deterministic conception can be subdivided into necessary and sufficient causes (or conditions). In a traditional deterministic view, a *necessary* condition is a condition that must be present to obtain an effect. One of the necessary conditions for the production of caries is the presence of bacteria. If a necessary condition for the production of an effect is removed, the effect can be prevented from happening. To prevent caries, we attempt to remove bacteria from teeth. A *sufficient* condition is a condition that automatically leads to an effect. Decapitation, for example, is a sufficient condition to cause death.

Probabilistic cause. A probabilistic cause is one that that increases the probability of an effect. For example, smoking increases an individual's probability of developing lung cancer, but the effect is not inevitable. Cigarette smoking causes about 90% of lung cancers, but the majority of smokers never develop lung cancer. Hume,[9] in fact, came to the conclusion that all causes were probabilistic causes, if the sequence of events were examined in sufficient detail.

Insufficient but nonredundant part of an unnecessary but sufficient (INUS) condition. This concept was developed by Mackie.[39] A commonly used illustration of an INUS condition is the initiation of a forest fire. Forest fires can be started in various ways—a lighted cigarette, a lighted match tossed from a car, lightning, a smoldering campfire, and so forth. The lighted match could be considered an INUS condition. By itself, it cannot necessarily cause a fire because it must combine with combustible material, such as dry leaves, and there must be oxygen to support combustion. Thus, by itself, the match is an insufficient condition. Nevertheless, it does add something that the other factors (such as dry leaves) do not, so it is nonredundant. It is an unnecessary condition, because there are ways, other than a match, to start a forest fire. Nevertheless, when the lighted match is combined with an appropriate set of other conditions, the larger combined set is sufficient to cause forest fires.

INUS conditions can explain failures to replicate experiments or clinical procedures. Technique-sensitive approaches to treatment in dentistry may be INUS conditions for a desired outcome, in that they work in the hands of some dentists but not others because of variation in the dentists' technical approach. For example, it has been estimated that more than 37% of composite resin restorations are clinically insufficiently cured.[40] However, light curing is a more complex process than first meets the eye, because successful curing involves the output power, spectrum, and tip design of the light; the exposure time; resin chemistry; the type of photoinitiator; the location and orientation of the restoration; the presence of any components that block light; and the clinician's ability to aim and maintain the light on target.[41] Attainment of optimal curing means getting all these INUS conditions right. In that sense, many factors that we interpret as deterministic causes are in effect INUS conditions, because we rarely know all the factors that are required to produce an effect and thus may not note conditions that are frequently present, such as the oxygen component of forest fires.

Patterns of causation

In practical terms, causality in epidemiology can be considered as a relationship between two variables, exposure and disease, that will always be observed under stable conditions. However, the relationship may change if new intervening or interacting variables are introduced. Dentistry and medicine have an abundance of possible factors involving host, agents, and environment that could influence outcomes, and these complex interrelationships give rise to the epidemiologic concept of the web of causation.[42] The web of causation has been described as a metaphor for the idea that causal pathways are complex and interconnected. A correspondingly large number of models have been developed to explain how causes can relate to effects (Fig 2-4).

Direct model. A single cause produces a single effect (see Fig 2-4a). The single-headed arrow in the diagram indicates that the association between cause and effect is directed forward in time (the cause precedes the effect). In biology and medicine, *direct causes* are defined as those that act at the same level of organization (ie, cell, organ, or organism) as the effect that is being measured. Such causes are most readily identified when the time between the introduction of the cause and observance of the effect is short and the cause is deterministic.

Treatment of dental abscesses by incision and draining would be considered a direct cause of pain relief from the perspective of the dentist. However, a neurophysiologist might view the treatment as a causal chain (discussed later), involving several steps in detection, neural pathways, and processing.

Pleiotropy. A single cause produces multiple effects (see Fig 2-4b). For example, cystic fibrosis is caused by a mutation in the gene that regulates the movement of chloride and sodium ions across epithelial membranes and thus has multiple effects in that the composition of sweat, digestive fluid, and mucus is altered. The effects of a single cause may not always be identical,

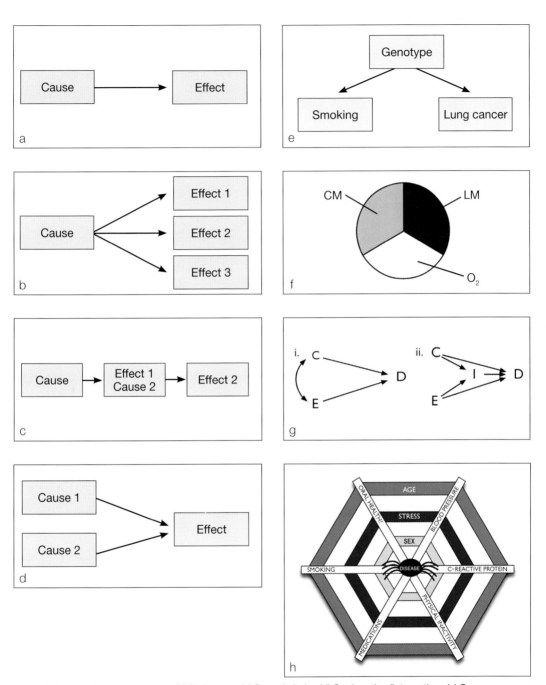

Fig 2-4 Causal models. *(a)* Direct. *(b)* Pleiotropy. *(c)* Causal chain. *(d)* Conjunction/interaction. *(e)* Common cause (R. A. Fisher's constitutional hypothesis). *(f)* Sufficient component model, illustrated by a three-component model of a forest fire, in which a lighted match (LM), combustible material (CM), and oxygen (O_2) equally contribute. *(g)* Graphic models. C, confounder; D, disease; E, exposure; I, child confounder. In part *i*, C is correlated with exposure and is a cause by itself, so C is a confounder. In part *ii*, I is a child of both E and C; therefore, both C and E would be expected to be associated at some level of I, and thus I becomes a confounder. *(h)* Web of causation for CHD (also see detailed explanations in the text).

depending on the intervening mechanisms; for example, the force generated by an orthodontic appliance can cause bone resorption of the socket wall where the vector of force is being applied but bone apposition of the socket wall opposite to where the vector of force is being applied.

Causal chain. A *causal chain* is an ordered series of events such that the first cause leads to the first effect, which is the cause of the second effect, and so forth (see Fig 2-4c). Migliorati[43] proposed a causal chain when he speculated, in a letter to the editor of a journal, that "bisphosphonates may cause oral avascular bone necrosis due to antiangiogenic effect leading to inhibition of osteoclasts." This argument came in a letter that presented only five cases in which bone necrosis had followed bisphosphonate administration. Such a small number of cases might not ordinarily seem convincing but, because a biologic pathway to explain the observation was demonstrated, thus fulfilling Hume's criterion 2 (a connection between the putative cause and the effect), the argument that bisphosphonates were a cause became much more plausible. Causal chain arguments are often important in buttressing the plausibility of many exposure-disease causal relationships, such as the role of infection in PD.

Conjunction/interaction. This model occurs when two or more causes, called *conjunctions* or *interactions*, necessarily occur together to produce an effect (see Fig 2-4d). For example, dental caries is thought to result from the conjunction of bacteria and diet in a susceptible host.

Interaction can change the direction and magnitude of an association between two variables. The interaction effect may be the result of a cumulative effect of multiple risk factors that are not acting independently, and interaction may produce an effect that is lesser or greater than the sum of the effects of each factor considered separately.

Confounding. Described earlier, confounding is also important in causal modeling and is managed in four ways: restriction, matching, stratifi-

cation, and randomization. Restriction or exclusion was discussed in the context of the study on ED and PD,[27] in which the effects of a confounder (smoking) was unlinked from its effects on the risk factor of interest (ie, the exposure) by simply excluding smokers from the study. Another method of controlling for confounding in case-control studies is matching, whereby the controls are selected so that the distribution of potential confounders is as similar as possible to the distribution found in the cases. A third strategy for dealing with confounding is stratification, in which the association between exposure and outcome is examined with the different levels (strata) of the confounding variable. The most effective means for controlling for confounding is randomization, as occurs in RCTs, because it produces groups in which both known and unknown confounders are distributed equally among the groups (and confounders by definition are unequally distributed among the exposure groups).

Confounding can also occur when there is a common cause or hidden variable between an exposure and a disease. R. A. Fisher,[44] perhaps the chief architect of modern statistical science, did not initially accept the linkage between smoking and lung cancer. Instead he invoked a common cause model and argued that there may be a genetic predisposition to smoke, some factor in a person's genotype or "constitution" that also influenced their predisposition to lung cancer (see Fig 2-4e). In Fisher's suggestion, the hidden variable was some aspect of the genotype that influenced both the tendency to smoke and the tendency to develop lung cancer and thereby produced an association between smoking and lung cancer. Evidence for his argument included data that monozygotic twins show closer similarity in their smoking habits than do dizygotic twins, indicating a genetic determinant to smoking behavior.

The second part of his argument was more rhetorical than substantive: "I believe that no one doubts the importance of the genotype in predisposing to cancers of all types."[44] Thus, if both smoking and cancer predisposition could be influenced by genotype, it became at least possible that the same factor influenced both.

Effect modification. Effect modification occurs when the effect of the risk factor on the outcome depends to some extent on the value of another variable. A moderator variable, which can be either qualitative (eg, race or sex) or quantitative, is one that affects the direction and/or the strength of the relationship between the independent variable and the dependent variable.[45]

Stratification, that is, separating the sample into several subsamples according to a criteria such as age, exposure, or income, is the method used to identify effect modifiers. The relative risks are then compared across the strata. For example, Hyman et al[46] stratified their sample into smokers and nonsmokers. They found that smokers with severe PD had 6 times the risk of heart attack that study participants with no PD had. However, nonsmokers with severe PD had no increased risk of heart attack. Thus, smoking modified the effect of PD on risk of heart attack, and the authors concluded that cigarette smoking is a necessary cofactor in the relationship between PD and CHD.[46]

Mediation. A mediator variable is one that explains the relationship between the independent and dependent variables. Unlike a confounder, which by definition is not part of the causal pathway between putative cause and effect, a mediator variable is part of the causal pathway. For example, a possible causal pathway for childhood caries is that poverty causes poor (sugar-rich) diet, which in turn causes caries in children. To put it another way, poverty causes caries, and the effect is mediated through poor diet. When the effect of the mediator variable (diet in this example) is removed, perhaps through some program subsidizing food purchases by poor families, the relationship between the independent variable (poverty) and the dependent variable (eg, caries) should disappear.[45]

Complex causal models. More complex models have been developed to deal with more complex situations where many possible causes and interacting factors are involved.

Counterfactuals (potential outcomes). The concept of counterfactual thinking can be illustrated by the use of what American writer Mercedes Lacky called the two saddest words in the world: "if only," as in "If only I hadn't married my ex-spouse," one of the many members of the "If-only-I-knew-then-what-I-know-now" family, with its implied regret about the dire consequences that ensued when the person did in fact marry the now ex-spouse. Another example is provided by "what if" thinking, in which a person calculates, for example, the potential wealth if he or she had purchased Apple stock at its low point. In that instance, the thinker is considering a potential but not an actual outcome.

Counterfactual comparison involves contrasting the outcome under certain conditions with what might be expected to be observed under alternative conditions that were never in fact employed or observed. For example, when a physician gives a patient a drug and observes the result, the intent is to determine whether the drug produced an effect on the patient. In effect, this is like a case study that has no control, and the difficulty is that the physician does not know what would have happened if the drug had not been given. The counterfactual is the observation that would have happened to the same patient if he or she had not received the drug at the precise same time. The true effect of the drug on the patient would be the difference between what did happen and the counterfactual. In fact, it is impossible to observe the counterfactual, because it is impossible to both give and not give the drug at the same time.

Maldonado and Greenland[47] commented that the fact that counterfactuals cannot be observed is disconcerting for some individuals and seems to contradict the common-sense notion that effects can be observed. They argued that basic problems of causal inference can be made logically precise by translating them into problems of inference about counterfactuals.

In any case, investigators design experiments that approximate what the expected result would be for the counterfactual condition. For example, investigators might alternate between treatment and nontreatment (ie, control) conditions, but the time of treatment and control conditions would be necessarily different, so that approach does not perfectly represent the counterfactual. Another approach would be to randomize a population into treated and nontreated groups, so that the nontreated (control) group represents the counterfactual. The observations could be done at the same time but to different people, so the control group does not represent a true counterfactual. It is, however, generally accepted that random assignment of patients into treatment and control groups is the best means of approximating the counterfactual.

The importance of counterfactual reasoning is that it underlies the logical foundation adopted by statisticians in developing quantitative statistical analysis of causation. Counterfactual reasoning appears in various forms such as Neyman's randomization model and potential outcomes models, structural equation models, and graphic models.[47]

Sufficient component cause. This approach refines the conception of a necessary cause to include causes that are neither specific nor strictly necessary to obtain an effect (see the discussion of INUS conditions). Rothman[48] recognized that disease outcomes have multiple contributing determinants that may act together to produce a given instance of disease and that conjunctions that formed a complete causal mechanism could be considered a sufficient cause. A sufficient component cause is made up of several components, no one of which is sufficient to produce the effect on its own, but a set of which can constitute a sufficient condition for an effect. Therefore, a given disease might be considered as arising from multiple causes. The sufficient component model can be illustrated as a pie chart in which the area is divided into wedges showing the approximate contribution of each individual component. For example, the forest fire example might be considered as a three-component model in which a lighted match, combustible material, and oxygen all contribute equally (see Fig 2-4f). Sufficient component cause models require specification of mechanisms, and there are rarely data to support such detailed specification in epide-

miology; therefore, these models have generally been limited to teaching examples.[49]

Graphic models. In these formal models (see Fig 2-4g), reviewed by Greenland and Brumback,[49] an edge or arc connects two variables. If there is an arrow pointing from one variable, say E (exposure), to another variable D (disease), then E is the parent of D and D is the child. A graph is causal if every arrow represents the presence of an effect of the parent on the child variable. If a variable has an arrow pointing into it (eg, I), it is called an *endogenous (response) variable*; otherwise, it is an *exogenous variable* (eg, E).

A path is a sequence of arcs connecting E, I, and D. There are many possible options for paths between variables and outcome, including backdoor paths, blocked paths, and directed paths. The graph itself is called *directed* if all the edges in it are arrows. A directed path indicates a potential causal pathway. A graph is acyclic if there is no cycle or closed path (ie, no variable is both an ancestor and a descendant of another). A curved line with arrows at each end that joins two variables indicates that a correlation exists between them. In part *i* of Fig 2-4f, C is correlated with exposure and is a cause by itself, so C is a confounder.

In a more complex case, (see part *ii* of Fig 2-4f), I is a child of both E and C; therefore, both C and E would be expected to be associated at some level of I, and thus I becomes a confounder. As more variables are introduced, the paths become numerous and complex. Nevertheless, causal graphs have proven useful as visual methods to check for confounding and the effectiveness of confounder adjustment.[49]

Streiner et al,[18] however, argued that in some instances it is possible to turn some of the arrows around and get exactly the same results. They cautioned that "Cause and effect can be established only through proper research design; no amount of statistical hand waving can turn correlations into conclusions about causation."

Structural equation models (SEMs). SEMs involve a system of equations and independence assumptions among variables to describe the web of causation. Each equation shows how a response (ie, outcome or dependent variable) changes as its direct (potentially) causal variable changes. SEMs can be used to test mediating effects of factors in overall patterns. Outcomes can be considered at the individual level or aggregate levels and can include consideration of potential outcomes, for example, if an individual stopped smoking or received a drug. This consideration of counterfactuals contrasts with regression equations that represent associations of actual outcomes with actual values of the covariates in a population.[49] Structural equations with unknown parameters go beyond graphic diagrams in specifying the functional form of effects but do not fully quantify causal relations.

SEMs have been extensively used in the social sciences but in epidemiology have been mainly utilized in teaching concepts,[50] with some exceptions. Aleksejūnienė at al,[51] for example, used an SEM to examine the path between lifestyle and levels of remaining periodontal support.

The web of causation. The statistical technique of multivariate analysis has demonstrated that multiple factors can be associated with some diseases. Krieger[42] has argued that one of the central concepts of epidemiology is that population patterns of health and disease can be explained by a complex web of interconnected risk and protective factors, "the web of causation." In this view, there is not necessarily any single cause, and causes of disease interact. When the strands of the web are distorted by these interactions, it brings forth the disease just as a fly trapped in a web brings forth the spider. In this view, the power of epidemiology to improve public health will depend on its ability to identify and predict the results of breaking selected strands of this causal web (see Fig 2-4h).

Problems include unknown effects of biomedical individualism as well as social determinants of disease. How widely the net of the web of causation is cast over the range of biomedical and social variables depends on the particular issue being investigated and the interests of the investigator. In any case, eliminating all possible plausible alternative explanations is a daunting task. Often investigators attempt to arrange comparisons so that only one factor differs between the groups, and its effects can be estimated. Alternatively, as noted earlier, statistical approaches are used to adjust for the effect of the factors that vary, but there are limitations to this approach, and some stubborn biases resist statistical adjustment. In the view of Bosco et al,[50] no adjustment method fully resolves confounding by indication because there is generally some reason that clinicians prefer one treatment over another for particular patients.

Assessing evidence for causation

Ultimately, the acceptance of some risk factor as a cause of a disease involves more than statistical calculations of association, no matter how sophisticated, and proponents for such causes must add other elements to their rhetoric to persuade the scientific community. Sackett et al[15] proposed a two-step process for assessing the evidence.

Strength of evidence. First, it is important to determine whether the basic methods were strong. The strongest evidence is an RCT followed by cohort study, case-control study, and case series. They suggested that readers can place considerable confidence in estimates of strength from an RCT, fair confidence in an estimate of strength from a cohort study, and little confidence in an estimate of strength from a case-control study.

Diagnostic tests for causation. The second step Sackett et al[15] suggested is to apply the diagnostic tests for causation. The pioneer English epidemiologist Sir Austin Bradford Hill proposed the following nine criteria[52]:

1. *Strength.* The larger the association, the more likely that it is causal. Sackett et al[15] stated that odds ratios of 4 or greater are considered strong. A meta-analysis of studies on PD and CHD incidence found PD to be an independent risk factor with risk estimates that ranged from 1.24 to 1.34. While the difference was statistically significantly different from 1 (ie, no effect), the strength of the association was relatively weak.[53]

However, there is the possibility that some individuals are particularly sensitive to the effects of oral health, and for them it might be a very important risk factor indeed. Genetic effects related to oral health have been previously noted even at the level of behavior. For example, dental care–related anxiety, fear of dental pain, and avoidance of dental care appear to be influenced by genetic variations.[54] Approaches such as mendelian randomization[55] and genome-wide associations,[56] though facing considerable computational and statistical challenges, would be expected to give new insights into the role of genetic constitution on disease susceptibility.

2. *Consistency.* The findings should be repeatedly observed by different persons in different places, circumstances, and times (the basic scientific principle of replication as a test of validity). Meta-analysis is often employed to assess consistency, and a key question of meta-analysis is whether the studies are similar enough to be grouped together. Heterogeneity can arise from differences in study design, exposure measurement, confounders, and bias. One meta-analysis of studies on PD and CHD incidence found that PD is a risk factor for CHD that is independent of traditional CHD factors, including socioeconomic status. Risk estimates were similar in subgroup analysis by sex, outcome, study quality, and PD assessment method.[53] On the other hand, Hujoel et al[57] did not find convincing evidence of a causal association between PD and CHD risk.

3. *Specificity.* The more specific an association between a factor and an effect is, the bigger the probability of a causal relationship.

4. *Temporality.* The effect has to occur after the cause (Hume's first criteria).

5. *Biologic gradient.* Greater exposure should generally lead to greater incidence of the effect.

6. *Plausibility.* To quote Hill, "It will be helpful if the causation we suspect is biologically plausible...what is biologically plausible depends on the biological knowledge of the day."[52] However, scientists are exceptionally adept in proposing possible mechanisms, so it is the exceptional epidemiologic association for which no mechanism can be proposed.[31] Nevertheless, there are biologic mechanisms by which PD could be associated with CHD (see chapter 7). Knowledge of a precise mechanism, although preferable, is not a necessary condition for epidemiologic information to be usefully applied. Identification of high-risk groups and modification of their behavior may be sufficient to curtail the incidence of disease.

7. *Coherence.* Cause-and-effect interpretations should not conflict with the known facts of the natural history and biology of the disease.

8. *Experiment.* In some instances, it may be possible to have experimental evidence that bears on the issue, such as having persons stop smoking and observing the decline in lung cancer.

9. *Analogy.* Hill illustrates this criterion as follows: "with the effects of thalidomide and rubella before us we would surely be ready to accept slighter but similar evidence with another drug or another viral disease in pregnancy."[52] Thus, the existence of a previously demonstrated relationship that shares features with the putative cause under consideration makes it more plausible.

Others have commented on these criteria and proposed modifications. Sackett et al,[15] for example, added evidence from true experiments in humans to the list and put that addition as first in order of importance. They also lowered specificity to eighth place in the importance rankings. Overall, though, application of Hill's criteria does not necessarily lead to unequivocal assessments of causation, and investigators can be expected to disagree on occasion.

Differences Among Studies

Because consistency is a major criterion of causation, epidemiologists, not to mention the general public, are naturally concerned about the issue of discrepancies where similar studies lead to opposing conclusions. There are a number of possible reasons for such differences.

Residual confounding

Statistical modeling can only work perfectly when all the measures in a model are measured perfectly. Residual confounding can occur when a confounder has not been adequately adjusted in the analysis, as is the case when the measurements of the confounding variable are inaccurate. Residual confounding can be suspected when there appear to be obviously spurious associations.

Risk factors tend to cluster; for example, in a study involving more than half a million people on meat intake and mortality,[58] those who consumed the most red meat were heavier, smoked more, were less educated, and consumed more calories and fat and fewer fruits and vegetables than those who consumed less red meat. Sophisticated statistical modeling led the researchers to conclude that red meat had an independent effect on mortality. However, a more detailed examination of the model by Sainani[59] found that it produced some other statistically significant but implausible associations. For example, death by infectious disease could not be plausibly explained by red meat consumption, and this spurious association indicated that the model has some unexplained (residual) riskiness that was unaccounted for.

Such residual confounding leads to spurious association. For example, if the amount of smoking were underestimated, some of the mortality that was actually attributable to smoking might be captured by some other variable that was associated with smoking, perhaps red meat consumption, and make that variable appear (mistakenly) to be independently associated with mortality. Because the risks for some implausible associations were similar to that found for consumption of red meat, Sainani[59] concluded that the study did not provide evidence of a causal relationship between consuming red meat and death.

Socioeconomic status is an important but difficult to measure variable that influences multiple health outcomes and can be a factor in residual confounding. What may be of particular importance in oral health epidemiology is general health awareness. Hujoel et al[60] found a dose-dependent association between two causally unrelated oral (lack of dental flossing) and general lifestyle (obesity) characteristics. They noted that good oral health may be the result of factors related to general health awareness rather than simply oral self-care patterns. They argued for more consideration of the hypothesis that general health awareness factors influence both oral and systemic diseases.

Some general rules for interpreting results from observational studies have been developed. First, the size of the effect should be considered. Sainani[59] suggested that in observational studies, when the ORs are small to moderate (ORs between 0.6 and 1.6 for a binary predictor), the observed effects could be entirely due to residual confounding when there are strong confounders in play. One of the major criticisms of many studies relating PD to cardiovascular disease has been that they adjusted for smoking (a strong confounder) by the use of multivariate analysis, an approach noted earlier, which is open to bias due to residual confounding.

Second, when the OR (or other risk measure) for the relationship being investigated is similar in value to ORs found for obviously implausible relationships in the same study, it becomes possible that the relationship may be a case of spurious association (eg, dental flossing and obesity).

Third, an obvious limitation of adjusting for confounding is that the confounder needs to have been measured and reported. Retrospective analysis of some data sets may be hampered because variables that are now thought to be important might not have been so considered when the study was done and thus were not measured.

Weak fundamental standards

An editor of a prominent epidemiologic journal, Feinstein[61] suggested that published epidemiologic studies sometimes fail to meet fundamental scientific standards used to specify hypotheses and groups. Moreover, some studies have low-quality data, do not analyze attributable actions, and exhibit detection bias so that overall these defects result in false-positive associations. These views have been challenged by other epidemiologists,[62] who argue that contradictory results do not necessarily indicate poor study methods. Feinstein, a passionate controversialist, responded to his critics.[63] Perhaps because of the importance of the issues to human health, the presence of strong interest groups, and the fact that people are exposed to some hazards in everyday life, disputes in epidemiology are more public and more intense than often occurs in science.

As noted earlier, a likely cause of spurious association is confounding. Associations reported in observational studies but not confirmed in RCTs tend to be associations of exposures that are related to many socioeconomic and behavioral measures that are in turn related to disease.[64] On the basis of an observational study,[65] hormone replacement therapy (HRT) was originally thought to protect against CHD because the risk ratio was calculated at 0.39. Because of that impressive result, an RCT on HRT was undertaken, but the results were disappointing to say the least; the risk for CHD was found to be substantially and significantly higher for participants taking HRT than untreated controls.[66]

It is noteworthy that the original study did not measure a number of important potential confounding variables, such as exercise, use of cholesterol-lowering drugs, and ethnicity, and residual confounding is now thought to be the reason for the aberrant relationship first reported.[67] The RCT does not suffer from residual confounding, because the randomization process distributes possible confounders equally among the groups.

Moreover, in the original study, HRT was found to confer almost as much protection against accidental or violent death as against CHD.[68] There does not appear to be a plausible biologic link to explain the association of HRT with accidental death, so it is possible that both associations were confounded with other risk factors. Beral et al[68] concluded that, "Previous claims that HRT protects against CHD should now be discounted." HRT users tended to be healthier and more affluent and tended to engage in healthier lifestyle habits, and observational studies examining the beneficial health effects of HRT are prone to selection bias.

Bias and chance

Other factors that can lead to discrepancies between studies include bias, such as measurement error in calculating exposures, and chance (or random error). False positives can also be generated by bias if the study methods systematically alter the research findings. For example, bias induced by self-reported smoking has been suggested to influence reported periodontitis–systemic disease associations.

Chance has a dominant role in producing false positives in studies that have a multiplicity of exposures and discrete outcomes because multiple comparisons can be made. In genetic epidemiologic studies, hundreds or hundreds of thousands of possible comparisons can be generated, and there is also abundant scope for subgroup analysis. If the data are not adjusted for the number of comparisons being made, a large number of statistically significant but false (ie, arising from chance) associations will be generated. In the epidemiology of occupational cancer, for example, the main determinants of false-positive associations have been (1) the absence of a specific, a priori hypothesis (a practice sometimes called *data dredging* or a *fishing expedition*); (2) a small magnitude of the association; (3) the absence of a dose-effect relationship; and (4) a lack of adjustment for tobacco smoking.[69]

Chance-induced false positives can be distinguished from bias-induced false positives by the criterion of replication. Chance-induced findings would not be expected to be replicated, whereas bias-induced findings might be replicated, because bias may operate in a consistent manner in different settings and populations and thus produce what appears to be consistent evidence for an association.

Divergent interpretations

Another source of discrepancy in conclusions among different studies lies in divergent interpretations that arise as different investigators focus on different aspects of the relationships in question. Cardiovascular diseases are an example of systemic chronic noncommunicable diseases, and PD is an example of a dental chronic noncommunicable disease. Clustering of chronic noncommunicable diseases occurs both within individuals and within populations. Hujoel[70] has noted that dental-systemic disease associations have been consistently identified, but the interpretation of these associations has been strongly influenced by the zeitgeist of the time they were introduced, so that the dominant medical hypothesis at the time was favored.

Informal Causal Fallacies

Informal logic can be thought of as the use of reason in everyday life. Causal arguments are often involved in everyday decision making and, as noted by Greene[11] for dentistry, incorrect cause-effect relationships can lead to treatment failure. In contrast to formal logical fallacies that only involve structure (eg, a categorical syllogism with a negative conclusion but positive premises), fallacies of informal logic generally require examination of the argument's content.

The discussion in the preceding sections has shown that establishment of causation is a complex business that requires satisfaction of four criteria and a detailed examination of content. It is therefore unsurprising that in everyday causal reasoning people often take shortcuts that entail ignoring some criteria; this process can lead to what may be called *informal causal fallacies*.

Some of these fallacies occur commonly. Perhaps the most famous is the post hoc fallacy, which uses only the criterion of temporality. This fallacy assumes that, just because B happened after A, A caused B. Widely used in the promotion of quack remedies, the argument is made that the treatment worked because the patients improved after treatment, but no comparison is made with what happens in the absence of treatment, nor is there any control for placebo effects. Thus, likely alternatives are not eliminated. Post hoc fallacy is also used by politicians who point to improvements in the economy after they take office or deteriorations in the economy after an opponent takes office, in both cases ignoring the host of other alternative explanations that may be involved.

The second criterion, contiguity, is frequently violated by quacks who suggest bizarre mechanisms often described by a jargon of their own invention and invoke principles unknown in physiology or biochemistry to explain the purported success of their methods.[18] For example, a number of bracelets, varying in composition and supposed mechanism, which have never been seriously investigated for their ability to cause positive health benefits, are sold widely to the public as a remedy for various ailments. These products likely are a waste of money and, more seriously, delay appropriate treatment. Poor causal reasoning about quack remedies has a public health price.

Other common types of fallacy have already been discussed, including the fallacy of confusing cause and effect, the fallacy of the common cause, and the belief that correlation proves causation.

Rhetoric

Because interpretation is to some extent a subjective process, it must be considered to be to some extent malleable to the interests of the interpreter. For example, Levis et al[71] contrasted the errors found in negative (no association) studies funded by industry and the reliability of positive (association demonstrated) studies funded by public bodies. Different interpretations in this field of research were apparently driven by "financial conditioning." There is some history to suggest that there is business bias, whereby epidemiologic studies that are funded by the potentially affected industry may underestimate or fail to detect increased risks.

Example: Smoking and lung cancer

A cause-effect relationship between smoking and lung cancer is now widely accepted but was once controversial, and acceptance was a slow process that involved arguments beyond statistics. The argument and the resolution of the controversy are briefly reviewed here because similar approaches will be required to resolve controversies about oral-systemic disease connections.

In brief, the tobacco industry and some prominent investigators held that proof that smoking caused lung cancer was insufficient. Holding the opposing view were, among others, Jerome Cornfield and his colleagues,[72] who introduced a number of technical and statistical innovations in epidemiology to buttress their arguments. An important development was the "Cornfield inequality," which answers a common criticism of epidemiologic studies, namely that an unknown and unobserved variable was the true cause of the outcome. For smoking and lung cancer, Cornfield et al[72] used the inequality as follows:

> [I]f cigarette smokers have 9 times the risk of nonsmokers for developing lung cancer, and this is not because cigarette smoke is a causal agent, but only because cigarette smokers produce hormone X, then the proportion of hormone-X producers among cigarette smokers must be at least 9 times greater than nonsmokers. If the relative prevalence of hormone-X-producers is considerably less than ninefold, then hormone-X cannot account for the magnitude of the apparent effect.

The Cornfield inequality was the first formal method of sensitivity analysis in observational studies and is of continuing use in providing a formal response to one of the most difficult criticisms of observational studies.[73] Subsequently, the focus on ORs was criticized, but the OR was still a practical approach given that the limitations of computers of the time meant that more sophisticated regression methods were not practical.[74]

Logic of hypothesis testing

However, despite the merits of the Cornfield inequality response, additional arguments were required. The normal practice in science is for the investigator to have a working hypothesis or provisional explanation of the available facts and to test the hypothesis by performing experiments or gathering new observations. Formally, the logic of hypothetical inference in science can be shown as follows, where H is the hypothesis and E are the observations that would be predicted by H under certain defined conditions:

Premise 1: If H, then E.
Premise 2: E is true.
Conclusion: It becomes more credible that H is true.

This form of inductive logic yields a conclusion that is not deductively certain. In fact in deductive logic, this form of argument is called the *fallacy of affirming the consequent*. In inductive logic, however, the conclusion states only that the hypothesis becomes more credible.

The traditional approach to criticizing such a hypothesis is to provide alternative hypotheses that would also predict the occurrence of E. A deductively valid form of hypothetical reasoning, the *modus tollens*, has the following structure:

Premise 1: If H, then E.
Premise 2: Not E.
Conclusion: H is false.

Cornfield et al[72] used both types of argument, as well as the disjunctive syllogism, to examine evidence in favor of the causal hypothesis (smoking causes lung cancer) as well as objections to the causal hypothesis made by critics, including some prominent authorities in statistics such as R. A. Fisher,[44] as well as spokespersons for the tobacco industry.

Assessment of alternative hypotheses

Cornfield et al[72] examined the alternative hypotheses put forth by the critics and showed that in each instance the alternative hypotheses did not fit with other data or could, on reasonable assumptions, be calculated to have effects that would be insufficient to explain the effect of smoking, whereas the consequents of the causal hypothesis were confirmed. They applied this approach to a broad range of criticism derived from mortality and population data, including the effect of aging, diagnostic factors, necropsy data, urban/rural differences, and sex differences as well as special population groups. They also reviewed retrospective and prospective studies and effectively discredited arguments based on the selection of study groups, accuracy of information, and inadequate consideration of other variables.

Cornfield et al[72] reviewed studies on the pathogenesis of lung cancer, including such factors as inhalation of smoke, studies on the effect of tobacco smoke on bronchial mucosa, laboratory studies on skin cancer in rodents, studies on bronchogenic cancer in various laboratory animals, and studies on the isolation and identification of specific chemical carcinogens in tobacco smoke. Then they considered the two major interpretations of the association of lung cancer and cigarette smoking: (1) the causal hypothesis that smoking causes lung cancer and (2) Fisher's common cause hypothesis[44] that smoking and lung cancer have a common cause, also known as the *constitutional hypothesis* because the common cause was often thought of as the person's constitution or genetic makeup. Cornfield et al[72] showed that the totality of the evidence, including changes to mortality from lung cancer with time, experimental carcinogenesis with tobacco tar, types of tobacco and cancer site, and mortality among discontinued smokers, argued against the constitutional hypothesis.

Finally, Cornfield et al[72] answered a popular criticism of the causal hypothesis, namely, "If cigarette smoke causes lung cancer, why do most heavy cigarette smokers fail to develop lung cancer?" They admitted that they had no answer to the question but compared the lack of inevitability of the smoking and lung cancer relationship to the lack of inevitability of tuberculosis in people exposed to tubercle bacilli, in particular babies in Lübeck, Germany, in 1929 to 1930. The infants were vaccinated with massive doses of tubercle bacilli in a contaminated vaccine, yet only 72 of 252 babies died. This tragic incident, however, did not cause anyone to doubt the causal role of the bacilli in the development of tuberculosis.

Altogether, the analysis by Cornfield et al[72] represents a brilliant example of the accumulation and assessment of wide-ranging evidence accompanied by a logical and forceful rhetoric calling for action by medical and public health authorities. Although there were flaws in their approach and their arguments did not completely refute all counterarguments, Cornfield et al[72] did demonstrate that the totality of the evidence indicated that the causal hypothesis was much more likely to be true than any other alternative hypothesis. They also pointed out that the higher standard of evidence, an RCT, was not feasible on ethical grounds.

Rhetorical tactics

Authors of scientific papers attempt to persuade reviewers, editors, peer scientists, and even on some occasions the general public of the truth of their conclusions. Issues concerning health hazards have many stakeholders: scientists, the media, regulators, affected industries, activist groups, regulators, and politicians, and all have axes to grind. Scientists, for example, have an incentive to propose more rigorous studies to evaluate risk that, if funded, may lead to their personal professional advancement; industry, in contrast, often wishes to downplay the risks associated with their products so that sales will not be impeded. To achieve their ends, stakeholders employ both logic and rhetoric in the court of scientific opinion.

Standards of proof

Many rhetorical strategies are employed, but two particularly important issues are the completeness of the evidence being considered and the appropriate standards of proof. Like lawyers arguing a case, authors will emphasize the facts that fit their case. Readers, on the other hand, expect that authors will cite relevant research in a balanced manner and not just provide facts for one side of the argument. Sometimes this expectation is not honored, and one role of referees is to monitor the cited references to ensure balance. The net result of this interplay is that the reader of well-refereed journals has a better chance of obtaining a balanced view of the evidence.

The choice of instances considered during analysis may be called the *causal field*. Different forms of causal reasoning may be adopted, depending on the causal field. White[14] used the example of a nuclear power plant where some of the workers have developed cancer. To investigate the cause, a researcher might apply Mill's method of agreement to those employees who developed cancer and by this means eliminate all risk factors not common to all cases. Perhaps exposure to a certain level of radiation is the only risk factor remaining. However, there is another choice of causal field that might better aid the owners of the power plant by helping them to avoid blame. Namely, they could focus on all the employees of the plant who were exposed to radiation and ask why some of those employees did not develop cancer. If the joint method of agreement and difference is employed, it may be possible to eliminate exposure to radiation from the list of causal candidates. Thus, choice of causal attribution method may be influenced by the practical interests of the parties concerned. (Neither of the choices of causal field outlined in the example contains all available relevant information, and reasoning from them violates one of the rules for acceptable use of inductive logic.)

Burden of proof

Like legal proceedings, scientific argument has the concept of burden of proof. The general rule is that the burden of proof is on the proponent; an author positing a causal relationship between oral health and systemic disease, for example, has to prove the relationship. In legal courts, there are different standards for proof: For criminal cases, the usual standard is beyond a reasonable doubt, but civil cases typically are decided on the balance of probabilities. In epidemiologic controversies, one tactic has been

to set the standard of proof to an impossible-to-achieve level.[75] This can be an effective tactic because the critics can defend their standards by noting they are only being rigorous.

For example, the tobacco firm Philip Morris mounted a multipronged "sound science" program in 1993 to discredit the evidence that secondhand tobacco smoke causes disease. The European "sound science" plans included a version of good epidemiologic practice that adopted standards of scientific proof (eg, that relative risks of less than 2 would be ignored) that would have made it impossible to prove that secondhand smoke or many other environmental agents were dangerous.[69]

Personal standards

The Cambridge logician A. Fisher[76] suggested that individuals set their own standards using the assertability question—"What evidence would it take to convince me of the truth of the conclusions?"—and compare the evidence offered with their personal standards.

When the information is sufficient to consider supporting action, a typical consideration is the risk-reward ratio. Because achieving oral health has benefits in and of itself and entails little risk, the decision to take action to improve oral health is often justified, even if the likelihood of the reward in the form of reduced systemic disease is deemed to be small. Thus, in the popular press, the general advice is to practice good oral hygiene even though the evidence for reducing a particular systemic disease may not be overwhelming.

Persuading with statistics

Abelson[77] suggested that the persuasive force of data and its analysis and presentation is governed by five properties ("MAGIC criteria"):

1. Magnitude
2. Articulation
3. Generality
4. Interestingness
5. Credibility

Magnitude refers to the strength of a statistical argument, which is enhanced with the quantitative magnitude of support for its quantitative claim. This aligns with Hill's criteria[52] for causation, strength of the association.

Articulation refers to the degree of comprehensible detail in which conclusions are phrased. Abelson[77] classified statements about research results as comprising *(1) ticks*, detailed descriptions of research results such as a claim of a specific comparative difference stemming from the rejections of a null hypothesis, typically a point in the summary; *(2) buts*, statements that qualify or constrain the ticks; and *(3) blobs*, which are clusters of undifferentiated research results.

The general goal in terms of clarity is to minimize the number of buts; however, buts are sometimes required to avoid misleading the reader. Abelson[77] suggested that it is more persuasive to minimize the number of ticks so that the most important one is emphasized.

Generality denotes the breadth of applicability of the conclusions. Generally, the context of any one study is narrow: particular groups of patients exposed to particular clinicians employing particularly (and sometimes locally) modified techniques. To support broadly applicable conclusions, it is generally necessary to include a wide variety of contexts, which can be a feature of studies employing meta-analysis.

Regarding *interestingness*, Abelson believes that, "[F]or a statistical story to be theoretically interesting, it must have the potential, through empirical analysis, to change what people believe about an important issue."[77] Cornfield et al[72] did that with their analysis of smoking and lung cancer, doubtlessly changing some people's views on the dangers of smoking and influencing their actions to the effect that multitudes of lives were saved.

Credibility refers to the believability of a research claim that rests on sound methodology and theoretical coherence; that is, the research must be capable of explaining a range of interconnected findings. Cornfield et al[72] did that by examining not only statistical issues but a number of related pathologic and experimental findings.

The author believes that a second C, *clarity*, should be added to form the MAGICC criteria; as a general rule in epidemiology, graphic techniques could be used to more persuasive effect. E. A. Tufte,[25] who has been called the "Da Vinci of data and the Galileo of graphics," has written extensively on the role of graphic design in explaining complex evidence effectively. Epidemiology illustrates his comment that "Human activities, after all, take place in intensely comparative and multivariate contexts filled with causal ideas…intervention, explanation, intention, action, prevention, diagnosis." Tufte[25] stated that the universal analytic issues are causality, comparison, and multivariate complexity. He wrote[25]:

> The analysis of cause and effect, initially bivariate, quickly becomes multivariate through such necessary elaborations as the conditions under which the causal relation holds, interaction effects, multiple causes, multiple effects, causal sequences, sources of bias, spurious correlation, sources of measurement error, competing variables and whether the alleged cause is merely a proxy or a marker variable.

Indeed, he might well be writing about the current debate on oral health–systemic disease connections.

Tufte[25] has developed six principles:

1. Show comparisons and contrasts.
2. Show causality, mechanism explanation, and systematic structure.
3. Show multivariate data that is more than one or two variables.
4. Completely integrate words, numbers, images, and diagrams.
5. Thoroughly describe the evidence.
6. Analytical presentations ultimately stand or fall depending on the quality, relevance, and integrity of their content.

Tufte's book *Beautiful Evidence*[25] illustrates how these principles can be applied.

General Suggestions for Assessing Causation

This chapter has presented background information about causality to enable dentists to assess current and future evidence on the associations between oral health and systemic disease. A better understanding of the principles involved in assessing evidence for causation will help dentists to apply the evidence reported in the literature to their everyday issues of problem solving in dentistry. To this end, dentists should consider the following suggestions for judging the data they read:

- Read the original article. Newspaper columns on health topics need to inform and entertain their readers and must do so in limited space. To be one step ahead of your patients, you would be well advised to read the original source and apportion your trust to some extent on the basis of the quality of the journal. Refereed journals provide the reader with a guarantee not of the truth of the conclusions but that at least reasonable current standards in the field have been met.
- Having identified the study design (by reading the original research), determine if the disadvantages, such as potential biases, apply to the study.
- Apply the criteria for causation. The basic criteria are that (1) the exposure preceded the appearance of disease; (2) there is a plausible mechanism that could explain the relationship; (3) there is a statistical association (such as OR or RR) between the exposure and the disease that is statistically significant (P value or confidence interval) and of reasonable size; and (4) there are no equally plausible alternative hypotheses that could explain the association. This requirement often entails assessing whether all confounders have been measured and measured well. Develop your own scientific standards for aspects such as the strength of the association that you think is required for an exposure to be considered a possible cause for an outcome.
- Follow the research forward and backward. Resources such as the Science Citation Index, Scopus, or Google Scholar can indicate if the study is finding acceptance, as evidenced by being cited positively in subsequent articles. However, it often takes considerable time for studies to be cited because of the time needed to complete research and publish. To assess research on a topic that has taken place in the past, look for systematic reviews or meta-analyses. These help you to develop a balanced view on the totality of the evidence and use the criterion of consistency. However, such reviews might have inclusion criteria or subjective judgments on research quality with which you might not necessarily agree.
- Pay particular attention to those paragraphs in the article where the authors discuss the limitations of their study. In some instances, this discussion of limitations is done in response to the criticisms of expert referees and should be considered seriously.
- Consider alternative explanations, such as confounding, for an observed association. An expert in informal logic, Walton,[78] suggested that readers ask seven critical questions about postulated causal relationships where A leads to B: (1) Is there a positive correlation between A and B? (2) Is there a significant number of instances? (3) Is there good evidence the relationship is A leading to B (and not B to A)? (4) Is there a possible common cause? (5) Is there an intervening variable, that is, is the relationship between A and B mediated through other causes? (6) Are the limits of the range over which A and B are related defined? (7) Is the relationship between A and B due to the way B is defined?
- Accept the Roman orator Cicero's advice and ask, "Cui bono?" This double-dative Latin adage asks you to consider who is going to benefit from a suggested course of action and whether the author (or speaker) is acting on the principle of self-interest rather than presenting an objective evaluation of the evidence.
- Have fun following the debates and disputes. The scientific enterprise can be considered

a major league sport involving major league intellects with true life-and-death outcomes. When disputes occur, the rhetorical gymnastics and innovative approaches used to resolve the issues are always interesting and can even be entertaining.

Acknowledgments

I would like to thank Dr C. A. G. McCulloch of the University of Toronto, as well as my colleagues at the University of British Columbia, Drs Carol Oakley, Batoul Shariati, Hugh Kim, and Ben Balevi, for their thoughtful comments and helpful corrections of this manuscript. I also appreciate the editorial assistance provided by Ms Claire Davies.

Glossary

absolute risk The probability of an event in the population being studied, it is a measure of the population impact. Although heavy smokers have a 20 times risk of lung cancer relative to nonsmokers and only a 2 times greater risk for heart disease, the effect on the burden of illness of the population is greater for heart disease, because heart disease is much more common than lung cancer.

absolute risk reduction (ARR) The difference between two absolute risks. If the incidence of stroke in an untreated (or placebo-treated) high-risk population is 5% for a given time period and the incidence for those taking an experimental drug is 1% for the same time period, the AAR is 5% − 1%, or 4%; that is, the drug has lowered the risk of stroke by 4%. The inverse of AAR (1/ARR) results in the number needed to treat to prevent one adverse event. In this example, clinicians would need to treat 1/0.04, or 25 people, to prevent one stroke.

association A relationship between an exposure (or a characteristic) and a disease that is statistically dependent; that is, the presence of one alters the probability of observing the presence of the other. Association is a necessary condition of a causal relationship, but many exposure-disease associations are not causal. If there is no association, the variables are said to be independent.

bias A systematic (as opposed to random) error leading to the deviation of results from the truth in one direction. Bias can result from many sources, including sample selection, measurement methods, and interpretation.

causation (causality) The relating of causes to the effects they produce. Epidemiologic evidence by itself is not sufficient to establish causation, but it can provide powerful circumstantial evidence.

confounding The error, sometimes described as a *bias*, that can occur when study groups that have been formed based on exposure to a risk factor (eg, periodontal disease) are being compared to determine their association with an outcome (eg, erectile dysfunction) but the groups differ in their exposure to risk or prognostic factors (eg, smoking) other than the factor being investigated. Confounding can cause overestimation or underestimation of the true association between an exposure and an outcome.

confounding variable A confounding variable is one that *(1)* has an association with disease; *(2)* is also associated with the exposure variable that is being investigated and is distributed differently among the different exposure levels; and *(3)* does not lie on the causal pathway between the exposure and the disease. If a confounding variable is known, appropriate research design can control for it.

correlation Linear association between two continuous or ordinal variables. The measure of the correlation is the *correlation coefficient*, which ranges from 1 (perfect positive association) through 0 (no association) to −1 (perfect negative association).

Cox regression (proportional hazards model) A regression method for modeling survival times in which the independent variables are described as *predictor variables* or *prognostic factors*. Cox regression makes no assumption about the distribution of survival times.

dose-response relationship (DRR) Change in the response (such as disease) as exposure to the factor of interest increases. The stronger the DRR, the more likely it is that the factor causes the disease.

hazard ratio (HR) Commonly used in reporting data on survival curves or other instances when time-to-event is the outcome variable, HR is the ratio of the risk of an event in one group to the risk in another group. If HR = 1, the groups are at equal risk. Unlike relative risk ratios, which are cumulative over an entire study using a defined endpoint, hazard ratios represent instantaneous risks.

incidence The number of new cases of a disease within a specified time period.

latency (latent period) Period between the onset of exposure and the appearance of clinically detectable disease. For chronic diseases, the latent period can range up to decades.

logistic regression A method to model the dependence of binary response variable (which takes a value of 1 or 0, such as presence [1] or absence of disease [0]) on one or more exploratory variables, which can be either continuous or categorical. It employs the logit function: logit $(p) = \ln (p/1-p)$, where p is the probability (having a value between 0 and 1) and ln is the natural logarithm to the base e. Logistic regression is typically used to calculate the odds ratio adjusted for some explanatory or predictor variables.

odds The ratio of the probability that an event will occur divided by the probability that it will not happen: Odds $= p/(1 - p)$, where p is the probability of the event.

odds ratio (OR) Measure of association obtained from a case-control study (see Table 2-1). OR > 1, increased risk; OR = 1, no difference in risk; OR < 1, decreased risk (protective effect). The OR is skewed; protective effects are seen between 0 and 1, while there is increased risk from 1 to infinity.

P value The probability that an outcome (such as a difference between the means of two groups) would occur by chance. P values range from 1 (absolutely certain) to 0 (absolutely impossible). $P < .05$ has been chosen as the value that establishes statistical significance.

prevalence Frequency of occurrence of a factor or condition in the population.

relative risk (RR) Used in the reporting of cohort studies and randomized controlled trials, the RR is the ratio of the incidence of disease or death among the exposed to the incidence of the unexposed $= p_1/p_2$, where p_1 is the probability of an event in group 1 (exposed) for a given period of time and p_2 is the probability in group 2 (unexposed). Although it uses a different calculation method from the odds ratio, RR approaches the same value when the probabilities are small. For example, among nonsmokers, people who drink more than 1.6 oz of alcohol per day have 2.33 times the risk of oral cancer compared with persons who do not drink alcohol. To put RR values in perspective, RR should be complemented by absolute risk and population impact information.

residual confounding In a regression model, the residual unexplained variance that remains after adjustment for confounders; that is, it represents inadequate control of confounding. It can occur because of failure to consider some confounders, inaccurate measurement of exposure (such as self-reports of tobacco use), insufficient data in some of the strata of confounders being adjusted for, and other violations of the model's assumptions.

risk The probability that an (often unfavorable) event, such as death or illness, will occur within a stated period of time.

risk factor A personal characteristic or exposure that is associated with the occurrence of disease.

spurious association A statistical relationship in which the variables have no causal connection, for example, obesity and use of dental floss.

statistical significance A measure of whether a particular result is unlikely to be due to chance. Statistical significance is generally specified by a value of $P < .05$, that is, less than 1 chance in 20.

References

1. Wilkinson E. Brush teeth to 'prevent' heart disease. BBC News Health 27 May 2010. http://www.bbc.co.uk/news/10176410. Accessed 24 September 2013.
2. Oz M, Roizen M. Brushing up boosts sex life. The Province, 20 January 2013:B9.
3. Lockhart PB, Bolger AF, Papapanou PN, et al. Periodontal disease and atherosclerotic vascular disease: Does the evidence support an independent association? A scientific statement from the American Heart Association. Circulation 2012;125:2520–2544.

4. Oz M. Breaking news: No link between gum disease and heart disease. 18 Apr 2012. http://www.doctoroz.com/videos/breaking-news-no-link-between-gum-disease-and-heart-disease. Accessed 24 September 2013.

5. Kabat GC. Hyping Health Risks: Environmental Hazards in Daily Life and the Science of Epidemiology. New York: Columbia University Press, 2008.

6. Bagnardi V, Blangiardo M, La Vecchia C, Corrao G. A meta-analysis of alcohol drinking and cancer risk. Br J Cancer 2001;85:1700–1705.

7. Glick M. Causation: A loosely founded concept in epidemiology [editorial]. J Am Dent Assoc 2007; 138:1532–1533.

8. Hume D. A Treatise of Human Nature (1739–40), ed 2. Oxford: Clarendon Press, 1978:173–175.

9. Hume D. An Enquiry Concerning Human Understanding, section 7 (1772). http://www.marxists.org/reference/subject/philosophy/works/en/hume.htm. Accessed 3 October 2013.

10. Mill JS. Of the four methods of experimental inquiry. In: A System of Logic, Ratiocinative and Inductive. Project Gutenberg, 2009:478–503. http://www.gutenberg.org/files/27942/27942-pdf.pdf. Accessed 19 October 2013.

11. Greene CS. The fallacies of clinical success in dentistry. J Oral Med 1976;31:52–55.

12. Bernard C. An Introduction to the Study of Experimental Medicine. New York: Collier Books, 1961.

13. Clark K. Civilization. A Personal View. London: BBC Books, 1969:259.

14. White PA. Causal attribution and Mill's methods of experimental inquiry: Past, present and prospect. Br J Soc Psychol 2000;39(pt 3):429–447.

15. Sackett DL, Haynes RB, Guyatt GH, Tugwell P. Clinical Epidemiology: A Basic Science for Clinical Medicine, ed 2. Boston: Little Brown, 1991.

16. Grimes DA, Shulz KF. An overview of clinical research: The lay of the land. Lancet 2002;359:57–61.

17. Concato J, Shah N, Horwitz RI. Randomized, controlled trials, observational studies and the hierarchy of research designs. New Engl J Med 2000;342:1887–1892.

18. Streiner PC, Norman GR, Blum HM. PDQ Epidemiology. Toronto: Decker, 1989:viii.

19. Huth EJ. How to Write and Publish Papers in the Medical Sciences. Philadelphia: ISI Press, 1982:58.

20. Venning GR. Identification of adverse reactions to new drugs. 4. Verification of suspected adverse reactions. Br Med J 1983;286:544–547.

21. Marx RE. Pamidronate (Aredia) and zoledronate (Zometa) induced avascular necrosis of the jaws: A growing epidemic [letter]. J Oral Maxillofac Surg 2003;61:1115–1118.

22. Ruggiero SL, Mehrotra B, Rosenberg TJ, Engroff SL. Osteonecrosis of the jaws associated with the use of bisphosphonates: A review of 63 cases. J Oral Maxillofacial Surg 2004;62:527–534.

23. Holm G. Smoking as an additional risk for tooth loss. J Periodontol 1994;65:996–1001.

24. Heaton B, Dietrich T. Analytic epidemiology and periodontal diseases. Periodontol 2000 2012;58:112–120.

25. Tufte E. Beautiful Evidence. Cheshire, CT: Graphics Press, 2006:122–139,156–185.

26. Brunette DM. Critical Thinking: Understanding and Evaluating Dental Research. Chicago: Quintessence, 2007.

27. Oğuz F, Eltas A, Beytur A, Akdemir E, Uslu MÖ, Güneş A. Is there a relationship between chronic periodontitis and erectile dysfunction? J Sex Med 2013;10:838–843.

28. Davies HTO, Crombie IK, Tavakoli M. When can odds ratios mislead? BMJ 1998;316:989–991.

29. Yip JK, Cho S-C, Francisco H, Tarnow DP. Association between oral bisphosphonate use and dental implant failure among middle aged women. J Clin Periodontol 2012;39:408–414.

30. Gilbert N. Biometrical Interpretation. Oxford: Clarendon Press, 1973:27–45.

31. Smith GD, Phillips AN. Confounding in epidemiological studies: Why "independent" effects may not be all they seem. BMJ 1992;305:757–759.

32. Kuchenhoff H. Misclassification and measurement error in oral health. In: Lasaffre E, Feine J, Leroux B, Declerck D (eds). Statistical and Methodological Aspects of Oral Health Research. Chichester, England: Wiley, 2009:279–294.

33. Janket SJ, Baird AE, Chuang SK, Jones JA. Meta-analysis of periodontal disease and risk of coronary heart disease and stroke. Oral Surg Oral Med Oral Pathol Oral Radiol Endod 2003;95:559–569.

34. Dietrich T, Garcia RI. Associations between periodontal disease and systemic disease: Evaluating the strength of the evidence. J Periodontol 2005; 76:2175–2184.

35. Sackett DL. Bias in analytic research. J Chronic Dis 1979;32:51–63.

36. Shrier I, Platt RW. Reducing bias through directed acyclic graphs. BMC Med Res Methodol 2008;8:70.

37. Straus SE, Richardson WS, Glasziou P, Hynes RB. Evidence-Based Medicine. How to Practice and Teach EBM, ed 3. Edinburgh: Churchill Livingstone, 2005:189–190.

38. Parascandola M, Weed DL. Causation in epidemiology. J Epidemiol Community Health 2001;55:905–912.

39. Mackie JL. The Cement of the Universe: A Study of Causation. Oxford: Clarendon Press, 1980.

40. Boksman L, Santos GC. Principles of light-curing. Inside Dent March 2012;8(3). http://www.dentalaegis.com/id/2012/03/principles-of-light-curing. Accessed 24 September 2013.

41. Price RB. Avoiding pitfalls when using a light-curing unit. Compend Contin Educ Dent 2013;34:304–305.

42. Krieger N. Epidemiology and the web of causation: Has anyone seen the spider? Soc Sci Med 1994; 39:887–903.

43. Migliorati CA. Bisphosphonates and oral cavity avascular bone necrosis [letter]. J Clin Oncol 2003; 21:4253–4254.

44. Fisher RA. Lung cancer or cigarettes [letter]? Nature 1958;182:108.

45. Baron RM, Kenny DA. The moderator-mediator variable distinction in social psychological research: Conceptual, strategic, and statistical considerations. J Pers Soc Psychol 1986;51:1173–1182.

46. Hyman JJ, Winn DM, Reid BC. The role of cigarette smoking in the association between periodontal disease and coronary heart disease. J Periodontol 2002;73:988–994.

47. Maldonado G, Greenland S. Estimating causal effects. Int J Epidemiol 2002;31:422–429.

48. Rothman KJ. Causes. Am J Epidemiol 1976;104: 587–592.

49. Greenland S, Brumback B. An overview of relations among causal modeling methods. Int J Epidemiol 2002;31:1030–1037.

50. Bosco JLF, Silliman RA, Thwin SS, et al. A most stubborn bias: No adjustment method fully resolves confounding by indication in observational studies. J Clin Epidemiol 2010;63:64–74.

51. Aleksejūnienė J, Holst D, Eriksen HM, Gjermo P. Psychosocial stress, lifestyle, and periodontal health. J Clin Periodontol 2002;29:326–335.

52. Hill AB. The environment and disease: Association or causation? Proc R Soc Med 1965;58:295–300.

53. Humphrey LL, Fu R, Buckley D, Freeman M, Helfand M. Periodontal disease and coronary heart disease incidence: A systematic review and meta-analysis. J Gen Intern Med 2008;23:2079–2086.

54. Binkley CJ, Beacham A, Neace W, Gregg RG, Liem EB, Sessler DI. Genetic variations associated with red hair color and fear of dental pain, anxiety regarding dental care and avoidance of dental care. J Am Dent Assoc 2009;140:896–905.

55. Smith GD, Ebrahim S. Mendelian randomization: Prospects, potentials, and limitations. Int J Epidemiol 2004;33:30–42.

56. Coughlin SC. Quantitative models for causal analysis in the era of genome wide association studies. Open Health Serv Policy J 2011;4:118–122.

57. Hujoel PP, Dransholt M, Spiekerman C, DeRouen TA. Periodontal disease and coronary heart disease risk. JAMA 2000;284:1406–1410.

58. Sinha R, Cross AJ, Graubard BI, Leitzmann MF, Schatzkin A. Meat intake and mortality: A prospective study of over half a million people. Arch Intern Med 2009;169:562–571.

59. Sainani K. The limitations of statistical adjustment. PM R 2011;3:868–872.

60. Hujoel PP, Cunha-Cruz J, Kressin NR. Spurious associations in oral epidemiological research; the case of dental flossing and obesity. J Clin Periodontol 2006;33:520–523.

61. Feinstein AR. Scientific standards in epidemiologic studies of the menace of daily life. Science 1988; 242:1257–1263.

62. Savitz DA, Greenland S, Stolley PD, Kelsey JL. Scientific standards of criticism: A reaction to "Scientific standards in epidemiologic studies of the menace of daily life" by A. R. Feinstein. Epidemiology 1990;1:78–83.

63. Feinstein AR. Scientific news and epidemiologic editorials: A reply to the critics. Epidemiology 1990; 1:170–180.

64. Smith GD, Ebrahim S. Data dredging, bias, or confounding. BMJ 2002;325:21–28.

65. Grodstein F, Stampfer MJ, Manson JE, et al. Postmenopausal estrogen and progestin use and the risk of cardiovascular disease. New Engl J Med 1996;335:453–461.

66. Rossouw JE, Anderson GL, Prentice RL, et al. Risks and benefits of estrogen plus progestin in healthy postmenopausal women: Principal results From the Women's Health Initiative randomized controlled trial. JAMA 2002;288:321–333.

67. Shaneyfelt T. Residual Confounding in Observational Studies [video]. http://www.youtube.com/watch?v=R6VwapsefRs. Accessed 24 September 2013.

68. Beral V, Banks E, Reeves G. Evidence from randomised trials on the long-term effects of hormone replacement therapy. Lancet 2002;360:942–944.

69. Swaen GG, Teggeler O, van Amelsvoort LG. False positive outcomes and design characteristics in occupational cancer epidemiology. Int J Epidemiol 2001;30:948–954.

70. Hujoel P. Dietary carbohydrates and dental-systemic diseases. J Dent Res 2009;88:490–502.

71. Levis AG, Minicuci N, Ricci P, Gennaro V, Garbisa S. Mobile phones and head tumours. The discrepancies in cause-effect relationships in the epidemiological studies—How do they arise? Environ Health 2011;10:59.

72. Cornfield J, Haenszel W, Hammond EC, Lilienfeld AM, Shimkin MB, Wynder EL. Reprints and reflections. Smoking and lung cancer: Recent evidence and a discussion of some questions. J Natl Cancer Inst 1959;22:173–203. Reprinted in Int J Epidemiol 2009;38:1175–1191 [erratum 2009;38:1751].

73. Greenhouse JB. Commentary: Cornfield, epidemiology and causality. Int J Epidemiol 2009;38:1199–1201.

74. Greenland S. Cornfield, risk relativism, and research synthesis. Stat Med 2012;31:2773–2777.

75. Ong EK, Glantz SA. Tobacco industry efforts subverting International Agency for Research on Cancer's second-hand smoke study. Lancet 2000; 355:1253–1259.

76. Fisher A. The Logic of Real Arguments. Cambridge: Cambridge University Press, 1988:22.

77. Abelson RP. Statistics as Principled Argument. Hillsdale, NJ: Laurence Erlbaum, 1995.

78. Walton D. Informal Logic, a Pragmatic Approach, ed 2. New York: Cambridge University Press, 2008: 277–278.

3 Mechanism-Based Salivary Diagnostics: Oral-Systemic Connectivity

David T. W. Wong, DMD, DMSc

With the recent advances made in basic and translational sciences, saliva has emerged as a potentially useful biofluid to screen and assess risk for oral and systemic diseases.[1,2] This chapter reviews and summarizes recent findings in the field of salivary diagnostics to encourage dental professionals to incorporate these tests into their practices.

Saliva is an inexpensive and noninvasive specimen that can be easily collected during a dental visit.[3] In addition to oral epithelial cells, oral flora, and nasopharyngeal discharge, saliva contains most of the molecules found in serum and other bodily fluids, such as electrolytes, proteins, steroid hormones, antibodies, cancer biomarkers, DNA, and RNA.[1,3] Analyses of saliva constituents have revealed the presence of thousands of proteins. More than 3,000 salivary RNA species, including messenger RNA (mRNA) and microRNA (miRNA), have also been identified.[1] Because of its rich composition of *omics* constituents (see next section), saliva is a source of numerous biomarkers of translational and clinical values.[2]

In the United States, 20% more Americans attend their dental appointments than their physician's appointments.[2] As more people regularly visit their dentists than their physicians, the availability of salivary diagnostic tests that can be implemented by dentists may increase early detection of diseases, which will allow initiation of early treatment.

On average, individual salivation can range from 0.3 to 0.7 mL of saliva per minute,[4] producing a range of 1.0 to 1.5 L of saliva daily. Saliva is generated within a population of cells called *acini*, collected in small ducts, and subsequently released into the oral cavity.[5] Three major and minor saliva-producing glands are located in and around the mouth and throat (Fig 3-1a). The three major glands—parotid, submandibular, and sublingual—contribute greater than 90% of total saliva, while the minor glands— labial, buccal, lingual, and palatal—supply the remainder.

Despite some commonalities, each gland is unique with regard to the composition of its respective fluids. Secretions from serous cells, a parotid and submandibular cell population, consist of a watery solution that is devoid of mucus. Saliva released from the mucous cells, present in both submandibular and sublingual glands, contains a viscous mucus-rich fluid. Depending on how it is collected, saliva can be obtained from the secretions of major or minor salivary glands or combined as whole saliva.[6] Saliva is largely a filtrate from the capillary bed that nourishes the salivary glands whereby ac-

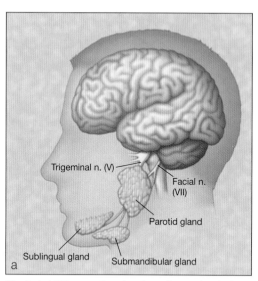
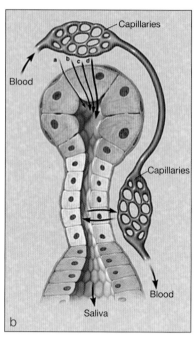

Fig 3-1 *(a)* Three pairs of major salivary glands (parotid, submandibular, and sublingual) surround the oral cavity. *(b)* Passive, active, and secretory mechanisms (a, b, c, d) transport fluid and analytes from the capillary bed to the ductal space in the salivary gland. n, nerve.

tive, passive, and secretory mechanisms are in place to provide passage of electrolytes, fluids, and molecular targets from the capillary bed to the salivary gland (Fig 3-1b).

State of the Science of Salivary Diagnostics

In 2002, initiatives by the National Institute of Dental and Craniofacial Research attracted researchers' interest in salivary diagnostics to advance the translational and clinical research of saliva.[3] The term *salivaomics*, or the study of biologic molecules present in saliva, emerged in 2008.[2] Salivaomics encompasses five categories known as the *diagnostic alphabets of saliva*.[2] These include the salivary proteome (or protein composition), transcriptome (mRNA), miRNA, metabolome (small molecular metabo-

lites such as metabolic intermediates and signaling molecules), and microbiome (microorganisms).[2] Methylomics is the latest omics to emerge in saliva.

To support salivary diagnostic research, researchers have designed a data management system and Web resource known as the *Salivaomics Knowledge Base* (available at http://hspp.ucla.edu/wonglab/).[2] This database was built on the basis of saliva ontology (known as *SALO*) and an open-source data portal (SDx-Mart) that hosts salivaomics data generated from studies of oral and systemic diseases.[2] The purpose of the Salivaomics Knowledge Base is to overcome data accessibility barriers and facilitate the use of salivary diagnostic data across research groups. Interactions and exchange of knowledge among researchers, diagnostic experts, and clinicians will help in the identification of salivary biomarkers and development of diagnostic tests.

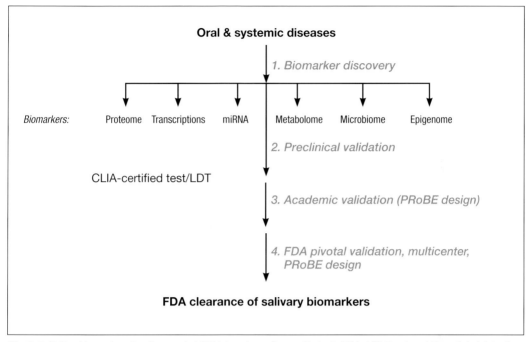

Oral & systemic diseases

1. Biomarker discovery

Biomarkers: Proteome Transcriptions miRNA Metabolome Microbiome Epigenome

CLIA-certified test/LDT

2. Preclinical validation

3. Academic validation (PRoBE design)

4. FDA pivotal validation, multicenter, PRoBE design

FDA clearance of salivary biomarkers

Fig 3-2 Saliva biomarker development. LDT, laboratory diagnostic test; FDA, US Food and Drug Administration; CLIA, Clinical Laboratory Improvement Amendments.

The rapid substantiation of the omics constituents of saliva enables researchers to design de novo biomarker development studies to discover and validate salivary biomarkers for early detection, treatment monitoring, recurrence prediction, and other translational and prognostic outcome assessments. The salivary diagnostic alphabets offer unparalleled advantages, because each disease may reflect differently in saliva through the proteome, genomics, miRNA, metabolome, microbiome, and methylomics. Informatics and statistical tools have been developed and are in place to harness the most discriminatory combination of salivary biomarkers that will detect oral and systemic diseases (Fig 3-2).

Salivaomics

Transcriptomics

Composed of coding (mRNA) and noncoding RNAs (small nucleolar RNAs [snoRNAs], miRNAs, and long noncoding RNAs [lncRNAs]), the transcriptome signifies a significant source of potentially relevant diagnostic information. MiRNAs are small (19 to 21 nucleotides) regulatory molecules that functionally interact with and potentially silence the translation of complementary antisense RNA sequences.[7] Similar to mRNAs, miRNAs can be aberrantly expressed in diseased cells and tissues.[8] These attributes suggest that transcriptomic evaluation may reveal highly specific disease-discriminatory indicators.

Both whole saliva and saliva supernatant harbor miRNAs and total RNA. Investigators probing the salivary transcriptome identified more than 1,000 miRNAs and more than 3,000 species of mRNA.[9] Suggesting that transcriptomic analysis yields biochemical data, these results support the utilization of saliva as an informative biofluid. With this in mind, investigators have discovered and are pursuing the identification of salivary biomarkers for oral, pancreatic, lung, and gastric cancers along with those for Sjögren syndrome, diabetes, and periodontal disease.[9-12]

Although gene chip arrays and quantitative polymerase chain reaction assays denote the most common methodologies for generating diagnostic values, the development of recent technologies promises to expand evaluative capacity. For example, the utilization of RNA sequencing platforms allows the quantitation of differentially represented transcripts in a solution.[13] Employing this and other global high-throughput technologies will permit a more thorough understanding of the salivary transcriptome and its role in diagnostics.

Proteomics

In 2004, the National Institute of Dental and Craniofacial Research provided funding to comprehensively decipher, catalog, and annotate the human salivary proteome, leading to the initial identification of 1,166 proteins in human saliva.[14] The salivary proteome contains a sizeable collection of diverse proteins.[15] The majority are synthesized and subsequently secreted into the oral cavity by the acinar cells of the salivary gland. This suggests that salivary proteomic constituents are a product of the salivary glands, which may be subject to internal and external factors. Consequently, the salivary proteome could be indicative of both local and distant diseases.

Traditional techniques used to evaluate salivary proteins include liquid chromatography, gel and capillary electrophoresis, nuclear magnetic resonance, mass spectrometry, immunoassays, and lectin probe analysis.[16] More contemporary methods, such as two-dimensional gel electrophoresis coupled with mass spectrometry, have allowed investigators to elucidate hundreds of salivary proteins.[15,17] Although its proteomic content is estimated to be only 30% of that of blood,[18] saliva is actively being investigated as a rich source of protein biomarkers capable of discerning between healthy and diseased subjects. In fact, researchers have reported unique proteomic profiles indicative of oral cancer, cystic fibrosis, endocrinologic and connective tissue disorders, dental caries, periodontitis, and even breast cancer.[19-21]

Methylomics

Epigenetics is the study of heritable changes in gene expression that are not reflected by changes in DNA sequence. While several epigenetic mechanisms, including DNA methylation, histone modification, and RNA interference, have been implicated in the pathogenesis of disease, none has been studied more than the methylome.[22]

Known to play a crucial role in cellular differentiation, DNA methylation allows cells to maintain unique characteristics by controlling and modulating gene expression.[23] Methylation patterns are typically established during embryogenesis and subsequently remain stable in normal tissues.[24] However, hypermethylation of CpG islands has been shown to be carcinogenic.[25] Identifying individuals with hypermethylated promoters may expedite the initiation of therapies and reveal the efficacy of screening high-risk populations.

It is not uncommon to find DNA within salivary secretions, and, as a result, several investigations have focused their efforts on elucidating patterns of promoter hypermethylation in salivary DNA. One study discovered gene panels capable of discerning oral squamous cell carcinoma patients from controls with 62% to 77% sensitivity and 83% to 100% specificity.[26] Additionally, two separate groups revealed regions of promoter hypermethylation in the saliva of patients with head and neck squamous cell carcinoma.[27] These reports suggest that saliva-based DNA may be an efficacious analyte for the detection and surveillance of head and neck squamous cell carcinoma and oral squamous cell carcinoma.

In addition, a number of studies have explored the effect of both local and global epigenetic alterations with regard to age.[28] In a recent study, researchers described a significant association between age and the methylation status of 80 genes in salivary samples.[29] Continued and future analyses in this area could serve as forerunners to the establishment of saliva-based predictive screenings for age-related disease.

Remarkably, salivary methylomic analysis techniques may also have a role in forensic science. Preliminary studies indicate that bisulfite sequencing of DNA from saliva and other biofluids could successfully discriminate five tissue-specific differentially methylated regions.[30] Altogether, results highlight the potential impact of utilizing saliva-based DNA not only as an indicator of disease but also as a discriminator of tissues between different individuals. These attributes may prove valuable in terms of discerning disease and identifying critical evidence.

Immunomics

Perhaps the most significant advancements in salivary diagnostics are the identification of immunologic markers useful in the assessment of systemic infections. Suspected to enter saliva from the blood through absorption and subsequent secretion by the salivary glands, these markers include the antigens, antibodies, and nucleic acids of infecting pathogens. The free exchange of blood-based molecules into saliva results in comparable concentrations of immunologic markers, a characteristic allowing for the noninvasive diagnosis and/or monitoring of systemic infections via oral fluids. In understanding this, the US Food and Drug Administration (FDA) has recently cleared enzyme-linked immunosorbent assay kits designed to probe saliva for indicators of human immunodeficiency virus type 1 (HIV-1) and type 2 (HIV-2).[31] Although further testing is required to confirm diagnosis, this represents a substantial step toward establishing saliva as a diagnostic medium.

Significant progress has also been noted with regard to hepatitis A, B, and C, whose antigens and antibodies are routinely detected in the saliva of infected individuals. In addition, recent investigations describe the efficacy of utilizing saliva to analyze hepatitis A virus (HAV) immunizations and evaluate acute exposures using immunoglobulin M, immunoglobulin A, immunoglobulin G, and HAV RNA tests.

Currently, diagnosis and monitoring of hepatitis B (HBV) and hepatitis C (HCV) are primarily blood based, yet researchers are now reporting quantifiable antibodies and antigens in saliva.[32,33] Accordingly, commercially available tests capable of identifying saliva-based HCV antibodies are under development. Although results obtained from this test draw parallels with serum immunoassays (97.5%), it has yet to obtain FDA clearance.

Because of the simplicity of saliva collection and its potential as a diagnostic medium, oral fluids have rapidly become the focus of investigation for several worldwide endemic microbes. Among these are malaria, dengue virus, Ebola virus, and *Mycobacterium tuberculosis* as well as herpes simplex virus, Epstein-Barr virus, cytomegalovirus, and human herpesvirus. Use of saliva to detect these disorders could decrease their associated mortality rates. Continued research is necessary, however, to expand beyond the now commercially available HIV and HCV tests to include a wider variety of microbes.

Microbiome

Microorganisms found in the human oral cavity have been referred to as the *oral microflora*, the *oral microbiota*, and more recently the *oral microbiome*.[34] While certain estimates state that approximately 500 to 700 bacterial species commonly inhabit the oral cavity, others suggest that the number may be as high as 10,000.[35] Not surprisingly, studies have shown that alterations in the oral microbial community have been correlated with the development of oral pathoses, malodor, and dental caries.[19–21]

The greater question is the relationship connecting the oral microbiome and systemic disorders. Although the mechanism linking salivary bacteria and distal disease currently eludes clarification, clinicians and basic scientists continue to explore this phenomenon. As a result, oral microbial candidate biomarkers are now being identified for Crohn disease, chronic pancreatitis, pancreatic cancer, and even obesity.[36] Nevertheless, while thought provoking, these studies have yet to be definitively validated and established as credible indicators. Continued efforts in this area could lead to the development of diagnostic measures capable of identifying early disease states, a truly impactful outcome.

Metabolomics

In general, a metabolome is composed of a variety of small molecules, including amino acids, organic acids, peptides, lipids, and nucleic acids. *Metabolomics* is the science of searching for the unique chemical fingerprints of these molecules within specific biologic samples.[37] Identifying discriminatory metabolomic alterations could aid in determining the selection, design, and modification of care plans.

In addition to tissues and cells, a number of biologic fluids, including saliva, contain metabolomic analytes.[38] As such, salivary metabolomics is an emerging and promising field that offers another unique perspective on the use of oral fluids in molecular diagnostics. In fact, researchers are now reporting significant discrepancies in several classes of metabolites (dipeptides, amino acids, carbohydrates, lipids, and nucleotides) when patients with periodontitis are compared with healthy subjects.[39] Similar studies analyzing the metabolic profiles discerned individuals with oral, pancreatic, or breast cancers from their respective healthy controls.[40–42] It can therefore be deduced that metabolomic signatures of both local and systemic diseases may be embedded in salivary secretions. Continued work in this arena could lead to the identification and employment of additional discriminatory metabolites useful in medical screening as well as disease diagnosis and monitoring.

Although the application of metabolomics is still in the early stages, its influence continues to grow each year. Integrating the knowledge obtained from different omics studies may help in understanding the biology of disease-specific metabolomic profiles and the mechanism of how individuals respond to therapies.

Future developments

The concurrent utilization of these omics libraries will be the canon of the future. This multi-tiered strategy will provide numerous layers of data revealing a clearer and perhaps more concise picture of a patient's disease state or potential response to treatments. The additive effect of these techniques may not only further the understanding of disease pathophysiology but also result in more favorable clinical outcomes.

It is in this spirit that the true value of salivary biomarkers reveals itself. De novo biomarker development studies can now be carried out in saliva. No longer is it necessary to be reliant on "me too"–type demonstrations of the clinical utility of a specific marker's presence in saliva when it has been demonstrated in blood or other biofluids. Now it is possible to harness the intrinsic treasures of salivary biomarkers for disease detection. Salivary biomarkers for early detection of diseases can be developed using inherent omics constituents, prospective study designs,[43] saliva-based bioinformatics, and statistical tools.

Oral-Systemic Connections

The revelation that oral fluids comprise biochemical and molecular data capable of reflecting health status simultaneously presents tremendous translation potential and a unique biologic question. While individual care plans based on the molecular and microbial constituency of saliva are constructed, what may be even more revealing is how biomarkers come to exist in saliva at all. In other words, what are the cellular and molecular mechanisms that drive the induction of salivary indicators for systemic disorders? With this question in mind, researchers are now focusing their efforts on communicative interplay between salivary glands and distant tissues.

Intercellular communication is a fundamental and imperative process in which individual cells molecularly correspond with neighboring and distant environments in an effort to coordinate physiologic activity within multicellular organisms.[44,45] Classically this phenomenon is considered to occur locally by means of direct cell contacts and remotely through juxtacrine, paracrine, and endocrine signaling modalities.[46] Typically enzymes, hormones, cytokines, and chemokines exemplify these long-range protein-based mechanisms. Each method is well studied and commonly results in a measurable cellular response in target cells.[46] The very nature of these processes and their effects emphasizes the regulatory complexity of the body and illustrates how tissues convey and react to information delivered via extracellular pathways. Although significant efforts have been applied to analyzing proteins in this capacity, recent studies have revealed a role for nucleic acids as major contributors to the communicative interaction of remote cell populations.[47–49]

Despite the ubiquity of ribonucleases, it is not uncommon to find RNA in the serum, plasma, breast milk, urine, and saliva of healthy and diseased patients.[50–52] Suggesting that secreted RNA can perpetuate in the extracellular milieu, these findings call into question the biologic significance of these molecules in this context. Alternatively, what role do these molecules serve outside their respective host cells?

To answer this question, it is necessary to understand that RNA innately possesses unique physiochemical properties that enable it to facilitate a number of biologic pathways.[53,54] As a product of transcription, both coding and noncoding RNAs efficiently store genetic information, a characteristic that highlights their potential impact on cellular dynamics. These attributes, in combination with its surprising extracellular stability, provide credence for the recent emergence of RNA as a possible mediator of long-distance extracellular communication.[53,54]

Including RNA as a potential effector of intercellular crosstalk adds an exciting and previously hidden dimension of molecular interplay and genetic regulation within a biologic system. However, its well-known propensity for degradation draws attention to the need for a protective vehicle that serves not only to shield the RNA from enzymatic destruction but also as a means for transport and delivery. Accordingly, studies have shown that certain microvesicular bodies called *exosomes* fulfill these parameters by encasing and delivering functional genetic information from donor to recipient cells.[55]

Measuring 30 to 100 nm in diameter, exosomes are small secretory lipidic assemblies formed by the invagination of intracellular vesicles. Exosomes are randomly secreted and routinely found in the conditioned media of multiple cell types as well as a number of biologic fluids, ranging from blood and saliva to breast milk and urine.[45,49,56,57]

Exosomes reportedly contain viable tissue-specific biochemical cargo that, on delivery, has been shown to induce unique molecular activity within target cells.[57–59] In fact, researchers are now showing that exosomal constituents may possess the capacity to manipulate immune responses, angiogenesis, coagulation, and numerous other complex physiologic mechanisms in recipient tissues.[60,61] Concertedly, these statements put forth the idea that exosomes may distinctively function as a means of protecting and shuttling biologically active information for the purposes of regulating cell communication.[55]

In considering the role of microvesicles in salivary diagnostics, it could be inferred that circulating exosomes derived from diseased tissues could interact with salivary glands (Fig 3-3). This event may alter the molecular constituency of saliva by modifying biochemical activity within saliva-secreting cells. In other words, salivary glands may be induced to generate and secrete discriminatory biomarkers by the circulating exosomes of diseased tissues.[62] Although the mechanistic details of such a phenomenon have yet to be explained, this exosomal inter-

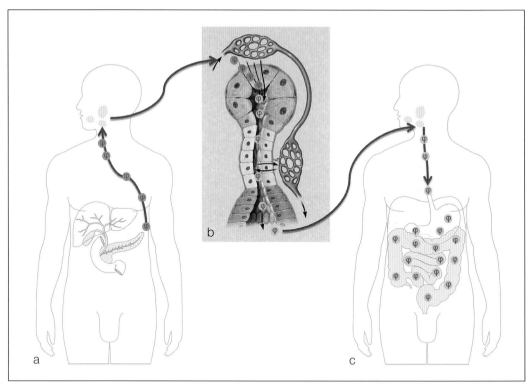

Fig 3-3 Mechanism-based salivary diagnostics. *(a)* Systemic disease development (pancreatic cancer) shedding disease-specific exosomes with shuttle through vasculature to the salivary glands. *(b)* Systemic disease-specific exosomes *(orange)* are taken up by salivary gland parenchymal cells, processed, and reintroduced into saliva as salivary biomarkers for the systemic disease embedded in exosomes *(green)*. *(c)* Systemic disease-specific salivary exosomes may exert systemic effects on the host, including mucosal immunity in the gastrointestinal tract.

play between distal tissues could account for the onset of disease-specific saliva-based biomarkers. While much remains to be proven, studies that further the understanding of the processes that yield these outcomes will not only help define the role of exosomes in extracellular communication but also lead to the development of novel strategies for disease diagnostics, monitoring, and therapeutics.

For example, using rodent models for pancreatic cancer development, researchers have shown that pancreatic cancer sheds tumor-specific biomarkers that are embedded in exosomes (see Fig 3-3a) and are shuttled to various parts of the body, including salivary glands, where they are taken up, processed, and reintroduced into saliva as disease-specific biomarkers (see Figs 3-3b and 3-3c).[63]

Mechanism-based salivary diagnostics must be pursued to provide the scientific credentials and to clarify how salivary biomarkers can develop during systemic disease pathogenesis. Of particular importance in these mechanistic developments is the emerging concept that RNA molecules are secreted in the extracellular spaces and act as endocrine signals to alter the phenotypes of target cells, both locally and at distant sites; this represents a novel paradigm in intercellular signaling. Recent advances in RNA sequencing technologies have identified a large and diverse population of extracellular RNA (exRNA), including miRNA and lncRNA. Given that approximately 60% to 80% of all protein-encoding genes are regulated by miRNA, and certain lncRNAs have been linked to regulation of the epigenome, extracellular delivery of these RNAs could have profound implications for a wide range of physiologic and pathologic processes.

In humans, exRNAs are found in all body fluids examined, including blood, saliva, urine, breast milk, cerebrospinal fluid, amniotic fluid, ascites, and pleural effusions. Recent reports in the literature suggest that exRNAs have both protective and pathogenic roles in a variety of human diseases. These findings highlight the transformative potential that secreted RNAs may have in the regulation of health and disease.

This emerging paradigm of cellular communication utilizing exRNA embedded in exosomes represents a scientifically credible mechanism in which disease-specific signals shed by a distal organ can serve as nanovectors and shuttle the information through the vasculature to different parts of the body, including the salivary glands, where they can be taken up, processed, and reintroduced into saliva as salivary biomarkers for the distal disease, thus giving credence to the connection between systemic disease or health and its oral manifestations.

Salivary Diagnostics in Current Practice

In the United States, a number of salivary tests are currently available to screen for viral infections such as HIV-1 infection[2] and human papillomavirus infection.[64] Furthermore, a number of saliva-based screening tests for HCV are available in Europe; FDA clearance for their commercialization in the United States is pending.[64]

Although salivary screening tests are common, saliva-based diagnostic tests for oral and systemic diseases are still lacking.[2] Promising research findings have been recently reported, particularly in oncology. Farrell et al[36] demonstrated the association between oral microbial

composition and pancreatic cancer. Comparison of salivary microflora identified 31 bacterial species that were found at higher levels among patients with pancreatic cancer or pancreatitis than among healthy subjects.[36] Among these species, the levels of two microbial markers, Neisseria elongate and Streptococcus mitis, were significantly different between healthy and diseased individuals. The diagnostic value of the two markers used in combination was validated; it had high sensitivity (96.4%) and specificity (82.1%).[36] Based on these results, development of a salivary diagnostic test for pancreatic disease is warranted.

Increased awareness among dental professionals will help to spread the implementation of salivary diagnostic tests in dental practice, provided that these specialists have a positive attitude toward salivary screening. Indeed, a national survey conducted among 1,945 US general dentists demonstrated that the majority (87%) of dental professionals were willing to incorporate salivary diagnostics into their practices.[65] Respondents thought it was important to screen for prevalent systemic diseases such as hypertension, cardiovascular disease, and diabetes in addition to screening for infectious diseases such as hepatitis and HIV. In addition, 83% of respondents were willing to perform medical screening using saliva samples or blood collected via fingerstick, and almost all respondents (96%) were willing to refer patients for physician consultation.

Conclusion

For salivary diagnostics to advance to clinical reality, two fundamental achievements must be in place: (1) the definitive and pivotal clinical validation of salivary biomarkers for systemic (nonoral) disease detection and (2) elucidation of the scientific underpinning of the mechanism whereby, on the development of a systemic disease, changes in salivary markers reflect the systemic disease. When these two foundational pillars are in place, salivary diagnostics will achieve clinical credibility and emerge as a promising landscape for molecular diagnostics.

Disclosure

David Wong is cofounder of RNAmeTRIX Inc, a molecular diagnostic company. He holds equity in RNAmeTRIX and serves as a company director and scientific advisor. The University of California also holds equity in RNAmeTRIX. Intellectual property that David Wong invented and was patented by the University of California has been licensed to RNAmeTRIX. Additionally, Dr Wong is a paid consultant to PeriRx.

References

1. Genco RJ. Salivary diagnostic tests. J Am Dent Assoc 2012;143(10 suppl):3S–5S.
2. Wong DT. Salivaomics. J Am Dent Assoc 2012;143(10 suppl):19S–24S.
3. Wong DT. Salivary diagnostics powered by nanotechnologies, proteomics and genomics. J Am Dent Assoc 2006;137:313–321.
4. Edgar WM. Saliva and dental health. Clinical implications of saliva: Report of a consensus meeting. Br Dent J 1990;169:96–98.
5. Tiwari M. Science behind human saliva. J Nat Sci Biol Med 2011;2:53–58.
6. Wong DT (ed). Salivary Diagnostics. Ames, IA: Wiley-Blackwell, 2008.
7. Lee RC, Feinbaum RL, Ambros V. The C. elegans heterochronic gene lin-4 encodes small RNAs with antisense complementarity to lin-14. Cell 1993;75:843–854.
8. Croce CM. Causes and consequences of microRNA dysregulation in cancer. Nat Rev Genet 2009;10:704–714.
9. Brinkmann O, Wong DT. Salivary transcriptome biomarkers in oral squamous cell cancer detection. Adv Clin Chem 2011;55:21–34.
10. Hu S, Vissink A, Arellano M, et al. Identification of autoantibody biomarkers for primary Sjögren's syndrome using protein microarrays. Proteomics 2011;11:1499–1507.
11. Lee H, Park M, Choi A, An J, Yang W, Shin KJ. Potential forensic application of DNA methylation profiling to body fluid identification. Int J Legal Med 2012;126:55–62.
12. Zhang L, Farrell JJ, Zhou H, et al. Salivary transcriptomic biomarkers for detection of resectable pancreatic cancer. Gastroenterology 2010;138:949–957.
13. Spielmann N, Ilsley D, Gu J, et al. The human salivary RNA transcriptome revealed by massively parallel sequencing. Clin Chem 2012;58:1314–1321.
14. Denny P, Hagen FK, Hardt M, et al. The proteomes of human parotid and submandibular/sublingual gland salivas collected as the ductal secretions. J Proteome Res 2008;7:1994–2006.
15. Hu S, Loo JA, Wong DT. Human saliva proteome analysis. Ann N Y Acad Sci 2007;1098:323–329.
16. Al Kawas SA, Rahim ZH, Ferguson DB. Potential uses of human salivary protein and peptide analysis in the diagnosis of disease. Arch Oral Biol 2012;57:1–9.
17. Hu S, Xie Y, Ramachandran P, et al. Large-scale identification of proteins in human salivary proteome by liquid chromatography/mass spectrometry and two-dimensional gel electrophoresis-mass spectrometry. Proteomics 2005;5:1714–1728.
18. Schulz BL, Cooper-White J, Punyadeera CK. Saliva proteome research: Current status and future outlook. Crit Rev Biotechnol 2013;33:246–259.
19. Paster BJ, Dewhirst FE. Molecular microbial diagnosis. Periodontol 2000 2009;51:38–44.
20. Takeshita T, Suzuki N, Nakano Y, et al. Relationship between oral malodor and the global composition of indigenous bacterial populations in saliva. Appl Environ Microbiol 2010;76:2806–2814.
21. Yang F, Zeng X, Ning K, et al. Saliva microbiomes distinguish caries-active from healthy human populations. ISME J 2012;6:1–10.
22. Vasilatou D, Papageorgiou S, Dimitriadis G, Pappa V. Epigenetic alterations and microRNAs: New players in the pathogenesis of myelodysplastic syndromes. Epigenetics 2013;8:561–570.
23. Ohgane J, Yagi S, Shiota K. Epigenetics: The DNA methylation profile of tissue-dependent and differentially methylated regions in cells. Placenta 2008;29(suppl A):S29–S35.
24. Grønbaek K, Hother C, Jones PA. Epigenetic changes in cancer. APMIS 2007;115:1039–1059.
25. Herman JG, Baylin SB. Gene silencing in cancer in association with promoter hypermethylation. N Engl J Med 2003;349:2042–2054.
26. Viet CT, Schmidt BL. Methylation array analysis of preoperative and postoperative saliva DNA in oral cancer patients. Cancer Epidemiol Biomarkers Prev 2008;17:3603–3611.
27. Carvalho AL, Henrique R, Jeronimo C, et al. Detection of promoter hypermethylation in salivary rinses as a biomarker for head and neck squamous cell carcinoma surveillance. Clin Cancer Res 2011;17:4782–4789.
28. Boks MP, Derks EM, Weisenberger DJ, et al. The relationship of DNA methylation with age, gender and genotype in twins and healthy controls. PLoS One 2009;4:e6767.
29. Bocklandt S, Lin W, Sehl ME, et al. Epigenetic predictor of age. PLoS One 2011;6:e14821.
30. Lee YH, Kim JH, Zhou H, Kim BW, Wong DT. Salivary transcriptomic biomarkers for detection of ovarian cancer: For serous papillary adenocarcinoma. J Mol Med (Berl) 2012;90:427–434.
31. United States Food and Drug Administration. First rapid home-use HIV kit approved for self-testing. FDA Consumer Health Information. http://www.fda.gov/downloads/ForConsumers/ConsumerUpdates/UCM311690.pdf. Accessed 6 May 2013.

32. Chen L, Liu F, Fan X, et al. Detection of hepatitis B surface antigen, hepatitis B core antigen, and hepatitis B virus DNA in parotid tissues. Int J Infect Dis 2009;13:20–23.

33. González V, Martró E, Folch C, et al. Detection of hepatitis C virus antibodies in oral fluid specimens for prevalence studies. Eur J Clin Microbiol Infect Dis 2008;27:121–126.

34. Dewhirst FE, Chen T, Izard J, et al. The human oral microbiome. J Bacteriol 2010;192:5002–5017.

35. Keijser BJ, Zaura E, Huse SM, et al. Pyrosequencing analysis of the oral microflora of healthy adults. J Dent Res 2008;87:1016–1020.

36. Farrell JJ, Zhang L, Zhou H, et al. Variations of oral microbiota are associated with pancreatic diseases including pancreatic cancer. Gut 2012;61:582–588.

37. Jordan KW, Nordenstam J, Lauwers GY, et al. Metabolomic characterization of human rectal adenocarcinoma with intact tissue magnetic resonance spectroscopy. Dis Colon Rectum 2009;52:520–525.

38. Walsh MC, Brennan L, Malthouse JP, Roche HM, Gibney MJ. Effect of acute dietary standardization on the urinary, plasma, and salivary metabolomic profiles of healthy humans. Am J Clin Nutr 2006; 84:531–539.

39. Barnes VM, Ciancio SG, Shibly O, et al. Metabolomics reveals elevated macromolecular degradation in periodontal disease. J Dent Res 2011;90:1293–1297.

40. Sugimoto M, Wong D, Hirayama A, Soga T, Tomita M. Capillary electrophoresis mass spectrometry-based saliva metabolomics identified oral, breast and pancreatic cancer-specific profiles. Metabolomics 2010;6:78–95.

41. Wei J, Xie G, Zhou Z, et al. Salivary metabolite signatures of oral cancer and leukoplakia. Int J Cancer 2011;129:2207–2217.

42. Yan SK, Wei BJ, Lin ZY, Yang Y, Zhou ZT, Zhang WD. A metabonomic approach to the diagnosis of oral squamous cell carcinoma, oral lichen planus and oral leukoplakia. Oral Oncol 2008;44:477–483.

43. Pepe MS, Feng Z, Janes H, Bossuyt PM, Potter JD. Pivotal evaluation of the accuracy of a biomarker used for classification or prediction: Standards for study design. J Natl Cancer Inst 2008;100:1432–1438.

44. Chen X, Liang H, Zhang J, Zen K, Zhang CY. Secreted microRNAs: A new form of intercellular communication. Trends Cell Biol 2012;22:125–132.

45. Théry C, Ostrowski M, Segura E. Membrane vesicles as conveyors of immune responses. Nat Rev Immunol 2009;9:581–593.

46. Pant S, Hilton H, Burczynski ME. The multifaceted exosome: Biogenesis, role in normal and aberrant cellular function, and frontiers for pharmacological and biomarker opportunities. Biochem Pharmacol 2012;83:1484–1494.

47. Bellingham SA, Guo BB, Coleman BM, Hill AF. Exosomes: Vehicles for the transfer of toxic proteins associated with neurodegenerative diseases? Front Physiol 2012;3:124.

48. Hood JL, San RS, Wickline SA. Exosomes released by melanoma cells prepare sentinel lymph nodes for tumor metastasis. Cancer Res 2011;71:3792–3801.

49. Yang C, Robbins PD. The roles of tumor-derived exosomes in cancer pathogenesis. Clin Dev Immunol 2011;2011:842849.

50. Fleischhacker M, Schmidt B. Circulating nucleic acids (CNAs) and cancer—A survey. Biochim Biophys Acta 2007;1775:181–232.

51. Kosaka N, Iguchi H, Yoshioka Y, Takeshita F, Matsuki Y, Ochiya T. Secretory mechanisms and intercellular transfer of microRNAs in living cells. J Biol Chem 2010;285:17442–17452.

52. O'Driscoll L. Extracellular nucleic acids and their potential as diagnostic, prognostic and predictive biomarkers. Anticancer Res 2007;27:1257–1265.

53. Dinger ME, Mercer TR, Mattick JS. RNAs as extracellular signaling molecules. J Mol Endocrinol 2008; 40:151–159.

54. Scott WG. Ribozymes. Curr Opin Struct Biol 2007; 17:280–286.

55. Lässer C, Eldh M, Lötvall J. Isolation and characterization of RNA-containing exosomes. J Vis Exp 2012;(59):e3037.

56. Record M, Subra C, Silvente-Poirot S, Poirot M. Exosomes as intercellular signalosomes and pharmacological effectors. Biochem Pharmacol 2011; 81:1171–1182.

57. Vlassov AV, Magdaleno S, Setterquist R, Conrad R. Exosomes: Current knowledge of their composition, biological functions, and diagnostic and therapeutic potentials. Biochim Biophys Acta 2012; 1820:940–948.

58. Dimov I, Jankovic Velickovic L, Stefanovic V. Urinary exosomes. Sci World J 2009;9:1107–1118.

59. Théry C, Zitvogel L, Amigorena S. Exosomes: Composition, biogenesis and function. Nat Rev Immunol 2002;2:569–579.

60. Lakkaraju A, Rodriguez-Boulan E. Itinerant exosomes: Emerging roles in cell and tissue polarity. Trends Cell Biol 2008;18:199–209.

61. Pegtel DM, van de Garde MD, Middeldorp JM. Viral miRNAs exploiting the endosomal-exosomal pathway for intercellular cross-talk and immune evasion. Biochim Biophys Acta 2011;1809:715–721.

62. Lau CS, Wong DT. Breast cancer exosome-like microvesicles and salivary gland cells interplay alters salivary gland cell-derived exosome-like microvesicles in vitro. PLoS One 2012;7:e33037.

63. Lau CS, Kim Y, Chia D, et al. Role of pancreatic cancer-derived exosomes in salivary biomarker development. J Biol Chem 2013;288:26888–26897.

64. Corstjens PL, Abrams WR, Malamud D. Detecting viruses by using salivary diagnostics. J Am Dent Assoc 2012;143(10 suppl):12S–18S.

65. Greenberg BL, Glick M, Frantsve-Hawley J, Kantor ML. Dentists' attitudes toward chairside screening for medical conditions. J Am Dent Assoc 2010; 141:52–62.

The Traveling Oral Microbiome

4

Wenche S. Borgnakke, DDS, MPH, PhD

Microbes are everywhere. Each time we breathe in, we inhale a million microbes or more, depending on where we are. Many remain trapped in our nostrils, but countless continue into our bodies; fortunately, the overwhelming majority cause no harm.

Science is now focused on identifying microbes and all other living organisms, thanks to novel technologies and computer capabilities of formerly unthinkable power. Collectively, the microorganisms in the oral cavity—bacteria, archaea (one-celled, nucleus-free organisms formerly classified as archaebacteria), fungi, viruses, and protozoa—have been referred to as the *oral microflora*, *oral microbiota*, and more recently, as the *oral microbiome*. Our understanding of the human oral microbiome is currently in a groundbreaking phase of development in which science has to rethink and rewrite large parts of what was hitherto known. High-throughput genetic-based assays, powerful, novel bioinformatics tools, and fast computers recently made it possible to comprehensively survey the human oral microbiome to identify and determine the prevalence of previously unknown or not culturable organisms.

The ability to fully describe the microbiome that inhabits the human body, including the oral microbiome, suggests a need to reexamine these microbes and their relationship to health and disease. The use of these methods sheds new light on the role of the oral microbiome in periodontal disease and in systemic diseases and conditions. This new insight will lead to future changes in clinical practice. We have yet only seen the very tip of the iceberg. The sky is the limit.

"I" Am Really "We"

Perhaps it is time for each of us to think of ourselves and our commensal microbes (usually present and living in or on our bodies) as constituting a "we" rather than an "I." That is, each of us can be considered a collective microbiome–human body "superorganism," in which microbes outnumber our roughly 100 trillion human cells by a ratio of 10:1, or $10^{14}:10^{13}$. In other words, of all the cells in this superorganism, only about 10% are human. Further knowledge regarding the human microbiomes that inhabit various body locations (nose, oral cavity, intestines, female reproductive tract, outer part of the urinary system, and skin) may in the future be used in combination with metagenomic information to identify high-risk individuals and thereby enable individualized preventive and therapeutic care, referred to as *personalized medicine*, in which the oral microbiome plays a pivotal role. Researchers are just now beginning to understand some aspects of this role.

Unlearn the Learned

Concept 1: "Periodontal pathogen" no more?

Old knowledge. Specific periodontal pathogens are especially "virulent" and cause periodontal disease.

New knowledge. Depending on the microbe-host environment interaction and the technique used for their detection, disease severity will vary, and different members of the oral microbiome will be identified in varying proportions in subgingival plaque.

Recently, Bizzarro and colleagues[1] studied subgingival plaque from 15 smokers and 15 nonsmokers. They used three different methods to identify the bacteria in subgingival plaque. With two of the methods, the researchers found no differences between smokers and nonsmokers in the proportions of the members of the microbiomes. In contrast, sequencing of the 16S ribosomal RNA (rRNA) revealed that some genera were more abundant in nonsmokers and others in smokers. This third method also showed that participants with more severe periodontal disease, particularly smokers, had fewer different kinds of microbes. Considering findings from previous studies as well as their own, Bizzarro et al wrote, "the 'pathogenic role' of few specific species is questionable. Thus, we consider now the identification of a few targeted species for diagnostic purposes to be an out-of-date procedure."[1]

Concept 2: Could periodontal bacteria actually be a consequence, and not the cause, of periodontal breakdown?

Old knowledge. Specific periodontal pathogens cause periodontal tissue breakdown. Mainly gram-negative, anaerobic bacteria cause periodontal disease. Clusters of microbes live in the plaque in the periodontal sulcus. They develop into a more mature ecosystem that eventually morphs into the most mature, complex, pathogenic biofilm that causes further breakdown of periodontal tissues.

New knowledge. Periodontal breakdown in susceptible individuals creates an environment suitable for particular oral microbes, which then flourish. Deep periodontal pockets provide an environment free of oxygen that enhances habitation by certain anaerobic bacteria.

Recently, Bartold and Van Dyke[2] questioned whether the so-called periodontal pathogenic bacteria really are the cause or may be a consequence of the chronic inflammation known as *periodontitis*. They agreed with Löe and colleagues,[3] who 50 years ago showed that the host-parasite interactions cause gingivitis. The oral microbiomes form an ecosystem that maintains health when in equilibrium. Bartold and Van Dyke[2] contended that the host is largely responsible for the complex alterations in the local periodontal environment that disturb this healthy homeostasis and facilitate the switch of commensal flora to an opportunistic pathogenic flora. Therefore, the authors concluded that such changes are caused mostly by the host, not by the bacteria.

Emerging evidence supports the major role of host responses modulated through genetic, immunologic, and inflammatory responses; stress; smoking; diet; social determinants; and general health—which have been identified as risk factors for periodontitis[4]—as being the major determinants of the outcomes of periodontitis. Therefore, the overgrowth of periodontal microbes may well be a result of the periodontal tissue breakdown and not the cause of periodontitis.

This concept is supported by the fact that currently there is no scientific evidence that identifies any particular bacteria as a cause of periodontitis. Only associations have been observed; that is, deep periodontal probing depths and an abundance of certain bacteria are detected simultaneously.

What does this mean for the dental practitioner?

The two aforementioned publications[1,2] express the current beliefs and synthesize sentiments that have been developing over the last few years. They actually make perfect sense. For many years, the search to identify the culprit bacteria that cause periodontal disease used methods that depended on growth and observation of bacteria in a laboratory. Now the members and communities of the oral microbiome in health and in disease can be explored without culturing the bacteria. They can now be detected from even small pieces of genetic material, so it is not necessary to examine the entire organism, let alone live ones that can be kept alive in the laboratory.

Detailed genetic analysis of bacteria is increasingly both available and economical and has demonstrated an unanticipated genetic diversity within species. This knowledge will guide future prevention and treatment protocols, which seem to point in the direction of personalized medical and dental care tailored to the individual, based on personal genetic, environmental, and clinical profiles.[5] The increasingly sophisticated molecular-level analytic tools and exploration of inflammatory responses and other host factors have shown that factors within the host may be at least as important as the potential pathogen.

For now, however, these new viewpoints on mechanisms will not change the need to keep the oral cavity as healthy and free of dental plaque as possible. Nevertheless, these perspectives indicate that dental professionals must constantly be vigilant and consider the possible existence of systemic health conditions and diseases in need of attention—and possibly even of discovery for the first time—especially in patients with severe periodontitis.[6]

What Is an Infection?

The term *infection* has various definitions. The main difference among definitions is that some include the reaction of host tissues to the infectious organisms and the toxins they produce while others regard merely the presence of the infectious agent in unusual amounts or places to be sufficient for application of the term, even in the absence of pronounced host responses. The latter state is what the former definition would regard as *carriage*; that is, the host acts as a carrier who does not necessarily show signs or symptoms of an infection but may do so if resistance is decreased. Still others regard an infectious agent as one that is not normally found in the body. These distinctions are important for how we think about infection in conjunction with periodontal disease and the identification of oral microbes in the rest of the body.

In this chapter, increased levels of oral microbes in the oral cavity are regarded as overgrowth of commensal microbes in environmental conditions conducive to their multiplication. The terms *infection*, *pathogen*, and *virulence* are not used in conjunction with organisms usually inhabiting the biofilm in the periodontium. The term *microbe* refers to both live and dead bacteria and their byproducts, as well as archaea, viruses, and fungi, unless specifically noted.

The Human Genome

Genomes and DNA

The term *genome* was adopted in 1920 and is a blend of the two words *gene* and *chromosome*. A genome consists of all the genetic material of a living entity. Genes are packaged chromosomes that consist of DNA, and DNA is made up of pairs of nucleotides in various sequences. The nucleotides are adenine (A), thymine (T), cytosine (C), and guanine (G). The nucleotides A and T are always bonded together as a pair, as are C and G, hence the expression *base pair*. The nucleic acid RNA uses uracil (U) instead of thymine, so its base pairs are A + U and C + G.

The Human Genome Project

The Human Genome Project was declared completed with the final mapping and sequencing of the human genome on April 14, 2003, which was 2 years ahead of the 15-year-long schedule.[7] For the first time, all 20,500 human genes were cataloged after sequencing of the 3 billion chemical base pairs that make up human DNA. This human genome is a "reference genome" from a combination of anonymous donors, but each human being has a unique gene sequence.

Knowledge about the human genome is pivotal to understanding how our bodies function so that preventive and curative measures can be devised to improve our patients' health and quality of life.

Metagenomics

Metagenomics is a sequence-based method that permits the genetic material from all the microbes harvested from a biologic sample to be analyzed simultaneously without the need for cultivating the microorganisms in a laboratory. Metagenomics provides vastly more information than the analysis of single, isolated microbes. It is possible not only to determine which organisms are present but also to deduce the relative abundance of the different species. Furthermore, it may be possible to discover which metabolic pathways are encoded by the organisms so that information can be obtained about their functions in the body. Metagenomics is used to analyze the human oral microbiome in unprecedented detail.

Sequencing of the 16S rRNA gene

The 16S rRNA gene has been sequenced to detect the order (sequence) in which the four nucleotides (A + U, C + G) appear. The entire length of the 16S gene of RNA from ribosomes has been sequenced, and this information is stored in the publicly accessible Human Microbiome Project database as a reference.[8] Scientists can now compare their findings to the reference RNA for identification. The bacterial 16S rRNA gene is the molecular marker most widely used to identify microbes to study the diversity of microbial communities.

The 16S rRNA gene is used as a reference for sequencing for a number of reasons:

- It is present in almost all bacteria.
- It is a highly conserved gene, preserved in its original form through various manipulations such as cell death and freezing.
- Its function has not changed over time, suggesting that random sequence changes are a more accurate measure of time (evolution).
- It is long enough (1,500 base pairs) for informatics purposes involving identification for comparisons to detect similarities and differences between genetic samples.

Importantly, as in metagenomics, the microbes do not have to be whole or alive for this method to be used. The DNA can stem from dead organisms or from only pieces thereof. Consequently, even bits of the cell walls (endotoxins) are sufficient for determining the identity of a certain microbe.

The Human Microbiome

A *microbiome* is the totality of microorganisms (also called *microbes*), their genetic elements (genomes), and environmental interactions in a particular environment. The term was coined in 2001, which indicates the novelty of this concept. Some consider the microbiome a "newly discovered organ," because its existence was not generally recognized until the late 1990s.

Researchers are beginning to understand its vast impact on human existence, health, and disease. The human microbiome consists of all the microbes that inhabit the human body (inside and on the surface). It contains about 100 trillion microorganisms, outnumbering human cells by 10:1 ($10^{14}:10^{13}$), and contains more than 2 million genes, outnumbering human genes by 100:1 (2,050,000:20,500). The human microbiome normally consists of beneficial, harmless, nonpathogenic organisms.

The microbiome is necessary for human survival. Its components digest food; synthesize essential nutrients and vitamins; educate and maintain the innate (inborn) and adaptive (acquired) immune system while maintaining self-tolerance to avoid autoimmunity; regulate immune homeostasis; fight off infections; and maintain homeostasis and healthy equilibrium.

Because of their small size, microorganisms make up only about 1% to 3% of body mass. For instance, 1.5 to 4.5 lb (0.7 to 2.0 kg) of microbes live in and on a 150-lb (68-kg) person.

The Human Microbiome Project

The Human Microbiome Project was launched by the US National Institutes of Health to characterize the human microbiome and subsequently analyze its role in health and disease.[9] The Human Microbiome Project is the largest ever 5-year project aimed at identifying and cataloging the human microbiome. Researchers sampled 300 healthy, 18- to 40-year-old individuals from two US cities. Even the presence of minor "gum disease" was enough to exclude a subject from the study.[10]

The study was focused on identifying the microbes residing in five body areas (Fig 4-1). Researchers sampled the following 15 body sites in each man and 18 sites in each woman:

- Nose: anterior nares (×1)
- Mouth: attached gingiva, hard palate, throat, palatine tonsils, dorsum of the tongue, buc-

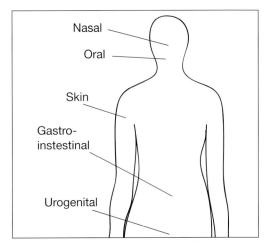

Fig 4-1 Body sites for sampling microbiomes for the Human Microbiome Project. (Adapted from National Institutes of Health.[9])

cal mucosa, supragingival and subgingival plaque, and saliva (×9)
- Skin: left and right retroauricular crease and left and right antecubital fossa (×4)
- Colon (gastrointestinal system, ie, lower gut): stool (×1)
- Urogenital: vagina (midvaginal, posterior fornix, and vaginal introitus) (×3)

Nine of the 15 or 18 sites sampled were located in the oral cavity, which is a testament to the immensely important role the oral microbiome plays in human health and disease.

The Human Oral Microbiome

Currently, about 700 different bacterial species are identified in the human oral cavity, but estimates suggest that the number may be as many as 1,200.[11] The oral cavity differs from all other human microbial habitats by the simultaneous presence of two types of surface for microbial colonization: shedding surfaces (mucosa) and solid surfaces (teeth, dentures, and orthodontic appliances). This intrinsic property of the oral cavity provides immense possibilities for a diverse range of microbiota. Saliva contains around 100 million bacteria and archaea per milliliter, by far the two most common types of microbe in the mouth.[12]

Currently, only about half of the microorganisms detected in the mouth are officially named, and only about three-quarters of those are indisputably oral commensals. The rest may represent transient colonization, but some may turn out to inhabit the mouth on a regular basis. Knowing which microbes live in the oral cavity is important for targeting measures to improve or attain oral health.

The Human Oral Microbiome Database

The human oral microbiome is the most studied human microflora. The Human Oral Microbiome Database was created to provide the scientific community with a comprehensive database of the oral bacterial species.[13] It is basically a ledger that provides information on the genomes of oral bacteria.

Although this chapter attempts to avoid technical terms as much as possible, here follows an example of the classification hierarchy of subgroups, namely for *Porphyromonas gingivalis*, formerly known as *Bacteroides gingivalis*:

- Domain: Bacteria
- Phylum: Bacteroidetes
- Class: Bacteroides
- Order: Bacteroidales
- Family: Porphyromonadaceae
- Genus: *Porphyromonas*
- Species: *gingivalis*

So far 12 different subgroups, known as *strains*, of the species *P gingivalis* have been identified, demonstrating its capability of adapting to new environments.[14]

The same order of classification hierarchy for *Streptococcus mutans* is Bacteria, Firmicutes, Bacilli, Lactobacillales, Streptoccaceae, *Streptococcus*, and *mutans*.

Does a core oral microbiome exist?

Researchers have wondered about the existence of a core set of oral microorganisms that are common to most humans. Only with these novel techniques is it possible to begin to look for possible answers to this question. When three healthy, unrelated individuals were studied, samples originating from shedding surfaces (mucosa of the tongue, cheek, and palate) were clearly distinguishable from the samples that were obtained from solid surfaces (teeth).[15] The three people had only one-quarter (26%) of the 6,315 unique bacterial genes sequences in common, but the families of bacteria to which these belonged were almost the same (99.8%) in the three persons. This supports the concept of a core microbiome in health.

However, the proportions of even the common microbes varied widely among the individuals (Fig 4-2). Moreover, the distribution and abundance of bacteria in the different oral sites sampled varied substantially among the three individuals (Fig 4-3). Interestingly, bacteria formerly regarded as causing periodontitis were harbored in the three subjects as well as in multiple participants in a larger study,[16] but typically only as a minor component of the plaque.

Several microorganisms that are common elsewhere in the body inhabit or are frequent guests in the oral cavity. For example, *Staphylococcus aureus* is frequently detected, although it is not a bacterium normally considered a regular member of the oral microbiome. In people with cleft lip and palate, transmission to the mouth can easily occur from the nasal microbiota. In a study of young children, those with fistulas had significantly more *S aureus* in the oral cavity than did those without fistulas, and those with larger fistulas had greater counts of *S aureus* than those with smaller fistulas.[17]

In 2010, a group of researchers characterized for the first time the "basal" fungal microbiome (*mycobiome*) of the oral cavity in healthy individuals. Figure 4-4 shows the fungi present in each of the 20 subjects examined, vividly illustrating the great diversity and individual differences in the composition of their mycobiomes.[18] The

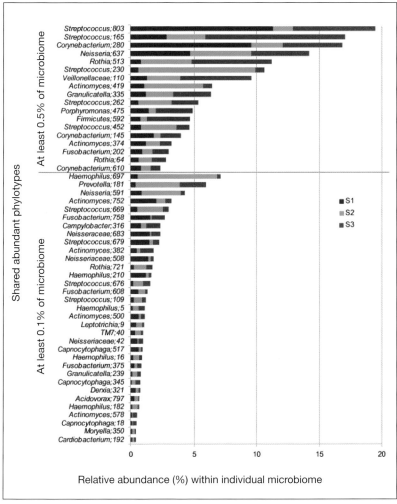

Fig 4-2 Shared abundant phylotypes in three oral microbiomes (S1, S2, and S3) and their relative abundance within an individual microbiome. (Only abundant phylotypes that contributed to at least 0.1% of the individual microbiome are shown.) The most abundant phylotypes (0.5% or more of the microbiome) are grouped separately in the upper panel. Phylotypes were defined as operational taxonomic units (OTUs) clustering sequences at a 3% genetic difference. The highest taxon (in most cases, genus) at which the OTU was identified is shown, together with the cluster identification number. Different colors indicate three different microbiomes: S1 (blue), S2 (green), and S3 (red). (Reprinted from Zaura et al[15] with permission.)

number of different fungi among the healthy subjects ranged from 3 to 16 fungi.

The dynamic oral microbiome

The teeth are unique in that they do not constantly renew their outer layer, shedding the old, as other human tissues do. Therefore, they allow a subgingival biofilm, consisting of a highly variable and complex community of microbes, to colonize, organize, and develop for extended periods. Bacteria within dental plaque biofilms are in a dynamic state and interact with each other, embedded within a self-produced matrix of extracellular polymeric substance. In con-

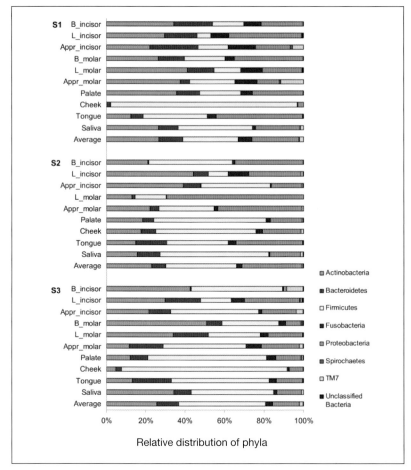

Fig 4-3 Average and site-specific relative distribution of bacterial phyla in three individuals (S1, S2, and S3). Unclassified bacteria were reads without a recognizable match in the full 16S rRNA reference database. B, buccal; L, lingual; Appr, approximal surface of either an incisor or a molar. (Reprinted from Zaura et al[15] with permission.)

trast to microorganisms growing in a planktonic state, the inhabitants of a biofilm are effectively protected within this dense structure from host defense mechanisms and from therapeutic agents, including antimicrobial agents.

Just like human microbiomes in other body locations, such a microcosm includes organisms of varying types and proportions, depending on whether its environment is in homeostasis. Once the milieu is altered, this delicate balance is interrupted to the benefit of certain commensal microbes, which subsequently exhibit opportunistic overgrowth to the detriment of other members of this biofilm community; the latter organisms then diminish in amount, possibly to rates below detection. Because the healthy state is so delicate, it can be questioned whether ardent use of bacteriostatic mouthrinse in the absence of periodontitis or gingivitis actually may do some harm and disturb the balance.

To enable researchers to explore the interactions between fungi and bacteria, 82 older Dutch community dwellers delivered unstimulated saliva (passive drooling into a sterile cup) samples first thing on awakening in the morning.[19] The

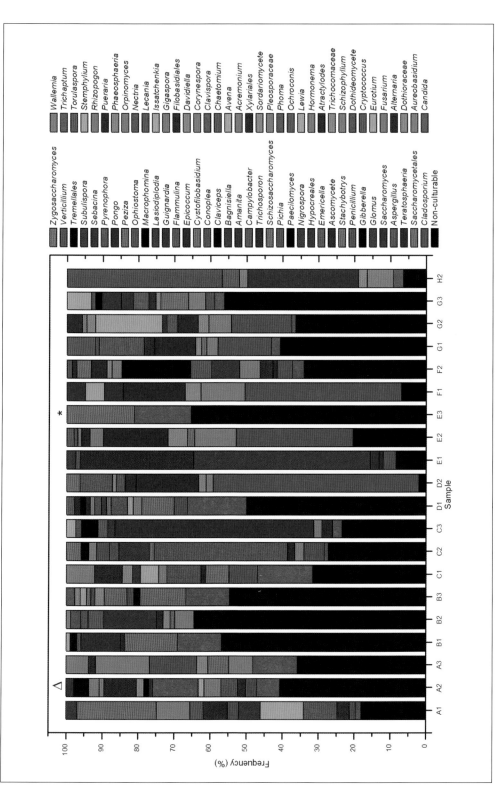

Fig 4-4 Overall distribution of fungi in oral rinse samples obtained from 20 healthy individuals. Δ, sample containing 16 fungal genera; *, sample containing 3 fungal genera. (Reprinted from Ghannoum et al[18] with permission.)

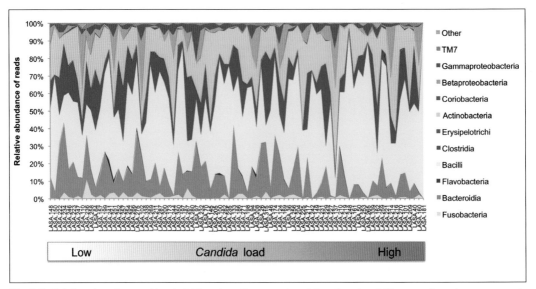

Fig 4-5 Relative abundance of bacterial taxa in saliva samples at the class level. The sample order corresponds to the increase in the *Candida albicans* load in the samples. The *Candida* load was measured as the proportion of internal transcribed gene (*Candida*) over 16S gene (bacteria) abundance by quantitative polymerase chain reaction. Increase in the *Candida* load was statistically significantly, positively correlated with reads classified as Bacilli (includes streptococci), while the *Candida* load correlated negatively with the classes Bacteroidia, Flavobacteria, and Fusobacteria. This shift in the composition of salivary bacteria to being dominated by sugar-loving and acid-producing bacteria, namely streptococci, is indicated by the increase in the proportion of yellow—namely the Bacilli class to which streptococci belong—with increasing proportions of *C albicans*. (Reprinted from Kraneveld et al[19] with permission.)

bacterial diversity of the salivary microbiome decreased significantly with increasing load of the yeast *Candida albicans*. Not only were there fewer kinds of bacteria present in persons with more *C albicans*, but their salivary bacteria composition also shifted markedly to being dominated by sugar-loving and acid-producing bacteria, namely streptococci (Fig 4-5). This leads to the question of whether controlling the oral environment to become less acidic may be a potential preventive measure for overgrowth of *Candida* as well as for prevention of caries, especially on the roots.

Numerous short- and long-lasting changes in a human's life cause more or less divergence from "normal" status in the oral cavity, in the gingival and periodontal tissues, in the gingivocrevicular fluid, and in the saliva. Many of their effects on the subgingival microcommunity are unknown. However, recent research provides a potential preventive and therapeutic use of existing knowledge of the effects of the oral microbiome on cancer. In 2013, Tezal and col-

leagues[20] reported for the first time an independent, inverse association between dental caries and head and neck squamous cell carcinomas (HNSCC). This relationship held up even among individuals who were never smokers and never drinkers. The notion that an acidic oral environment seems to protect against HNSCC was demonstrated by decreased levels of caries, crowns, and endodontic treatment in individuals with HNSCC compared with higher levels of such caries experience among those without HNSCC. This is a counterintuitive finding, because caries is normally associated with poor health.

When various measures for caries prevention, such as vaccinations or antimicrobial and gene therapy, are conceived in the future, the balance of the oral environment should be considered; for example, therapy should take into account the potential prevention of HNSCC and preserve the beneficial effects of lactic acid bacteria.

Distribution of oral microbes

Intraoral diversity

Within the oral cavity, groups of microbial species arrange themselves into surface-localized communities that vary considerably in composition according to their exact location. Even adjacent oral sites "only millimeters or less" apart exhibited "strikingly different" microbial community compositions.[21]

Another study found that there were considerable differences in bacterial composition among teeth at different intraoral locations and even among different surfaces of the same tooth.[22] The most pronounced differences were observed in incisors and canines, where *Streptococcus* species were found on 40% to 70% of the vestibular surfaces but were almost absent on the lingual surfaces. The bacterial composition of saliva samples was not representative of supragingival and subgingival plaque samples. The dorsum of the tongue specifically harbored several bacterial species detected in ventilator-associated pneumonia.

In summary, proportions of bacterial species differ markedly on different intraoral surfaces. Even within streptococci, there are differences in colonization patterns by the various species. Therefore, sites for sampling and for local therapeutic measures should be carefully chosen for determination of oral microbial composition. Importantly, microbes in saliva do not necessarily represent the biofilm in either supragingival or subgingival plaque. Furthermore, the different methods used to sample the saliva, for instance passive drooling, active swishing with a liquid, insertion of paper points, or oral swabs, may affect the representativeness of the salivary composition.

Oral epithelial cells: Hostels for traveling microbes from elsewhere. A variety of visiting (transient) bacterial species are harbored in oral epithelial cells, which therefore together could be considered a reservoir for these bacteria. *Enterococcus faecalis* was the most prevalent visiting species found in oral epithelial cells (20.6%) but was identified only in people with deep periodontal pockets.[23] No correlation was found with age, sex, bleeding on probing, and supragingival biofilm. Half of those with great attachment loss also harbored *Pseudomonas aeruginosa*.

Another study found that subgingival plaque samples contained DNA from those two bacteria as well as two more nonoral pathogenic bacteria (*Escherichia coli* and *S aureus*). DNA from these four bacteria was found—alone or together with DNA from bacteria usually associated with periodontitis—to be strongly associated with periodontitis.[24]

The finding that the prevalence of the opportunistic bacteria *E coli*, *E faecalis*, *S aureus*, and *P aeruginosa* is correlated with presence and severity of periodontal disease could be regarded as confirmation that host factors are important in such invasion by common inhabitants of other body sites that multiply in the mouth under certain favorable conditions. The discovery further supports the new concepts that, in periodontitis, *(1)* bacteria (and viruses) interact with microbes that do not normally inhabit the mouth and *(2)* groups of several microbes, not only one bacterium, are found in periodontitis.

Intraindividual and interpersonal diversity

The composition of the salivary microbiome varies both within and among persons and over time. Figure 4-6 presents the relative proportions of the most frequently identified bacterial phyla for each of five individuals at different time points. The salivary microbial community appeared to be stable over at least 5 days.[23] However, samples taken up to 29 days after baseline showed that the microbiome compositions of samples taken at closer time intervals were not necessarily more similar than those obtained over longer intervals in any individual. The saliva samples were dominated by the seven major groups (phyla), but only five groups were found in all participants at all times (see Fig 4-6). The remaining two were also found in all participants but not every time.

Time will tell whether a core universal human salivary microbiome will emerge.[25] It should

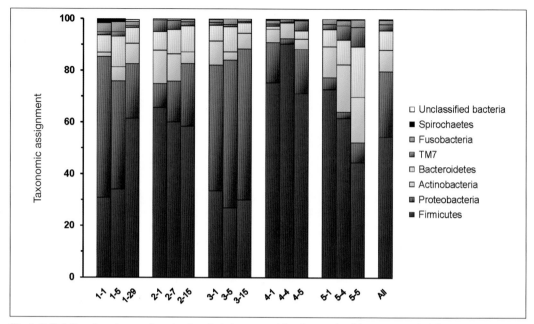

Fig 4-6 Relative abundance of predominant phyla across 15 salivary microbiomes, namely 3 from each of five individuals on 3 different days. Sample numbers include participant ID and the follow-up day after the first sampling time point (day 1). The days are indicated by the number after the hyphen (-) on the horizontal axis. For instance, the saliva samples from the left-most participant were taken on days 1, 5, and 29. Bacterial phyla are indicated by color. The rightmost column, designated as *All*, displays the average phyla proportions when the individual samples were pooled. Both *Streptococcus* and *Staphylococcus* species belong to the order Bacilli, which are part of the phylum Firmicutes *(blue)*. (Reprinted from Lazarevic et al[25] with permission.)

be kept in mind that the saliva may not represent similar microbiome compositions in dental plaque or in biofilm on oral mucosal surfaces.

Geographic diversity

Several research teams have explored whether various populations in different countries and of different racial backgrounds indeed share a core oral microbiome, despite their individual variation. There is scant evidence that some evolutionary lineages of bacteria have adapted to particular ethnic groups.[26] With the limited information available, few of these differences can be directly related to differences in prevalence of periodontal disease. Asian populations are regularly colonized with *Actinobacillus actinomycetemcomitans (Aa)* serotype c with

questionable pathogenic potential. On the contrary, the JP2 clone of *Aa* causes significantly higher prevalence of aggressive periodontitis in adolescents whose descent can be traced back to the Mediterranean region and Western parts of Africa.[26]

In adult Koreans with advanced periodontitis, all diseased sites harbored *Fusobacterium* species, while *P gingivalis, Treponema* species, and *Tannerella forsythia* were detected in more than 96% of the sites.[27] Even in periodontally healthy subjects, *Fusobacterium* species were present in the highest proportion (58%) of sites, while *Treponema* species, *P gingivalis,* and *T forsythia* each were detected in about one-fifth of healthy sites.

The oral mucosa microbiota in cheek swabs from six Amazon Amerindians of Guahibo ethnicity living in Venezuela was highly dominated by four bacterial groups (phyla).[28] These Amerindians shared only 23% of the subgroups (genera) with non-Amerindians from previous studies and had a lower richness of genera (51 versus 177 genera reported in non-Amerindians). In addition, their microbiota included some bacteria common in soil.

In another study, saliva samples were obtained from 10 individuals from each of 12 worldwide locations.[29] Overall, approximately 13.5% of the total variance in the composition of genera was due to differences among individuals. Investigation of some environmental variables revealed a significant association between the genetic distances among locations and the distance of each location from the equator.

There is high diversity in the salivary microbiome within and among individuals, indicative of an enormous geographic diversity in the human salivary microbiome. Microbial community diversity in the Batwa Pygmies, a former hunter-gatherer group from Uganda, is significantly higher than that in agricultural groups from Sierra Leone and the Democratic Republic of Congo.[30] Forty microbial genera previously not described in the human oral cavity were identified in the Batwa. Their distinctive composition of the salivary microbiome may have been influenced by recent changes in lifestyle and diet.

Knowledge regarding geographic variations in the oral microbiome and their relationship to periodontal disease and other oral conditions would be clinically important for providing individualized periodontal treatment in the future.

Traveling Oral Microbes

The effects of oral microbes on the rest of the body may be categorized as indirect and direct. The indirect effects consist of the body's general cascade of inflammatory reactions to those microbes and bacterial endotoxins. The direct effect is observed as the consequences of specific oral organisms traveling to and colonizing body locations outside the oral cavity. Therefore, the particular microbes need to be identified via detection of the microorganism itself or specific antibodies to it. The rest of this chapter focuses on the direct effect of oral microbes venturing outside the oral cavity and emphasizes the logistics of their travels. Only systemic consequences not specifically addressed in other chapters are described.

Travel destinations

In addition to the mouth and connected spaces, oral microbes have been identified in the following body sites:

- Neck
- Atherosclerotic plaque in the cardiovascular system (coronary arteries, carotid arteries, and coronary thrombi in myocardial infarction)
- Heart valve prostheses
- Surfaces of intracardiac devices (pacemakers and implantable cardioverter-defibrillators)
- Brain (atherosclerotic thrombi in ischemic stroke, brain tissue, and meninges)
- Respiratory tract (lungs)
- Liver
- Gastrointestinal system
- Pancreas
- Joints (synovial fluid)
- Vertebrae
- Vertebral disc
- Mother-infant unit in pregnancy with adverse pregnancy outcomes (fetal brain tissue, amnion, chorion, amniotic fluid, umbilical cord, and placenta)
- Breast milk
- Vagina, including the cervix
- Voice prostheses
- Bite marks or wounds (human bites on human skin)

Travel options

Dissemination of oral microbes occurs in various ways. First, travel within a human body via different avenues and by various vehicles is described. This is considered *domestic* or *intrapersonal travel*. In the next section, interpersonal transfer between humans is depicted as *interpersonal* or *international travel*.

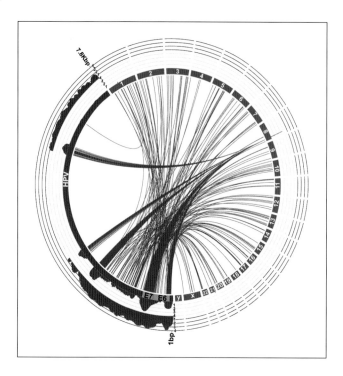

Fig 4-7 Identification of HPV integration into the HeLa genome. The integration of human papillomavirus genome HPV NC_001357 *(red)* into chromosome 8 in the HeLa cell genome represented by human genome version 19 *(blue)* is supported by read pairs with one read mapping to HPV and the other mapping to the human genome *(purple lines)*. The log-transformed coverage of the reads supporting integration *(purple histogram:* axis minimum = 0; axis maximum = 4) is consistent with the known integration of the HPV E6 and E7 genes shown in pink on the HPV genome. The log-transformed coverage of the viral mate pairs is also shown *(red histogram)*. bp, base pair. (Reprinted from Riley et al[31] with permission.)

Domestic/intrapersonal

By air: Aspiration. *Pulmonary aspiration* refers to the entry of material from the oropharynx (upper respiratory tract) or gastrointestinal tract into the lungs via the larynx and lower respiratory tract, which is the part of the respiratory system from the trachea to the lungs. When food or drink is aspirated, people use the expression that the particle or liquid "went down the wrong (wind) pipe."

By direct transfer: Genetic material. In the human superorganism, the bacteria are in frequent, intimate contact with human cells. Bacterial DNA integrates into the human somatic genome, including bacteria that often are part of the oral microbiome. Figure 4-7 shows integration of genetic material from the human papillomavirus (HPV) into human chromosome 8.[31] Such transfer occurs more frequently in cancer.

By blood: Bacteremia. Each time the integrity of the oral cavity is compromised, it presents an opportunity for bacteremia, which is the presence of bacteria in the normally sterile blood. Oral bacteria slip into the bloodstream during most professional dental procedures. However, such bacteremias are short lived and transient, and the highest intensity is limited to the first 30 minutes after a triggering episode.[32] This is the conclusion of a review of 50 pertinent reports. Yet some individuals are not able to clear the bacteria before they lodge themselves in new garages on their journey, such as arterial walls and organs. The current consensus is that bacteremia is caused by everyday activities to a much greater extent than occasional procedures by dental professionals.[30]

By blood: Fungemia? *Fungemia* is the term used to describe the situation in which fungi or yeasts are present in the blood. *C albicans* has been implicated in some cases of infective endocarditis. However, the *C albicans* organisms that invade the bloodstream do not seem to originate in the oral cavity.[33] A Brazilian team simultaneously examined the palatal mucosa, the palatal surface of the maxillary denture, and the blood of patients with denture stomatitis for presence of *C albicans*.[34] The researchers found a strong relationship between denture stomatitis and *Candida* species from the palatal mucosa and maxillary denture. Despite abundant amounts of the yeast in these two locations, however, use of a novel DNA identification method detected no *C albicans* in the blood.

Bloody entryways and access roads. Routes of possible entry by oral microorganisms into the systemic circulation include:

- Root canal: periapical and lateral lesions into the alveolar and adjacent blood vessels, including those in the maxillary sinus
- Periodontium: into capillaries and other small blood vessels in junctional epithelium and gingival connective tissues or into the alveolar blood vessels
- Mucosal lesions with injury to capillaries in the oral cavity: injuries caused by mastication of hard food items or biting of tongue or cheek; denture-related ulcers; candidiasis; and pierced tissue (with jewelry): tongue, lip, and maybe face via saliva

Bloody travel vehicles. Various mechanisms for the systemic dissemination of oral microbes via the circulating blood have been suggested. These include flowing freely in the bloodstream; catching a ride with a "raft" of lipoproteins, sometimes along with medium-sized cholesterol molecules; adhering to red blood cells; and hiding intracellularly. The last mechanism is an especially effective mode of transport that can be likened to the Trojan horse model. The microbes are engulfed or cloaked in a phagocytosis-like fashion, thereby not only being transported but also evading discovery and attacks by the host defense system (circulating phagocytes) and antibiotics. *P gingivalis*, the "atherogenic bacterium," especially uses this method. Bacteria internalized in white blood cells (phagocytes) can persist in the circulation for extended periods.

International/interpersonal

By direct transfer: Direct contact between humans. Oral microbes are transmitted via kissing, sharing of utensils, parents licking or cleaning a pacifier or prechewing food for their babies, oral sex, biting, and so on. Unquestionably, the most important microbe transmitted by direct contact between people is HPV, which is described in a later section.

Cariogenic bacteria are transmitted from parents or caregivers to the child whose oral cavity is sterile at birth. There is limited contemporary evidence for parent-to-child transmission of bacteria usually associated with periodontal disease. A study genetically identifying *Aa* and *P gingivalis* in subgingival plaque in families with periodontitis revealed interspousal transmission of *Aa* in 4 of 11 married couples (36%) and of *P gingivalis* in 2 of 10 married couples (20%).[35] Parent-to-child transmission of *Aa* was seen in 6 of 19 families (32%), whereas *P gingivalis* was not transmitted from parent to child in any of the study families.

When salivary DNA in edentulous infants and their mothers was compared, it became clear that even the young, predental baby hosted a wide variety of bacteria.[36] A total of 397 bacterial genera were identified. Only 28 were different between the adult and the child, 27 of them seen in the adults. *Streptococcus* was the predominant genus in infant saliva, significantly more abundant than in the mothers (62.2% in infants versus 20.4% in adults). This study demonstrated that a diverse bacterial community exists in the oral cavity of infants even before tooth eruption. It remains to be seen which environmental factors affect the further colonization and subsequent risks for oral and gastrointestinal disease.

Growing evidence supports an oral origin for bacteria that cause chorioamnionitis, an inflammation of the fetal membranes (amnion and chorion). While bacteremia is the main suspected travel mode, receptive oral sex from a partner with periodontal disease can also be the cause.[37-39]

Bite marks in humans by humans mostly are seen in violent crime, especially in rape attacks and child abuse. The use of morphology of the bite mark has been abandoned, and instead identification via the culture-independent DNA analysis is generally accepted as hard evidence in court. A research team found that streptococcal DNA from bite mark samples aligned significantly more closely with profiles generated from the teeth responsible for the bite than with those from other teeth in the same individual. Hence, streptococcal DNA can be used directly from bite marks.[40]

Another team examined three genomic regions of streptococcal DNA to discriminate between swabs from bite marks and teeth from 16 participants.[41] Using three different techniques, the researchers found probabilities of 92%, 99%, and 100%, respectively, for correct identification of the tooth whose plaque was in the bite mark.

Bacterial DNA is preserved for a longer time in bite marks than in, for instance, decomposing human cells in a corpse and may therefore be useful if collected a longer time after the bite occurred. Bacterial DNA is more convenient in such cases because it could be difficult to distinguish human DNA between the biter and the bitten. Consequently, oral bacterial DNA may be used in forensic dentistry to provide documenting information on the identification of the biter.

By indirect transfer: Via pacifier. Many parents clean their infant's pacifier with their own saliva by sucking it. In so doing, parents transfer their oral microbes to the child.[42] Based on a study of 184 infants, pediatricians concluded that vaginal delivery and parents' cleaning of pacifiers with their saliva generated independent and additive, significant protective effects against development of asthma (88% decrease) as well as eczema and sensitization (63% decrease for each) at age 18 months. The authors speculated that the child's immune system is stimulated by microbes in the mother's birth canal and the parents' saliva.

However, various professional dental organizations have strongly opposed recommendation of this practice because of the risk of transfer of oral organisms that contribute to the development of caries and periodontal disease.

By indirect transfer: Layover in dental laboratory or hospital equipment. Removable dentures are often in need of adjustment and repair due to resorption of the edentulous alveolar ridges after extraction of teeth. Bacteria that inhabit the oral microbiome and can turn into opportunistic pathogens in a favorable milieu have been found in pumice samples from dental laboratories. Additionally, studies have shown that the pumicing procedure produces splatter and aerosols, through which the bacteria can spread.

By air: Sneeze propelled. Although periodontal bacteria are reported to be part of atmospheric air high above the ocean, it is not known whether such high flyers actually can infect a new host on landing and multiply in the adopted environment. Moreover, the literature currently seems devoid of confirmed colonization through human-to-human transmission of oral microbes after sneezing or coughing. However, such transmission may be possible.

By water: Sink drain. A first of its kind report was published in April 2013: DNA from *P gingivalis* was identified in the complex biofilm in the drain of a sink in a hospital bathroom. Applying a novel technique of generating genomic DNA from single cells, the researchers recovered a nearly complete genome representing a new strain of the periodontal bacterium, namely *P gingivalis* JCVI SC001.[43]

Travelers

Oral bacteria easily penetrate the bloodstream when the periodontium is inflamed due to infection. The ease with which this occurs seems to depend on the severity and extent of the periodontal infection and inflammation and is higher in people with poor oral hygiene. That is, the worse the periodontal disease, the more easily will bacteria penetrate the bloodstream. Once in the blood, the microbes from the periodontal biofilm and their byproducts—such as live or dead microbes and pieces of bacterial cell walls (lipopolysaccharides)—will travel to various destinations in the body. Lipopolysaccharides are large molecules that are also known as *endotoxins*. They are a major constituent of the outer cell membrane of gram-negative bacteria, for instance those often associated with periodontal destruction.

Endotoxins can elicit strong immune responses. Humans are much more sensitive to them than are other mammals, such as mice. A dose of 1 µg/kg induces shock in humans, but mice will tolerate a dose up to 1,000 times higher.[44] This is a major reason why findings from research conducted in mice with experimental periodontal disease should be viewed with caution, because the results may not transfer directly to humans.

Travel qualifications

Through the use of powerful novel techniques, an unexpected genetic diversity within the bacterial species has recently come to light. In many cases, the evolution of specific species and their subspecies is disproportionately associated with infection or overgrowth.[26] Only a limited number of species and strains are detected in bacteremias so far. It may be that certain microbial attributes play a role in the ability of certain bacterial species to penetrate and survive in the bloodstream, invade distant tissues and organs, and ultimately multiply there. Reportedly, some species exhibit innate attributes that enhance such activities, including the ability to:

- Adhere to multiple different surfaces (microbes, tissues, immune cells, and salivary molecules)
- Decrease the activity of cells that would engulf them (impede phagocytic activity)
- Penetrate between cells in tissue and into host cells
- Initiate, maintain, and ensure long-term survival of an intracellular localization for transportation, defense, and multiplication (Trojan horse model)

Because only certain subspecies (strains) of bacteria seem to travel systemically, it is necessary to identify exactly which strains cause harm in order to target those organisms in future therapy and prevention.[45]

Travel share: The mouth, the gut, and atherosclerosis

Recently, a landmark study was designed to test the hypothesis that bacteria from the mouth and/or the gut could end up in atherosclerotic plaque and thus contribute to the development of cardiovascular disease.[46] Using 16S rRNA genes to survey and compare the bacterial diversity of oral, gut, and atherosclerotic plaque samples from 15 individuals with atherosclerosis and 15 healthy controls, Koren and colleagues[41] found the following:

- Bacterial DNA was present in the atherosclerotic plaque.
- *Veillonella* and *Streptococcus* species were detected in the majority of the atherosclerotic plaque samples.
- The combined abundances of *Veillonella* and *Streptococcus* species in atherosclerotic plaques correlated with their abundance in the oral cavity.
- DNA from several additional bacteria was common to the atherosclerotic plaque and oral or gut samples within the same individual.

Certain *S mutans* strains have been detected in specimens from heart valves and atheromatous plaque from individuals undergoing surgery, and certain strains are shown to be able to attach to, enter, and survive for several hours in human coronary artery endothelial cells.

Overall, these findings strongly support the hypothesis that the oral cavity and the gut can be sources for atherosclerotic plaque–associated bacteria.[46] These bacteria may contribute to further inflammation and eventual destabilization and rupture of the plaque, ultimately causing a heart attack or stroke. More studies are needed to confirm these initial, intriguing results.

Frequent traveler: Human papillomavirus

Although HPV might not be thought of as part of the normal human oral microbiome, the US Centers for Disease Control and Prevention (CDC) estimates that up to 80% of Americans will harbor HPV at some time during their lifetime.[47] HPV is the most common sexually transmitted virus in the United States. The vast majority of infections go unnoticed, so most infected persons do not realize that they are passing the virus on to a sex partner. No HPV test for men has been approved by the CDC.[47] About 90% of the infections (others would regard this as carriage, not infection) will resolve within 2 years, and the majority are undetectable after 1 year, except in some immunocompromised individuals, such as those infected with human immunodeficiency virus (HIV).

HPV does not multiply in saliva or blood. It establishes productive infections only in keratinocytes of the skin or mucous membranes. More than 40 HPV types can infect the mouth and throat as well as the genital areas of males and females. HPV is not disseminated via bacteremia but is easily transferred by direct contact, most often during vaginal and anal sex; it may also be passed on during oral sex and genital-to-genital contact. HPV may also be transmitted via kissing. Whether the exact means of transmission is direct contact or via saliva remains to be determined. There is as yet no evidence that saliva acts as an HPV transmission vehicle for oral or genital contamination. However, given the presence of shed epithelium cells in oral fluids, this route is quite possible.

In addition to causing cancer, which will be discussed in a later section, HPV infections can cause other health problems, including 100% of genital warts; recurrent respiratory papillomatosis, a rare condition in which warts grow in the throat; and juvenile-onset recurrent respiratory papillomatosis seen in babies infected by their mothers during delivery. The types of HPV that can cause genital warts are not the same as the types of HPV that can cause cancers. Warts can appear from weeks to months after HPV is contracted.[48]

World traveler: Prevalence of HPV. There are more than 100 different kinds of HPV, but not all of them cause health problems. According to the World Health Organization (WHO), the two most prevalent HPV types are HPV-16 (3.2%) and HPV-18 (1.4%).[49] The global prevalence of infection with HPV in women without cervical abnormalities is 11% to 12%; rates are higher in sub-Saharan Africa (24%), Eastern Europe (21%), and Latin America (16%). Particularly high prevalences are seen in Eastern Africa and the Caribbean, where rates exceed 30%. In general, higher rates are observed in less developed regions of the world.[49] For instance, 75.3% of the population in a study in India was infected by HPV.[50]

HPV was detected in 4.0% of oral rinse obtained from 1,688 healthy men, aged 18 to 74 years (median 31 years), from the United States, Mexico, and Brazil. The HPV types were similar in the three countries, except that HPV-55 was more often seen in Mexico.[51] The strongest predictor for presence of oral HPV was smoking. However, the prevalence of oral HPV in these men was only one-tenth that of infection at genital sites (4% versus approximately 40%). The reason is not evident, but the authors speculated that the mouth may be more resistant to infection than the anogenital area. Over 12 months, 4.4% of these men acquired new oral HPV. However, most were cleared within a year, after a median infection period of less than 7 months.[52]

In the United States, approximately 79 million individuals are currently infected with HPV.[47] That is a full quarter of the entire US population of 313.9 million, including all ages. About 14 million people will contract the infection each year, and about 360,000 men and women develop genital warts. Around 7% of the US adult population, namely 10.1% of males and 3.6% of females, have one or more of 37 types of oral HPV, detected in purified DNA from oral exfoliated cells obtained from oral rinse.[53,54]

Vaccination and testing for HPV. The CDC recommends three doses of HPV vaccine for all girls and boys aged 11 or 12 years, as well as for older unvaccinated individuals. However, by July 2013, the vaccination coverage of adolescent girls aged 13 to 17 years remained unchanged since 2012. Only about half (53.8%) of girls received one or more doses of HPV vaccine, and only one-third (33.4%) received all three doses of the recommended series (Fig 4-8).[55] Vaccines against other diseases were received by 92.6% of these adolescents. Despite the availability of safe and effective HPV vac-

Fig 4-8 Estimated vaccination coverage with selected vaccines and doses among adolescents aged 13 to 17 years, by survey year (National Immunization Survey–Teen) in the United States, from 2006 to 2012. Tdap, tetanus toxoid, reduced diphtheria toxoid, and acellular pertussis; MenACWY, meningococcal conjugate; HPV, human papillomavirus. *≥ 1 dose Tdap vaccine at or after the age of 10 years. †≥ 1 dose MenACWY vaccine. §HPV vaccine, either bivalent or quadrivalent, among females. Advisory Committee on Immunization Practices recommends either bivalent or quadrivalent vaccine for females. ¶HPV vaccine, either bivalent or quadrivalent, among males. Advisory Committee on Immunization Practices recommends the quadrivalent vaccine for males; however, some males might have received bivalent vaccine. (From Centers for Disease Control and Prevention.[55])

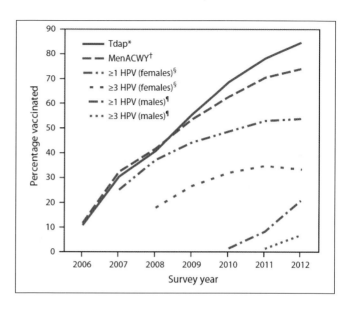

cines, the vast majority missed the opportunity to obtain them during their medical visit.

As an aside, a study conducted among 10% of Danish dentists showed that they had no increased risk of being infected with HPV.[56] Dental practitioners are in an eminent position to be alert to any signs of epithelial changes in the oral mucosa. As partners of the patient-centered health care team, dental professionals can also contribute to their patients' general health care by educating and encouraging them to obtain HPV vaccination as part of overall health.

Intermittent traveler: Herpes simplex virus

Several types of viruses inhabit the oral cavity and are more often associated with periodontal pockets than gingivitis. The role of these viruses as causative agents for periodontitis has been questioned. Nevertheless, herpes simplex virus (HSV) merits mention as a frequent, although intermittently dormant, member of the oral microbiome.

After infecting an individual, HSV takes up permanent residence in the host. HSV spreads easily between humans, mostly via direct contact such as kissing and caressing but also through shared utensils and towels, lip balm, and razors as well as via sexual contact. The carrier from whom the virus is transferred needs not have signs or symptoms of the infection, such as cold sores. Such transmission is termed *asymptomatic viral shedding*.

Herpes simplex type 1 is usually acquired in childhood, whereas type 2 typically spreads through sexual contact, and about 20% of sexually active adults in the United States are infected. However, type 1 can also be transmitted via oral sex and cause genital cold sores. Likewise, type 2 is increasingly seen in the oral cavity; about 15% of oral infections are caused by HSV-2. HSV-1 is estimated to affect more than half the US population, and 80% to 90% are affected by the age of 50 years.

About 50 million US adults experience between one and three symptomatic episodes every year. After the first outbreak of a herpetic lesion, the virus moves from the skin to the central nervous system. There it will stay dormant until a triggering event, such as stress, illness, fever, sun exposure, menstrual periods, or surgery, interrupts the host's homeostasis and decreases resistance. The outbreaks may occur in the buccal and gingival mucosa or on the tonsils, as well as on the lips.

Many dental professionals refrain from treating a patient during the active phase of an outbreak. This is due to concern about potential viral transmission either via direct contact between dental personnel and a patient's cold sores or via a virus-containing aerosol created by air blown into the mouth and bounced back over the lips of an infected patient.

Lifelong lurking traveler: Epstein-Barr virus

The Epstein-Barr virus (EBV), also known as *human herpesvirus 4*, is a common member of the human herpesvirus family and as such lingers in the human body for life.[57] Ironically, the EBV infects not only epithelial cells but also the B cells of the immune system that are supposed to combat this virus. It stays dormant in the B cells until a triggering event causes it to proliferate. Worldwide, more than 90% of adults are EBV seropositive.

EBV is usually acquired in early childhood or adolescence. Children are susceptible as soon as the antibodies inherited from their mother wear off, and about half of 5-year-olds in the United States were exposed to the virus. If infection instead occurs during adolescence or during the teen years, infectious mononucleosis will manifest itself in one-third to one-half of the cases in the United States. Because the virus is transferred via saliva (and genital secretions), infectious mononucleosis is known as the *kissing disease* (or *mono*). EBV is also identified in oral diseases such as oral lichen planus.

Reverse traveler: *Helicobacter pylori* bacterium

Although not discovered until 1984,[58] *Helicobacter pylori* is the bacterium responsible for stomach and duodenal ulcers. *H pylori* is one of the most common pathogenic infective agents; about half the world's population is affected. Its prevalence correlates closely with socioeconomic and hygienic conditions. Developing countries have a prevalence of 80% to 90%, whereas that of developed countries usually is less than 40%.[59]

After pooling results from different studies, a meta-analysis concluded that there is a close relation between infection with *H pylori* in the oral cavity and in the stomach; in pooled data, 45.0% of gastrically infected individuals and 23.9% of individuals without stomach infection have oral *H pylori*.[60] Initial infection with *H pylori* usually occurs in childhood and is observed in primary endodontic infections, even in live, cultivable form.[61]

Even in the absence of gastritis, *H pylori* is frequently detected in the oral cavity, especially in people with periodontitis; in dental plaque in up to 88% of people; in benign laryngeal lesions; on the surface of oral cancer; and in salivary gland secretions. Additionally, the same type of *H pylori* was identified in the mouth (saliva and plaque) and in the stomach, and in one study nobody had oral *H pylori* infection without gastric infection.[59]

There is no consensus whether *H pylori* should be regarded as a transient or a common member of the oral biofilm. The mechanism by which *H pylori* reaches the oral cavity is unknown. It is possible that occasional reflux or vomit from the gastric (juice) reservoir allows colonization of the oral cavity. It is also possible that the reverse is true. As well, oral presence of *H pylori* could even present a mode of interpersonal transmission, including transmission from mother to child.[59]

Pooling of findings from 26 studies showed that aggressive systemic antibiotic therapy resolved the presence of *H pylori* in the stomach in about 90% of individuals but in the mouth in only 6%.[60] That is, 94% still harbored the bacterium in the mouth (tongue dorsum, supragingival and subgingival plaque, and the saliva) after the intensive antibiotics course. The oral cavity may act as a permanent or transient reservoir or sanctuary for *H pylori* and may be the source of reinfection of the stomach. It has been suggested that professional removal of plaque and calculus as well as home oral hygiene procedures be performed along with the systemic triple antibiotic treatment of *H pylori*. Close collaboration with the patient's gastroenterologist or other medical care provider is pivotal.

Because a large proportion of adults harbor *H pylori* in the oral cavity, dental treatment could result in frequent exposure of the dental care providers via aerosols. Some studies have found dental personnel to be at greater risk, whereas others have not. Polish dentists who had practiced longer than 15 years had a much elevated rate of infection in their gingival sulci, and male dentists were much more often infected than female dentists.[62] Moreover, a serologic study at a dental school in Japan showed that clinical dental professionals were at 2.7 times greater risk for contracting *H pylori* infection over a 6-year period than were non-clinical employee controls.[63]

Travel interruption: Antibiotics

Microbial susceptibility to antibiotics

Subgingival plaque. Periodontitis patients in Spain and The Netherlands showed striking differences in the bacterial composition of their subgingival plaque: *Aa* was significantly more prevalent (23% versus 3%) in the subgingival plaque of Dutch patients, while *P gingivalis* was significantly more prevalent (65% versus 37%) in the Spanish patients.[64] In addition to possible associations with the genetic background of the patients, a factor potentially contributing to these differences is the significant difference in medical use of antibiotics in the two countries. While The Netherlands is the most restrictive country in Europe, Spain is among the countries that use the highest number of doses of antibiotics per inhabitant.

This hypothesis is supported by the observation by the same research group that the minimum inhibitory concentration of common antibiotics determined against selected periodontal bacteria was significantly higher in Spain than in The Netherlands.[65] Therefore, many more different bacterial species grew in the Spanish patients, and bacteria were resistant to penicillin, amoxicillin, metronidazole, clindamycin, and tetracycline. Especially, five Spanish patients, but no Dutch patients, harbored three or more tetracycline-resistant periodontal microbes. Hence, the widespread use of antibiotics in Spain is reflected in the level of resistance of the subgingival microflora of adult patients with periodontitis.

Another research group in Colombia tested in vitro susceptibility of *P gingivalis*, *Fusobacterium nucleatum*, black-pigmented *Prevotella species,* and *Aa* to metronidazole, amoxicillin, amoxicillin/clavulanic acid, clindamycin, and moxifloxacin in patients with chronic periodontitis.[66] The authors found that periodontal microorganisms from patients with chronic periodontitis can be highly resistant to the antimicrobial agents commonly used in anti-infective periodontal therapy.

Saliva. The first study on the long-term effects of amoxicillin treatment of acute otitis media on the salivary microbiota compared children with this condition who used and who did not use antibiotics.[67] All children had recovered by the follow-up visit, regardless of the treatment regimen. The antibiotics resulted in reduced species richness and diversity as well as a significant shift in the relative abundance of 35 groups of bacteria. Some salivary bacteria decreased posttreatment, whereas one phylum, namely the Proteobacteria, gained a higher relative abundance. A substantial recovery of the salivary bacterial community from the antibiotic did occur but was still incomplete 3 weeks posttreatment.

Guts. Antibiotics use may also play a role in development of irritable bowel diseases, of which the major conditions are Crohn disease and ulcerative colitis. Both are chronic immunologically mediated diseases caused by a dysregulated immune response to intestinal flora in a genetically susceptible host. In analyses of data from national registries in Denmark, individuals diagnosed with irritable bowel disease in childhood had a 15-fold greater risk of developing Crohn disease and extensive ulcerative colitis 44 years later.[68] Importantly, after 26 years follow-up, there was also a trend toward an increased risk of colorectal cancer.

Guts: A gas station for tanking up with antibiotic resistance genes. The human gut microbiome is a reservoir of antibiotic resistance genes.

Researchers identified a total of 1,093 antibiotic resistance genes, accounting for 0.3% of the total human gut microbiome gene set of 4.1 million genes, which they established by sequencing gut microbiome genes from 85 Danish, 39 Spanish, and 38 Chinese individuals.[69] By far, the Chinese harbor the greatest diversity and abundance of antibiotic resistance genes, with more than twice the abundance of the Danes but only about 10% more than the Spaniards. Tetracycline resistance genes amounted to about half of all the antibiotic resistance genes in each of the three populations. Single-nucleotide polymorphism-based analysis indicated that antibiotic resistance genes from the two European populations are more closely related while the Chinese ones are clustered separately. These human antibiotic resistance genes were found to be clearly unique when compared with other natural environments, such as soil, marine, lake, and so on, indicating that these changes did not occur by random mutation.

Traveling genes: Ferried by gut viruses. Rather recently, researchers have begun to appreciate the important role the gut plays in the immune system and in teaching it which cells are good (host's own) and which are bad (foreign) and should be eradicated. However, the mechanisms applied in the guts are not yet explored to any great extent. A recent landmark study reported that a mouse experiment showed for the first time that viruses in the gut help confer antibiotic resistance to bacteria.[70] The viruses seem to protect the gut bacteria from antibiotics by acting like reservoirs for snippets of genetic material that are then given to bacteria in need of protection. In other words, viruses hand to the gut bacteria genes that enable them to survive the attack of the drug. This resistance is promoted not only toward one drug but also to other types of antibiotics, thus possibly contributing to the development of superbugs.

Prophylactic use of antibiotics

Whereas preventing bacteremia following invasive procedures was the pathophysiologic (non–evidence-based) rationale for prior guidelines for antibiotic prophylaxis, everyday life activities such as chewing, toothbrushing, and flossing are now regarded as more responsible for bacteremia than occasional events such as dental procedures. Consequently, new guidelines have been developed and published in 2006 to 2009 by various bodies,[71–79] taking all available evidence into consideration. These revisions are intended to define more clearly for dental clinicians when antibiotic prophylaxis is or is not recommended and to provide more uniform and consistent global recommendations.

Increasingly, scientists and health care professionals understand the immense importance of avoiding the use of antibiotics unless absolutely needed. This constraint is necessary not only because there is a risk that the patient will develop allergies and resistance to the medication and that microbes will develop resistance but also because antibiotics cause harm to the body's microbiomes, the duration of which has been underappreciated until now. For example, a systematic review and meta-analysis concluded that antibiotics were consistently associated with resistance of bacteria to future antibiotics in an individual for up to 12 months.[80] Furthermore, the likelihood of detecting resistant bacteria increased with the number or duration of antibiotic courses the previous year.

Thorough literature reviews have not identified any evidence that taking antibiotics before dental treatment prevents infections of the heart or orthopedic implants. Hence, the risks of using antibiotics would probably outweigh the potential benefit in almost all individuals. In a randomized controlled trial in which 414 immunocompromised patients with cancer or solid organ transplants were given one 500-mg dose of amoxicillin prior to an invasive dental procedure but only half of whom were given postoperative antibiotics, no difference was found in postoperative surgical site infection between patients who were treated with postoperative antibiotics and those who were not.[81]

The adverse clinical symptoms potentially experienced by the patient when taking antibiotics include upset stomach, allergic reactions including life-threatening anaphylactic shock, and overgrowth by *Clostridium difficile*. This bacterium releases toxins that can cause bloating, diarrhea, and abdominal pain, which may be-

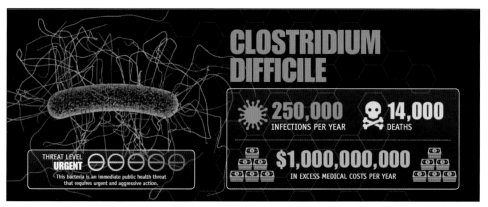

Fig 4-9 *Clostridium difficile* has been assigned the label *urgent threat level*, which means, "This bacteria is an immediate public health threat that requires urgent and aggressive action." (From Centers for Disease Control and Prevention.[82])

come severe. Infection with *C difficile* is the most common cause of pseudomembranous colitis. This can progress to toxic megacolon that is potentially fatal.

Traditionally, older adults in hospitals or long-term care facilities were infected, but younger and healthy individuals without a history of antibiotic use or exposure to health care facilities are increasingly affected. Each year, more than half a million people get sick from *C difficile* in the United States alone; about 250,000 people require hospitalization, and about 14,000 people die from the infection (Fig 4-9).[82] In the year 2000, a more dangerous, antibiotic-resistant strain emerged in Europe and the United States, where it has spread and killed. From 2000 to 2007, deaths related to *C difficile* increased by 400%.[82] Although about half of the infections happen in people younger than 65 years, 90% of the associated deaths occur in seniors aged 65 years and older. Among patients who survive and recuperate, about one in five experiences relapse. Antibiotic treatment options are lacking, but transplantation of stools from healthy donors is highly effective in reestablishing homeostasis in the guts.[83]

Destination: Heart—Infective endocarditis.
Background. *Endocarditis* is an inflammation of the inner layer of the heart, or endocardium. Usually, the heart valves, whether natural or prosthetic, are involved, although other cardiac structures and the surface of intracardiac devices may be affected. The following factors increase the individual's risk of developing infective endocarditis (IE):

- Older age and frailty
- Male sex
- Low levels of white blood cells
- Immunodeficiency or immunosuppression
- Malignancy
- Uncontrolled diabetes
- Hemodialysis
- Alcohol abuse[84]

IE has evolved over time; socioeconomic changes and medical progress have led to an increase in age of onset, number of comorbidities, and attribution to a health care–associated staphylococcal cause. The incidence in non-US Western countries has been stable the past few decades, at about 25 to 50 cases per year per 1 million inhabitants aged 20 years or older. This is less than 4 cases per 100,000 individuals or 0.04/1,000.[85,86] A nationwide study from 1998 to 2009 of about 8 million hospitalized patients in the United States identified 12.7 cases of IE annually per 100,000 population, that is, 127 cases per 1 million (0.13/1,000) in 2009 with an annual mean increase of 2.4%.[87] Hitherto, the IE incidence was estimated at 4 cases per

100,000. Importantly, the increased level is device and hospital associated.[87] The incidence has not increased since the 2007 to 2008 publication of the American Heart Association Guidelines for Prevention of Infective Endocarditis.[71,72,86,87]

Eighty-five percent of patients with IE have positive blood cultures; the causative microorganisms are staphylococci, streptococci, and enterococci.[88] About 80% of cases are related to *S aureus* and streptococci (but not the oral *Streptococcus viridans* [*viridans streptococci*] associated with endodontic infection) when bacteria seem to be responsible.[87]

Based on epidemiologic studies demonstrating changes in the profile of IE, science has moved away from the notion that IE is a streptococcal infection caused by commensal oral bacteria in patients with previously known heart disease. IE is now regarded as a predominantly staphylococcal health care–associated disease in elderly patients who suffer from much comorbidity.[84,89] This finding is of great significance for all health care providers.

Roadmap: Guidelines for prophylactic antibiotics use for IE. Various professional review committees have conducted thorough analyses of the existing literature related to IE and the prophylactic use of antibiotics in order to prepare evidence-based recommendations for clinical practice. All the review groups largely reviewed the same body of literature and unanimously agreed on the lack of evidence for any efficacy of premedication prior to dental procedures. However, the only body that took the full consequence of the realization of the lack of such evidence was the British National Institute for Health and Care Excellence (NICE), which made the evidence-based decision to never recommend premedication for dental procedures for anyone.[73]

Based on the same body of literature, the other groups designed slightly different guidelines, realizing that their recommendations are not appropriately evidence based but rather created by expert consensus. Some write that their rationale is based on the expectation that clinicians and patients alike are not ready for the dramatic change to completely abandon the traditional practice of premedication altogether. Seven teams published their guidelines between 2006 and 2009.[71–79]

The review committees realized that usual, everyday life activities such as chewing, flossing, and toothbrushing cause more bacteremia than occasional dental procedures. The committees also first and foremost emphasized prevention of oral disease, especially for those at risk of IE, and of course urged provision of any needed dental care for those patients.

The changes in recommendations for prophylactic use of antibiotics prior to dental procedures represent a drastic reduction in the use of antibiotics compared with prior guidelines. This is in agreement with the recommendation of the CDC, which urges health care providers to practice good stewardship of antibiotics as long as any of them are still effective.[82]

Most review groups concluded the following:

- Only an extremely small number of cases of IE might be prevented by premedication before dental procedures, even if such prophylactic therapy were 100% effective.
- There is great risk of harm in developing bacterial resistance.
- There is substantial risk of developing allergy and insensitivity in the host.
- Use of antibiotic prophylaxis for IE before dental procedures is reasonable only for patients with underlying cardiac conditions that are associated with the highest risk of adverse outcomes from eventual contraction of IE (Boxes 4-1 to 4-3).
- Antibiotic prophylaxis is not recommended based solely on an increased lifetime risk of acquisition of IE.

Box 4–1	The only cardiac conditions for which it is reasonable to use prophylactic antibiotics for prevention of IE, namely those with the highest risk of adverse outcome from endocarditis*

AHA,[71] AHA/ADA,[72] and ACC/AHA[74,75] (2007–2008)

- Prosthetic cardiac valve or prosthetic material used for cardiac valve repair
- Previous IE
- Congenital heart disease (CHD)
  - Unrepaired cyanotic CHD, including palliative shunts and conduits
  - Completely repaired congenital heart defect with prosthetic material or device, whether placed by surgery or by catheter intervention, during the first 6 months after the procedure (because endothelialization of prosthetic material occurs within 6 months after the procedure)
  - Repaired CHD with residual defects (which inhibit endothelialization) at the site or adjacent to the site of a prosthetic patch or prosthetic device
- Cardiac transplantation recipients who develop cardiac valvulopathy

BSAC[78] (2006)

- Previous IE
- Cardiac valve replacement surgery (mechanical or biologic prosthetic valves)
- Surgically constructed systemic or pulmonary shunt or conduit

Australian[73] (2008)

- Prosthetic cardiac valve or prosthetic material used for cardiac valve repair
- Previous IE
- CHD, but only if it involves:
  - Unrepaired cyanotic defects, including palliative shunts and conduits
  - Completely repaired defects with prosthetic material or devices, whether placed by surgery or catheter intervention, during the first 6 months after the procedure (after which the prosthetic material is likely to have been endothelialized)
  - Repaired defects with residual defects (which inhibit endothelialization) at or adjacent to the site of a prosthetic patch or device

- Cardiac transplantation with the subsequent development of cardiac valvulopathy
- Rheumatic heart disease in Indigenous Australians only

NICE[77] (2008)

- Acquired valvular heart disease with stenosis or regurgitation
- Valve replacement
- Structural CHD, including surgically corrected or palliated structural conditions but excluding isolated atrial septal defect, fully repaired ventricular septal defect, fully repaired patent ductus arteriosus, and closure devices that are judged to be endothelialized
- Hypertrophic cardiomyopathy
- Previous IE

ESC[79] (2009)

- Similar to AHA,[71] AHA/ADA,[72] and ACC/AHA[74,75]
- Prosthetic valve or a prosthetic material used for cardiac valve repair
- Previous IE
- CHD:
  - Cyanotic CHD without surgical repair or with residual defects, palliative shunts, or conduits
  - Congenital heart defect with complete repair with prosthetic material whether placed by surgery or by percutaneous technique, up to 6 months after the procedure
  - Residual defects persisting at the site of implantation of a prosthetic material or device by cardiac surgery or percutaneous technique

Irish Dental Association[76] (2008)

- Same as AHA,[71] AHA/ADA,[72] and ACC/AHA[74,75]

*All guidelines specifically state: **No other cardiac conditions than those listed, including any congenital defects, are recommended for antibiotic prophylaxis.**

AHA, American Heart Association; ADA, American Dental Association; ACC, American College of Cardiology; BSAC, British Society for Antimicrobial Chemotherapy; Australian, Infective Endocarditis Prophylaxis Expert Group; ESC, European Society of Cardiology.

Box 4–2	Dental procedures for which prophylaxis to prevent IE *is reasonable* ONLY for patients suffering from conditions listed in Box 4-1

AHA,[71] AHA/ADA,[72] and ACC/AHA[74,75] (2007–2008)
- All dental procedures that involve manipulation of gingival tissue or the periapical region of teeth or perforation of the oral mucosa*

BSAC[78] (2006)
- All dental procedures involving dentogingival manipulation or endodontics

Australian[73] (2008)
Always/routine
- Extraction
- Periodontal procedures including surgery, subgingival scaling, and root planing
- Replanting avulsed teeth
- Other surgical procedures (eg, implant placement, apicoectomy)

Consider prophylaxis for the following procedures if multiple procedures are being conducted, the procedure is prolonged, or periodontal disease is present
- Full periodontal probing for patients with periodontitis

- Intraligamentary and intraosseous local anesthetic injection
- Supragingival calculus removal/cleaning
- Rubber dam placement with clamps (where there is risk of damaging gingiva)
- Restorative matrix band/strip placement
- Endodontics beyond the apical foramen
- Placement of orthodontic bands
- Placement of interdental wedges
- Subgingival placement of retraction cords, antibiotic fibers, or antibiotic strips

NICE[77] (2008)
- None

ESC[79] (2009)
- Dental procedures requiring manipulation of the gingival or periapical region of teeth or perforation of the oral mucosa†

Irish Dental Association[76] (2008)
- Same as AHA,[71] AHA/ADA,[72] and ACC/AHA[74,75]

*Endorsed by the Infectious Diseases Society of America and by the Pediatric Infectious Diseases Society.
†Endorsed by the European Society of Clinical Microbiology and Infectious Diseases (ESCMID) and by the International Society of Chemotherapy (ISC) for Infection and Cancer.
AHA, American Heart Association; ADA, American Dental Association; ACC, American College of Cardiology; BSAC, British Society for Antimicrobial Chemotherapy; Australian, Infective Endocarditis Prophylaxis Expert Group; ESC, European Society of Cardiology.

Box 4–3	Dental procedures for which prophylaxis to prevent IE *is NOT reasonable* for patients suffering from conditions listed in Box 4-1

AHA,[71] AHA/ADA,[72] and ACC/AHA[74,75] (2007–2008)
- Routine anesthetic injections through non-infected tissue
- Dental radiographs
- Placement of removable prosthodontic or orthodontic appliances
- Adjustment of orthodontic appliances
- Placement of orthodontic brackets
- Shedding of primary teeth
- Bleeding from trauma to the lips or oral mucosa

BSAC[78] (2006)
- N/A (not applicable due to the recommendation to never use prophylactic antibiotics)

Australian[73] (2008)
- Oral examination
- Infiltration and block local anesthetic injection
- Restorative dentistry
- Supragingival rubber dam clamping and placement of rubber dam
- Intracanal endodontic procedures
- Removal of sutures

- Impressions and construction of dentures
- Orthodontic bracket placement and adjustment of fixed appliances
- Application of gels
- Intraoral radiographs
- Supragingival plaque removal

NICE[77] (2008)
- All dental procedures

ESC[79] (2009)
- Local anesthetic injections in noninfected tissue
- Removal of sutures
- Dental radiographs
- Placement or adjustment of removable prosthodontic or orthodontic appliances or braces
- Following shedding of primary teeth
- Trauma to the lips and oral mucosa

Irish Dental Association[76] (2008)
- Same as AHA,[71] AHA/ADA,[72] and ACC/AHA[74,75]

AHA, American Heart Association; ADA, American Dental Association; ACC, American College of Cardiology; BSAC, British Society for Antimicrobial Chemotherapy; Australian, Infective Endocarditis Prophylaxis Expert Group; ESC, European Society of Cardiology.

Table 4-1	Prophylactic regimens to prevent IE recommended ONLY in adults with conditions listed in Box 4-1 and ONLY for dental procedures listed in Box 4-2		
Association or group	First choice	Patients with allergy to penicillin or ampicillin	Additional notes
AHA,[71] AHA/ADA,[72] and ACC/AHA[74,75] (2007–2008)	Amoxicillin, 2 g	Cephalexin, 2 g* Clindamycin, 600 mg Azithromycin, 500 mg Clarithromycin, 500 mg	*Or other first- or second-generation oral cephalosporin in equivalent dosage.[72] Cephalosporins should not be used in a person with a history of anaphylaxis, angioedema, or urticaria after intake of penicillin or ampicillin.[72]
BSAC[78] (2006)	Amoxicillin, 3 g	Clindamycin, 600 mg	Preoperative mouthwash of chlorhexidine gluconate (0.2%), held in mouth for 1 min.
Australian[73] (2008)	Amoxicillin, 2 g	Clindamycin, 600 mg	
NICE[77] (2008)	None	None	Do not offer chlorhexidine mouthwash as prophylaxis against IE to people at risk undergoing dental procedures.
ESC[79] (2009)	Amoxicillin, 2 g	Clindamycin, 600 mg	Cephalosporins should not be used in a patient with anaphylaxis, angioedema, or urticaria after intake of penicillin and ampicillin.
Irish Dental Association[76] (2008)	Amoxicillin, 3 g	Clindamycin, 600 mg	

AHA, American Heart Association; ADA, American Dental Association; ACC, American College of Cardiology; BSAC, British Society for Antimicrobial Chemotherapy; Australian, Infective Endocarditis Prophylaxis Expert Group; ESC, European Society of Cardiology.

Table 4-1 summarizes the recommended regimens of antibiotic prophylaxis to prevent IE in adults prior to dental procedures. All groups recommended roughly that, as the first choice, adults be given 2 g of amoxicillin orally or intravenously between 30 and 60 minutes prior to the procedures. If patients are allergic to penicillin, adults should be given 600 mg of clindamycin. The Irish group suggested that the patient use chlorhexidine mouthwash 5 minutes before the beginning of a procedure,[76] whereas the NICE group explicitly stated that the dentist should not offer any such mouthwash.[77]

This major reduction of indications for antibiotic prophylaxis has not given rise to an increase in development of oral streptococci–related IE. This fact supports a posteriori the recommended limitations, assuming that at least some clinicians are following the current recommendations to drastically decrease use of antibiotics.[84]

Destination: Artificial joints.

Background. After a thorough literature review, the American Academy of Orthopaedic Surgeons (AAOS) and the American Dental Association (ADA) published a report regarding premedication in conjunction with dental procedures in patients with artificial joints.[90] The report described the evidence and concluded with recommendations developed based thereon. Importantly, the conclusion was that there is no evidence that oral microbes infect prosthetic implants or for the efficacy of any preventive measures for such potential infection.[90,91]

Roadmap: Guidelines for prophylactic antibiotics use for artificial joints. Unfortunately, the AAOS/ADA group did not act on their own clear conclusions of their own thorough review of all the existing evidence.[90] The group could have declared that the review found no evidence for infection of prosthetic joints by microbes originating in the mouth; no evidence for the efficacy of taking prophylactic antibiotics; and no evidence for the efficacy of using antimicrobial mouthrinse. Instead, the group listed recommendations for consideration that, in their own words, are based on "limited, unconvincing evidence" and "inconclusive evidence." Finally, the group offered the following advice based on "consensus, lacking evidence": "Individuals with artificial joints and other orthopedic prostheses should attain and maintain proper oral hygiene as part of general health."[90]

Bumps in the road from the clinician's perspective. All updated recommendations immensely limit the use of prophylactic antibiotics and hence differ dramatically from long-time practices for physicians, cardiologists, dentists, and their patients. Individuals who took prophylactic antibiotics in the past, but no longer need to, include those with mitral valve prolapse, rheumatic heart disease, bicuspid valve disease, calcified aortic stenosis, and congenital heart conditions, such as ventricular septal defect, atrial septal defect, and hypertrophic cardiomyopathy.[92] In addition, nobody with prosthetic joints should receive any premedication.

Despite the lack of any definitive scientific evidence, until recently it was believed necessary to attempt to prevent IE and infections of joint replacement with antibiotics before many invasive procedures were started. Because the old guidelines were highly accepted by clinicians and patients alike, with the attitudes, "Better safe than sorry" and "Prevention is better than cure," it may take some time, maybe several years and possibly decades, for the new guidelines to become fully implemented. "I cannot afford to have a single patient contract infection after my services," is a common theme among practicing dentists. Dissemination of information about the harm done by overuse or misuse of antibiotics to medical and dental clinicians, as well as to patients, is essential but will take time.

Clear and concise information from the dentist is pivotal to obtaining the reassurance and trust of patients. Especially for patients who "needed" prophylactic antibiotic coverage in the past, it is important that dentists, hygienists, cardiologists, and other medical care providers deliver the explanation in a consistent manner. It is crucial to provide an explanation of why antibiotic prophylaxis is no longer recommended, discussing with the patients the lack of demonstrated ("proven") benefits and the potentially serious risks of antibiotic prophylaxis.

The legal system—especially in the United States—prompts clinicians to practice "defensive dentistry" in fear of litigation, even if this means disregard for the scientific evidence and current clinical guidelines for standard of care. However, adherence to recognized, evidence-based guidelines affords robust legal protection.[79] Consequently, fear of litigation should not be an issue and certainly ought not place patients at risk for the potentially life-threatening consequences of unnecessary and ineffective antibiotic use.

Antibiotic resistance. An authoritative report by the Centers for Disease Control and Prevention was published on September 16, 2013.[82] The report, *Antibiotic Resistance Threats in the United States, 2013*, for the first time prioritized 18 bacteria into three levels of antibiotic resistance threat in the United States: *urgent* (3 bacteria), *serious* (12 bacteria), and *concerning* (3 bacteria)

The report did not specify the exact strains of the drug-resistant bacteria, nor did it specifically list any bacteria that inhabit the mouth, but several groups of bacteria that are commensal or frequent visitors in the oral cavity were listed.[82] For instance, members of the following bacterial groups represent serious antibiotic resistance threats: *Acinetobacter*, *Campylobacter*, *Candida*, *P aeruginosa*, and *S aureus*.

The report cited conservative estimates of the number of known serious infections with each of the 18 bacteria as well as the number of subsequent deaths.[82] Figure 4-10 shows methicillin-resistant *S aureus* (MRSA) as an example.

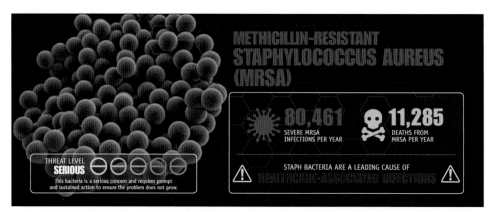

Fig 4-10 MRSA has been assigned the threat level of *serious*, which means, "This bacteria is a serious concern and requires prompt and sustained action to ensure the problem does not grow." (From Centers for Disease Control and Prevention.[82])

MRSA is a much dreaded source of serious, even fatal infections that occur mostly in hospitals but also in care facilities and in the community. In the United States alone, it is estimated that there are more than 80,000 cases of invasive MRSA infection annually, resulting in more than 11,000 deaths.[82] Those infections cannot be treated because of the development of species that are resistant to antibiotics. The report commented that an unknown, but much higher, number of less severe infections are caused by MRSA in both health care settings and the community.[82]

The report cautioned about the looming "postantibiotic era" that is on the horizon because bacteria are rapidly developing resistance to antibiotics and doing so faster than science can develop new types of effective medications. Therefore, the CDC urged all health care providers to prescribe antibiotics wisely and carefully weigh their potential benefits and risks in each case. The CDC suggested four core actions to prevent antibiotic resistance[82]:

1. Prevention of infections and the spread of resistance
2. Tracking of resistant infections and their causes and risk factors
3. Improvement of antibiotic prescription practices and stewardship

4. Development of new drugs and diagnostic tests

Medical care professionals, including dental care providers, can contribute to at least the first three activities.

The most important way to slow the development of resistance is to change the ways in which antibiotics are used. The CDC estimated that, in the United States, up to 50% of antibiotic use in humans and much of that in animals is unnecessary and inappropriate and makes everyone less safe. The commitment to always use antibiotics appropriately and safely—prescribing them only when they are needed to treat disease and selecting the right antibiotics and administering them in the right way in every case—is known as *antibiotic stewardship*. Promotion of antibiotic best practices is a first step in antibiotic stewardship. These practices include[82]:

- Ensuring that all orders have dose, duration, and indications
- Obtaining cultures before prescribing antibiotics
- Taking an "antibiotic timeout" to reassess the need for antibiotics after 48 to 72 hours

Final travel destinations: Cancer caused by oral bacteria and viruses

Increasingly, scientists realize that cancer to a great extent is related to tissue injury, infection, and inflammatory processes and not only to genetics. Given the travel activities of oral microbes and the inflammatory host responses they stimulate, it is not surprising that oral organisms are also associated with cancers outside the oral cavity, especially in the digestive tract and the lungs. Several oral microorganisms can convert alcohol to carcinogenic acetaldehyde that in conjunction with other mucosal irritants can help explain the known associations between heavy drinking, tobacco smoking, use of snuff, poor oral health, and the prevalence of oral and upper gastrointestinal cancers.[93]

Oral microorganisms are identified in oral and gastrointestinal cancers. However, it is not always possible to determine whether the oral bacteria and viruses play a causative role in initiation and development of tumors or secondarily infect already existing lesions.[94,95] Figure 4-11 provides a conceptual illustration of bacteria that colonize cancerous tissue.[94]

Periodontal disease has been associated with cancer of the breast only in epidemiologic studies; that is, any microbiologic evidence is lacking. Moreover, EBV is suggested to be implicated in tumorigenesis in breast carcinomas, renal cell carcinomas and nephroblastomas (Wilms tumors), bladder cancer, and thyroid cancers. However, these studies did not explore whether EBV was also present in the mouth.

The World Health Organization (WHO) has specifically designated the following bacterium and two viruses, commonly present in the oral cavity, as human carcinogens: *H pylori*,[96] HPV,[97] and EBV.[98]

Human papillomavirus

As already discussed, HPV infects several sites of the human body, resulting in various clinical manifestations ranging from warts and benign hyperplastic lesions to neoplasias of the ano-

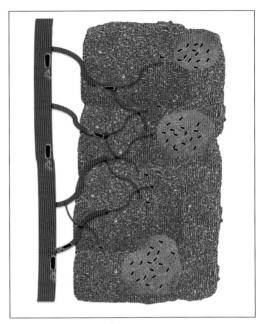

Fig 4-11 Proposed mechanism of bacterial entry into and proliferation within tumors. Tumor *(pink/purple)* development leads to recruitment of new blood supply, involving disorganized and leaky vasculature, permitting circulating bacteria *(black)* to enter the tumor. Bacteria replicate primarily within hypoxic *(pink)* tumor regions, which feature immune suppression, abundant nutrients, and low oxygen concentrations. (Reprinted from Cummins and Tangney[94] with permission.)

genital area, the skin, the oral cavity, and the pharynx.

The authors of a large study on oral cancers in Croatia recommended that clinicians carefully observe and monitor lesions in the following particular oral locations from which samples were most often HPV positive, especially with the HPV types that carry high risk for development of cancer: the vermilion border, the labial commissures, and the hard palate.[99]

Worldwide, about 610,000 or 4.8% of the 12.7 million cancers that occurred in 2008 were attributed to infection with HPV.[44] According to the WHO, the world's two most prevalent types of HPV are HPV-16 (3.2%) and HPV-18 (1.4%), the same two types most prone to cause cancer.[49]

Infections with HPV are strongly associated with increased risks of developing the following malignancies (shown with the proportion of cases caused by HPV):

- Oropharyngeal cancer, including the base of the tongue and the tonsils (60%)[100]
- Genital cancers other than cervical: vulva (50%), vagina (65%), penis (35%), and anus (90%)[48]
- Cervical cancer (~100%)[48]

After HPV-16 and HPV-18, the six most common HPV types are the same in all world regions, namely types 31, 33, 35, 45, 52, and 58; these types account for an additional 20% of cervical cancers worldwide.[49] According to the WHO, there were more than half a million new cases of and 274,883 deaths from cervical cancer in the world in 2008.[101] About 86% of cases occur in developing countries, representing 13% of female cancers.[101]

Each year in the United States, about 12,000 women are diagnosed with cervical cancer.[42] The CDC recommends the Papanicolaou (Pap) test for cervical cancer screening for women between the ages of 21 and 65 years, including during pregnancy.[47]

Cervical cancer often develops years, even decades, after the infection. Among Swedish HPV-16–positive women, the median time from infection to development of carcinoma in situ was between 7 and 12 years.[48] Swedish women with consistently high HPV-16 loads had 30 times higher risk for cervical carcinoma, and 1 in 4 (25%) of women infected with a high viral load before the age of 25 years developed cervical carcinomas.[102]

A study of saliva and the cervix in 43 sexually active women showed that the abundance of HPV is lower in saliva than in the cervix when HPV is present in the cervix.[100] However, the same HPV types were detected in saliva and the cervix, and all women with high salivary amounts of HPV also had cervical infection.

Whereas HPV-16 and HPV-18 cause about 70% of cervical cancers, the most dangerous subtype for oral cancer is HPV-16. Having antibodies against the HPV-16 types E6 and E7 is associated with a very high risk of oropharyngeal cancer and hypopharyngeal/laryngeal cancer, namely a 179- and 15-fold risk, respectively.[103] Otherwise, HPV DNA and serum antibodies to HPV were rarely found in patients with head and neck cancers in Central Europe and Latin America.[103] Each year, more than 30,000 people in the United States are diagnosed with cancers in the oral cavity and pharynx, and about 8,000 deaths occur. Roughly 8,400 people in the United States are diagnosed annually with cancers of the oropharynx that are attributed to HPV-16.[47] Cancers of the oropharynx are about three times more prevalent among men than among women.

Typically, oral cancers that are not related to HPV are located at the front part toward the tip of the tongue, the floor of the mouth, and the buccal and gingival mucosa, whereas HPV-related malignant lesions are found in the back of the throat, on the base of the tongue, and on or near the tonsils. These latter locations are consistent with the observed change in sexual behavior toward oral sex, especially among the younger generations and after the appearance of HIV and AIDS.

HPV-positive oropharyngeal cancers are less likely to occur among moderate to heavy drinkers than are HPV-negative oropharyngeal cancers. Consequently, a different segment of the US population is now at risk, namely younger individuals and more frequently white people. The target population of public health preventive measures therefore needs to change. When specimens from oropharyngeal cancers resected from 1984 to 2004 were examined, the population-level incidence (new cases) of HPV-positive cancers increased by 225% from 1988 to 2004, whereas incidence for HPV-negative cancers declined by 50%.[104] The authors ominously predicted that if this incidence trend continues, the annual number of HPV-positive oropharyngeal cancers might surpass that of cervical cancers in the United States by year 2020. No HPV test is currently approved for detecting oropharyngeal cancers, which unfortunately is the fastest-growing cancer in young women who do not smoke cigarettes or drink alcohol in excess.

It is expected that HPV vaccination will decrease the prevalence of premalignancies and malignancies in all affected areas, such as the oropharynx. This is important because the 5-year survival expectancy for oral cancer is still only about 50%, despite modern surgical and other medical advances. However, such HPV-associated cancers have a better prognosis than do non–HPV-related cancers. Dental and medical health care providers have important and potentially life-saving roles to play in early detection, treatment, and educational prevention of HPV-associated malignancies.

Other bacteria and viruses

Oral malignancies. Oral cancer tissue specimens and healthy controls differ in their content of bacteria; four bacteria are specific for tumorigenic tissues.[105] These bacteria can break down sugar molecules and tolerate acid. Additionally, *P gingivalis* is abundantly present in malignant gingival epithelium and hence may be implicated in oral squamous cell carcinomas.[106] Other bacteria and viruses that usually live in the oral cavity, with extra high abundance in periodontitis, are also present in oral cancerous and precancerous lesions.

H pylori seems to be involved in the pathogenesis of cancerous lesions of the upper gastroesophageal tract, including the oral cavity.[107,108]

EBV is present in oral diseases such as oral squamous cell carcinoma, as demonstrated by oral cells expressing EBV genes.[109] Also, EBV was found in 100.0% of specimens from 36 oral squamous cell carcinomas, in 77.8% of 9 premalignant lesions, and in 8.3% of 12 specimens of clinically normal oral mucosa in a study.[103] EBV is also implicated in oral hairy leukoplakia. Smoking, alcohol use, and age do not seem to be risk factors for EBV infection.[110]

Nonoral cancers.
Cancer of the larynx, pharynx, and esophagus. Figure 4-12 shows the phyla and genera of bacteria found in laryngeal cancerous tissue (see Figs 4-12a and 4-12d)and adjacent normal tissue (see Figs 4-12b and 4-12e) from 29 patients with laryngeal carcinoma and of normal tissue (see Figs 4-12c and 4-12f) from 31 control patients with vocal cord polyps.[111]

Fusobacterium and *Fusobacteria* (phylum and genus) were abundant in patients with squamous cell carcinoma of the larynx. The bacterial composition of 15 genera of oral bacteria was significantly different between the laryngeal cancer and control groups and hence may be associated with laryngeal cancer. Gong et al[111] speculated that interactions occur between the bacterial communities and laryngeal cancerous tissue, with the roles of cause and effect switching at different stages as the tumor develops. There was considerable overlap in proportions of oral bacteria between the three types of tissues, and 871 species were detected in all three (Fig 4-13). In contrast, 1,547 species were found in cancerous tissue only. *Streptococcus anginosus* is commonly linked with esophageal and pharyngeal cancers but not with oral cancers.[105]

EBV may also be involved in neoplastic transformation in nasopharyngeal squamous cell carcinomas.[57,109] Such EBV-associated nasopharyngeal cancer is found predominantly in Southern China and in people of Chinese ancestry but also occurs in Africa and was detected in Japanese people as well.[109]

The presence of certain bacteria in the dental plaque of patients scheduled to undergo surgery for thoracic esophageal cancer is a risk factor for postoperative development of pneumonia. Preoperative toothbrushing can reduce such risk.[112]

Dental professionals have important roles to play as members of the health care team. They not only may be the first primary health care providers to discover cancerous or precancerous lesions in spaces adjacent to the oral cavity but also may provide guidance regarding the importance of good oral hygiene before any surgery.

Colorectal cancer. Several bacterial species are present in great abundance in colorectal cancer. Surprisingly, these bacteria are not pathogens from external sources but rather commensals, usually living in the digestive tract, including the mouth.[113] The oral microbes *F nucleatum, Campylobacter concisus,* and *S mutans* are implicated in cancer of the colon and the rectum[39]; much higher levels of *F nucleatum* have

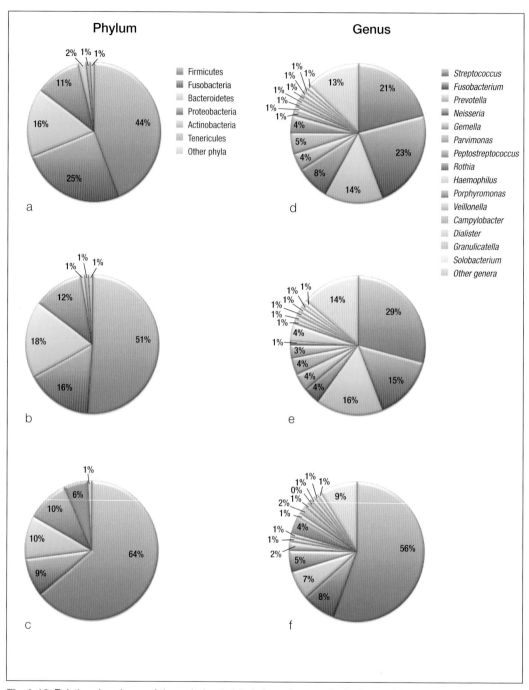

Fig 4-12 Relative abundance of the main bacterial phyla and genera in the larynx. Microbial profiles within the laryngeal squamous cell carcinoma (LSCC) tumor *(a)*, normal tissue adjacent to tumor *(b)*, and control groups *(c)* at the level of phyla. Microbial profiles in the LSCC tumor *(d)*, normal tissue adjacent to tumor *(e)*, and control groups *(f)* at the level of genera. The values are mean sequence abundances in each group and each level. (Reprinted from Gong et al[111] with permission.)

Fig 4-13 Venn diagram for overlap of observed operational taxonomic units among tissue samples taken from three groups: patients with laryngeal squamous cell carcinoma (LSCC) tumor *(green)*, normal tissue adjacent to tumor *(blue)*, and control patients with vocal cord polyps *(red)*. The three groups shared 871 species; the LSCC tumor and control groups shared 1,138 species; the normal tissue adjacent to tumor and control groups shared 1,162 species; and the LSCC tissue and normal tissue adjacent to tumor groups shared 1,520 species. (Reprinted from Gong et al[111] with permission.)

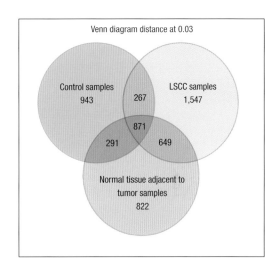

Fig 4-14 Representative fluorescence in situ hybridization targeting *Fusobacterium* species in colorectal mucosal biopsy sections using bacterial 16S rRNA probes. *(a and b)* Composite images of Cy3- and DAPI-stained views of sections hybridized with a *Fusobacterium*-specific probe. A *Fusobacterium* species *(arrows)* is localized within the mucus layer of colorectal sections in *(a)* and within the crypts of colorectal sections in *(b)*. *(c)* Positive control showing sections stained with a general bacterial probe (Eub 388). General bacteria, including most *Eubacteria* species *(arrows)*, are localized to the mucus layer above the epithelium. (Reprinted from McCoy et al[118] with permission.)

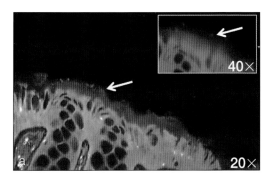

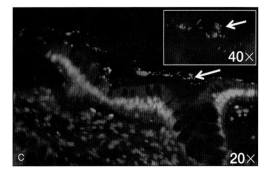

been found in colorectal lesions than in normal colon tissue in the same individuals.[113,114] The recent identification of mechanisms for the tumorigenic ability of certain strains of *F nucleatum* support its causal role.[115,116] Fusobacteria are also implicated in irritable bowel disease[117] and precancerous adenomas in the colon,[118]

both strong risk factors for colorectal cancer. The *Fusobacterium* species penetrate the mucus layer (Fig 4-14a) and within the crypts (Fig 4-14b) in the colorectal tissue, whereas nonpathogenic bacteria stay in the mucus layer above the epithelium (Fig 4-14c).[118]

A systematic review and pooling of findings from 27 studies with about 7,300 cancer cases concluded that infection with *H pylori* is a risk factor for colorectal neoplasms.[119] People infected with *H pylori* had about 50% higher risk for developing cancer of the colon or rectum.

Hence, the dental practitioner can play an important role in management and potential prevention of these diseases by keeping the oral cavity as free of bacteria as possible.

Pancreatic cancer. Long-term epidemiologic studies show periodontal disease to be significantly associated with development of cancer of the pancreas in US male health professionals[120] and in Europe.[121] The latter study assessed levels of antibodies to 25 specific oral bacteria and identified elevated levels of specific antibodies to some of the bacteria most often present in periodontal disease. For instance, people with high levels of antibodies against *P gingivalis ATTC 53978* had more than a twofold higher risk of pancreatic cancer than did those with low levels. Interestingly, those with high levels of antibodies to oral bacteria associated with periodontal health had a 45% lower risk of pancreatic cancer than did people with low levels. This indicates a potentially protective effect of healthy oral bacteria. Therefore, periodontal disease might increase the risk for pancreatic cancer. Moreover, increased levels of antibodies against specific commensal oral bacteria that can inhibit growth of pathogenic bacteria might be used in the future to reduce the risk of pancreatic cancer.

Gastric and duodenal cancers. The bacterium *H pylori* is frequently found in the oral cavity (gingival sulcus, dental plaque, and saliva). *H pylori* is etiologically associated with 63% of gastric cancers and 5.5% of the world's total cancer deaths but with 25% of infection-linked cancer deaths.[59] It is implicated in development of cancers of the stomach and the duodenum. The WHO designation of *H pylori* as a type I carcinogen in humans was mostly due to its involvement in developing gastric adenocarcinoma, the world's second most commonly diagnosed fatal cancer.[96]

H pylori seems to be involved in the pathogenesis of cancerous lesions of the upper gastroesophageal tract, including the oral cavity.[107,108] *H pylori* is also the primary agent causing gastric cancer. However, EBV is a contributing cause in up to about 10% of these tumors globally.[122] Being of male sex and smoking appear to strengthen this link, whereas drinking alcohol does not seem to have any effect on the association between EBV and stomach cancer.

In persons with periodontitis, positive associations were found between various periodontal bacteria and precancerous lesions of the stomach.[123] However, the relationship between the cumulative burden of these periodontal bacteria and gastric precancerous lesions was much stronger than that between any individual bacterium and lesions. This supports the emerging concept that the bacterial community functions like a unit.

Lung cancer. Chronic infection with *Chlamydophila* (formerly *Chlamydia*) *pneumoniae* is a risk factor for lung cancer. Those infected with *C pneumoniae* have about 50% higher risk for cancer than do those without *C pneumoniae* infection, as calculated by a meta-analysis that pooled results from 12 studies.[124] When data from 8 studies that looked back in time were pooled, the risk was more than doubled. Although *C pneumoniae* is not considered a common member of the oral microbiome, this bacterium has been detected in subgingival plaque in periodontitis.[125]

Despite the lack of microbiologic information, a longitudinal, nationally representative US epidemiologic study supports this relationship.[126] Among fatal cancers occurring over a 17-year span among 11,328 adults aged 25 to 74 years, lung cancer demonstrated the strongest association with periodontal disease. Those with periodontitis had 73% and edentulous individuals had 37% higher risk of dying of lung cancer than did people with a healthy periodontium, even after researchers controlled for other risk factors, such as smoking.

Lymphomas. A lymphoma is a type of cancer that is created when B or T lymphocytes assume a state of uncontrolled cell growth and multiplication. The bacterium *H pylori* is implicated in development of gastric mucosa–associated lymphoid tissue lymphoma. EBV can cause non-Hodgkin lymphomas, namely *(1)* endemic Burkitt lymphoma (also called *Burkitt tumor*), occurring mostly in equatorial Africa; *(2)* immunodeficiency-associated Burkitt lymphoma in individuals with HIV infection or transplant patients and others taking immunosuppressive medication; and *(3)* a variety of other lymphomas.

Future Travels

The oral microbiome in humans is extraordinarily complex; such communities of microbes, along with those of the gut, have the greatest diversity and abundance of all human microbiomes. Now that more rapid, reliable, and affordable molecular techniques are available—and many more are in speedy development or refinement—the genomes of individual microbial communities can be identified. In addition to studying individual microbial communities, researchers must study the interaction, organization, and communication (eg, cell-to-cell signaling) of these communities. There are still many microbes in the human mouth and the rest of the body whose identity and function are largely or completely unknown. These long-time or transient members of the human microbiomes and the interactions between them must be studied over time and under myriad internal conditions and external influences within the host and from the greater surrounding environment to learn about their function, flexibility, and reactions to conditions and stimuli such as diseases and antibiotics present in the host. Not until these and other mechanisms are better understood will it be possible to successfully manipulate individual human microbiomes in the quest for improved oral health.

Exciting and exotic travels continue to clear new paths on which to walk wherever they lead into the unexplored lands of the microbes inhabiting the human body. This journey will be bursting with new discoveries that help improve the future understanding of interactions among the host genome, epigenome, and oral microbiome. Medical and dental professionals have the duty and privilege to skillfully apply these discoveries in a personalized manner to promote the health, including the oral health, of each individual human being.[127,128]

References

1. Bizzarro S, Loos BG, Laine ML, Crielaard W, Zaura E. Subgingival microbiome in smokers and non-smokers in periodontitis: An exploratory study using traditional targeted techniques and a next-generation sequencing. J Clin Periodontol 2013;40:483–492.
2. Bartold PM, Van Dyke TE. Periodontitis: A host-mediated disruption of microbial homeostasis. Unlearning learned concepts. Periodontol 2000 2013;62:203–217.
3. Löe H, Theilade E, Jensen SB. Experimental gingivitis in man. J Periodontol 1965;36:177–187.
4. Genco RJ, Borgnakke WS. Risk factors for periodontal disease. Periodontol 2000 2013;62:59–94.
5. Garcia I, Kuska R, Somerman MJ. Expanding the foundation for personalized medicine: Implications and challenges for dentistry. J Dent Res 2013;92:S3–S10.
6. Borgnakke WS, Glick M, Genco RJ. Periodontitis: The canary in the coal mine. J Am Dent Assoc 2013;144:764–766.
7. Collins FS, Morgan M, Patrinos A. The Human Genome Project: Lessons from large-scale biology. Science 2003;300:286–290.
8. HOMD 16S rRNA Gene Sequence Download. Human Oral Microbiome Database. 8 May 2013. http://www.homd.org/modules.php?op=modload&name=seqDownload&file=index&type=R. Accessed 23 September 2013.
9. National Institutes of Health. Human Microbiome Project. 28 Jun 2013. http://commonfund.nih.gov/hmp/. Accessed 23 September 2013.
10. Aagaard K, Petrosino J, Keitel W, et al. The human microbiome project strategy for comprehensive sampling of the human microbiome and why it matters. FASEB J 2013;27:1012–1022.
11. Dewhirst FE, Chen T, Izard J, et al. The human oral microbiome. J Bacteriol 2010;192:5002–5017.
12. Wade WG. Characterisation of the human oral microbiome. J Oral Biosciences 2013;55:143–148.
13. Human Oral Microbiome Database. 20 September 2013. http://www.homd.org/index.php. Accessed 23 September 2013.

14. Tribble GD, Kerr JE, Wang BY. Genetic diversity in the oral pathogen *Porphyromonas gingivalis*: Molecular mechanisms and biological consequences. Future Microbiol 2013;8:607–620.

15. Zaura E, Keijser BJ, Huse SM, Crielaard W. Defining the healthy "core microbiome" of oral microbial communities. BMC Microbiol 2009;9:259.

16. Paster BJ, Boches SK, Galvin JL, et al. Bacterial diversity in human subgingival plaque. J Bacteriol 2001;183:3770–3783.

17. Tuna EB, Topcuoglu N, Ilhan B, Gençay K, Kulekçi G. *Staphylococcus aureus* transmission through oronasal fistula in children with cleft lip and palate. Cleft Palate Craniofac J 2008;45:477–480.

18. Ghannoum MA, Jurevic RJ, Mukherjee PK, et al. Characterization of the oral fungal microbiome (mycobiome) in healthy individuals. PLoS Pathog 2010;6:e1000713.

19. Kraneveld EA, Buijs MJ, Bonder MJ, et al. The relation between oral candida load and bacterial microbiome profiles in Dutch older adults. PLoS One 2012;7:e42770.

20. Tezal M, Scannapieco FA, Wactawski-Wende J, et al. Dental caries and head and neck cancers [epub ahead of print 12 September 2013]. JAMA Otolaryngol Head Neck Surg doi: 10.1001/jamaoto .2013.4569.

21. Zijnge V, Ammann T, Thurnheer T, Gmür R. Subgingival biofilm structure. Front Oral Biol 2012;15:1–16.

22. Simón-Soro A, Tomás I, Cabrera-Rubio R, Catalan MD, Nyvad B, Mira A. Microbial geography of the oral cavity. J Dent Res 2013;92:616–621.

23. Colombo AV, Barbosa GM, Higashi D, et al. Quantitative detection of *Staphylococcus aureus*, *Enterococcus faecalis* and *Pseudomonas aeruginosa* in human oral epithelial cells from subjects with periodontitis and periodontal health. J Med Microbiol 2013;62;1592–1600.

24. da Silva-Boghossian CM, do Souto RM, Luiz RR, Colombo AP. Association of red complex, *A. actinomycetemcomitans* and non-oral bacteria with periodontal diseases. Arch Oral Biol 2011;56:899–906.

25. Lazarevic V, Whiteson K, Hernandez D, François P, Schrenzel J. Study of inter- and intra-individual variations in the salivary microbiota. BMC Genomics 2010;11:523.

26. Rylev M, Kilian M. Prevalence and distribution of principal periodontal pathogens worldwide. J Clin Periodontol 2008;35:346–361.

27. Choi BK, Park SH, Yoo YJ, et al. Detection of major putative periodontopathogens in Korean advanced adult periodontitis patients using a nucleic acid-based approach. J Periodontol 2000;71:1387–1394.

28. Contreras M, Costello EK, Hidalgo G, Magris M, Knight R, Dominguez-Bello MG. The bacterial microbiota in the oral mucosa of rural Amerindians. Microbiology 2010;156:3282–3287.

29. Nasidze I, Li J, Quinque D, Tang K, Stoneking M. Global diversity in the human salivary microbiome. Genome Res 2009;19:636–643.

30. Nasidze I, Li J, Schroeder R, Creasey JL, Li M, Stoneking M. High diversity of the saliva microbiome in Batwa pygmies. PLoS One 2011;6:e23352.

31. Riley DR, Sieber KB, Robinson KM, et al. Bacteria-human somatic cell lateral gene transfer is enriched in cancer samples. PLoS Comput Biol 2013;9: e1003107.

32. Parahitiyawa NB, Jin LJ, Leung WK, Yam WC, Samaranayake LP. Microbiology of odontogenic bacteremia: Beyond endocarditis. Clin Microbiol Rev 2009;22:46–64 [erratum 2009;22:386].

33. Meurman JH, Siikala E, Richardson M, Rautemaa R. Non–*Candida albicans* candida yeasts of the oral cavity. In: Mendez-Vilas A (ed). Communicating Current Research and Educational Topics and Trends in Applied Microbiology, vol 2 [online book]. Badajoz, Spain: Formatex, 2007:719–731. http:// www.formatex.org/microbio/. Accessed 23 September 2013.

34. de Oliveira CE, Gasparoto TH, Dionisio TJ, et al. *Candida albicans* and denture stomatitis: Evaluation of its presence in the lesion, prosthesis, and blood. Int J Prosthodont 2010;23:158–159.

35. Asikainen S, Chen C, Slots J. Likelihood of transmitting *Actinobacillus actinomycetemcomitans* and *Porphyromonas gingivalis* in families with periodontitis. Oral Microbiol Immunol 1996;11:387–394.

36. Cephas KD, Kim J, Mathai RA, et al. Comparative analysis of salivary bacterial microbiome diversity in edentulous infants and their mothers or primary care givers using pyrosequencing. PLoS One 2011; 6:e23503.

37. Hansen LM, Dorsey TA, Batzer FA, et al. *Capnocytophaga* chorioamnionitis after oral sex. Obstet Gynecol 1996;88:731.

38. Lopez E, Raymond J, Patkai J, et al. *Capnocytophaga* species and preterm birth: Case series and review of the literature. Clin Microbiol Infect 2010;16:1539–1543.

39. Alanen A, Laurikainen E. Second-trimester abortion caused by *Capnocytophaga sputigena*: Case report. Am J Perinatol 1999;16:181–183.

40. Hsu L, Power D, Upritchard J, et al. Amplification of oral streptococcal DNA from human incisors and bite marks. Curr Microbiol 2012;65:207–211.

41. Kennedy DM, Stanton JA, Garcia JA, et al. Microbial analysis of bite marks by sequence comparison of streptococcal DNA. PLoS One 2012;7:e51757.

42. Hesselmar B, Sjoberg F, Saalman R, Aberg N, Adlerberth I, Wold AE. Pacifier cleaning practices and risk of allergy development. Pediatrics 2013; 131:e1829–e1837.

43. McLean JS, Lombardo MJ, Ziegler MG, et al. Genome of the pathogen *Porphyromonas gingivalis* recovered from a biofilm in a hospital sink using a high-throughput single-cell genomics platform. Genome Res 2013;23:867–877.

44. Warren HS, Fitting C, Hoff E, et al. Resilience to bacterial infection: Difference between species could be due to proteins in serum. J Infect Dis 2010;201:223–232.

45. Han YW, Wang X. Mobile microbiome: Oral bacteria in extra-oral infections and inflammation. J Dent Res 2013;92:485–491.

46. Koren O, Spor A, Felin J, et al. Human oral, gut, and plaque microbiota in patients with atherosclerosis. Proc Natl Acad Sci U S A 2011;108:4592–4598.

47. Centers for Disease Control and Prevention. Human papillomavirus (HPV). 1 Feb 2013. http://www.cdc.gov/hpv/. Accessed 23 September 2013.

48. Ylitalo N, Josefsson A, Melbye M, et al. A prospective study showing long-term infection with human papillomavirus 16 before the development of cervical carcinoma in situ. Cancer Res 2000;60:6027–6032.

49. Forman D, de Martel C, Lacey CJ, et al. Global burden of human papillomavirus and related diseases. Vaccine 2012;30(suppl 5):F12–F23.

50. Kulkarni SS, Kulkarni SS, Vastrad PP, et al. Prevalence and distribution of high risk human papillomavirus (HPV) types 16 and 18 in carcinoma of cervix, saliva of patients with oral squamous cell carcinoma and in the general population in Karnataka, India. Asian Pac J Cancer Prev 2011;12:645–648.

51. Kreimer AR, Villa A, Nyitray AG, et al. The epidemiology of oral HPV infection among a multinational sample of healthy men. Cancer Epidemiol Biomarkers Prev 2011;20:172–182.

52. Kreimer AR, Pierce Campbell CM, Lin HY, et al. Incidence and clearance of oral human papillomavirus infection in men: The HIM cohort study. Lancet 2013;382:877–887.

53. Sanders AE, Slade GD, Patton LL. National prevalence of oral HPV infection and related risk factors in the U.S. adult population. Oral Dis 2012;18:430–441.

54. Gillison ML, Broutian T, Pickard RK, et al. Prevalence of oral HPV infection in the United States, 2009–2010. JAMA 2012;307:693–703.

55. Centers for Disease Control and Prevention. National and state vaccination coverage among adolescents aged 13–17 years — United States, 2012. MMWR Morb Mortal Wkly Rep 2013;62:685–693.

56. Genner J, Scheutz F, Ebbesen P, Melbye M. Antibody to human papilloma virus in Danish dentists. Scand J Dent Res 1988;96:118–120.

57. Cruz I, Van den Brule AJ, Steenbergen RD, et al. Prevalence of Epstein-Barr virus in oral squamous cell carcinomas, premalignant lesions and normal mucosa—A study using the polymerase chain reaction. Oral Oncol 1997;33:182–188.

58. Marshall BJ, Warren JR. Unidentified curved bacilli in the stomach of patients with gastritis and peptic ulceration. Lancet 1984;1(8390):1311–1315.

59. Silva DG, Tinoco EM, Rocha GA, et al. Helicobacter pylori transiently in the mouth may participate in the transmission of infection. Mem Inst Oswaldo Cruz 2010;105:657–660.

60. Zou QH, Li RQ. Helicobacter pylori in the oral cavity and gastric mucosa: A meta-analysis. J Oral Pathol Med 2011;40:317–324.

61. Hirsch C, Tegtmeyer N, Rohde M, Rowland M, Oyarzabal OA, Backert S. Live Helicobacter pylori in the root canal of endodontic-infected deciduous teeth. J Gastroenterol 2012;47:936–940.

62. Loster BW, Czesnikiewicz-Guzik M, Bielanski W, et al. Prevalence and characterization of Helicobacter pylori (H. pylori) infection and colonization in dentists. J Physiol Pharmacol 2009;60(suppl 8):13–18.

63. Matsuda R, Morizane T. Helicobacter pylori infection in dental professionals: A 6-year prospective study. Helicobacter 2005;10:307–311.

64. Sanz M, van Winkelhoff AJ, Herrera D, Dellemijn-Kippuw N, Simón R, Winkel E. Differences in the composition of the subgingival microbiota of two periodontitis populations of different geographical origin. A comparison between Spain and The Netherlands. Eur J Oral Sci 2000;108:383–392.

65. van Winkelhoff AJ, Herrera D, Oteo A, Sanz M. Antimicrobial profiles of periodontal pathogens isolated from periodontitis patients in The Netherlands and Spain. J Clin Periodontol 2005;32:893–898.

66. Ardila CM, Granada MI, Guzman IC. Antibiotic resistance of subgingival species in chronic periodontitis patients. J Periodontal Res 2010;45:557–563.

67. Lazarevic V, Manzano S, Gaia N, et al. Effects of amoxicillin treatment on the salivary microbiota in children with acute otitis media. Clin Microbiol Infect 2013;19:E335–E342.

68. Jakobsen C, Paerregaard A, Munkholm P, Wewer V. Paediatric inflammatory bowel disease during a 44-year period in Copenhagen County: Occurrence, course and prognosis—A population-based study from the Danish Crohn Colitis Database. Eur J Gastroenterol Hepatol 2009;21:1291–1301.

69. Hu Y, Yang X, Qin J, et al. Metagenome-wide analysis of antibiotic resistance genes in a large cohort of human gut microbiota. Nat Commun 2013;4:2151.

70. Modi SR, Lee HH, Spina CS, Collins JJ. Antibiotic treatment expands the resistance reservoir and ecological network of the phage metagenome. Nature 2013;499:219–222.

71. Wilson W, Taubert KA, Gewitz M, et al. Prevention of infective endocarditis: Guidelines from the American Heart Association: A guideline from the American Heart Association Rheumatic Fever, Endocarditis, and Kawasaki Disease Committee, Council on Cardiovascular Disease in the Young, and the Council on Clinical Cardiology, Council on Cardiovascular Surgery and Anesthesia, and the Quality of Care and Outcomes Research Interdisciplinary Working Group. Circulation 2007;116:1736–1754 [erratum 2007;116:e376–e377].

72. Wilson W, Taubert KA, Gewitz M, et al. Prevention of infective endocarditis: Guidelines from the American Heart Association: A guideline from the American Heart Association Rheumatic Fever, Endocarditis and Kawasaki Disease Committee, Council on Cardiovascular Disease in the Young, and the Council on Clinical Cardiology, Council on Cardiovascular Surgery and Anesthesia, and the Quality of Care and Outcomes Research Interdisciplinary Working Group. J Am Dent Assoc 2008;139(suppl): 3S–24S [erratum 2008;139:253].

73. Infective Endocarditis Prophylaxis Expert Group. Prevention of endocarditis. 2008 update from Therapeutic guidelines: Antibiotic version 13, and Therapeutic guidelines: Oral and dental version 1. Melbourne: Therapeutic Guidelines Limited, 2008. http://www.tg.org.au/uploads/PDFs/Prevention%20of%20endocarditis.pdf. Accessed 23 September 2013.

74. Bonow RO, Carabello BA, Chatterjee K, et al. 2008 focused update incorporated into the ACC/AHA 2006 guidelines for the management of patients with valvular heart disease: A report of the American College of Cardiology/American Heart Association Task Force on Practice Guidelines (Writing Committee to revise the 1998 guidelines for the management of patients with valvular heart disease). Endorsed by the Society of Cardiovascular Anesthesiologists, Society for Cardiovascular Angiography and Interventions, and Society of Thoracic Surgeons. J Am Coll Cardiol 2008;52:e1–e142.

75. Nishimura RA, Carabello BA, Faxon DP, et al. ACC/AHA 2008 Guideline update on valvular heart disease: Focused update on infective endocarditis: A report of the American College of Cardiology/American Heart Association Task Force on Practice Guidelines endorsed by the Society of Cardiovascular Anesthesiologists, Society for Cardiovascular Angiography and Interventions, and Society of Thoracic Surgeons. J Am Coll Cardiol 2008;52:676–685.

76. Stassen L, Rahman N, Rogers S, et al. Infective endocarditis prophylaxis and the current AHA, BSAC, NICE and Australian guidelines. J Ir Dent Assoc 2008;54:264–270.

77. National Institute for Health and Care Excellence (NICE). NICE clinical guideline 64: Prophylaxis against infective endocarditis: Antimicrobial prophylaxis against infective endocarditis in adults and children undergoing interventional procedures. London: NICE, 2008. http://publications.nice.org.uk/prophylaxis-against-infective-endocarditis-cg64. Accessed 23 Sept 2013.

78. Gould FK, Elliott TS, Foweraker J, et al. Guidelines for the prevention of endocarditis: Report of the Working Party of the British Society for Antimicrobial Chemotherapy. J Antimicrob Chemother 2006; 57:1035–1042.

79. Habib G, Hoen B, Tornos P, et al. Guidelines on the prevention, diagnosis, and treatment of infective endocarditis (new version 2009): The Task Force on the Prevention, Diagnosis, and Treatment of Infective Endocarditis of the European Society of Cardiology (ESC). Endorsed by the European Society of Clinical Microbiology and Infectious Diseases (ESC-MID) and the International Society of Chemotherapy (ISC) for Infection and Cancer. Eur Heart J 2009;30:2369–2413.

80. Costelloe C, Metcalfe C, Lovering A, Mant D, Hay AD. Effect of antibiotic prescribing in primary care on antimicrobial resistance in individual patients: Systematic review and meta-analysis. BMJ 2010; 340:c2096.

81. Lopes DR, Peres MP, Levin AS. Randomized study of surgical prophylaxis in immunocompromised hosts. J Dent Res 2011;90:225–229.

82. Centers for Disease Control and Prevention. Antibiotic resistance threats in the United States, 2013. Published online 16 Sep 2013. http://www.cdc.gov/drugresistance/threat-report-2013/pdf/ar-threats-2013-508.pdf. Accessed 23 Sept 2013.

83. van Nood E, Vrieze A, Nieuwdorp M, et al. Duodenal infusion of donor feces for recurrent Clostridium difficile. N Engl J Med 2013;368:407–415.

84. Chirouze C, Hoen B, Duval X. Infective endocarditis prophylaxis: Moving from dental prophylaxis to global prevention? Eur J Clin Microbiol Infect Dis 2012;31:2089–2095.

85. Duval X, Leport C. Prophylaxis of infective endocarditis: Current tendencies, continuing controversies. Lancet Infect Dis 2008;8:225–232.

86. Duval X. Simplification of the prophylaxis of endocarditis: We were right! Arch Cardiovasc Dis 2013; 106:69–71.

87. Bor DH, Woolhandler S, Nardin R, Brusch J, Himmelstein DU. Infective endocarditis in the U.S., 1998–2009: A nationwide study. PLoS One 2013;8: e60033.

88. Murdoch DR, Corey GR, Hoen B, et al. Clinical presentation, etiology, and outcome of infective endocarditis in the 21st century: The International Collaboration on Endocarditis-Prospective Cohort Study. Arch Intern Med 2009;169:463–473.

89. Chatterjee S, Sardar P. Early surgery reduces mortality in patients with infective endocarditis: Insight from a meta-analysis. Int J Cardiol 2013;168:3094–3097.

90. American Academy of Orthopaedic Surgeons, American Dental Association. Clinical Practice Guideline Unit. Prevention of orthopaedic implant infection in patients undergoing dental procedures; evidence-based guideline and evidence report, version 0.2 2.2.2012. Rosemont, IL: American Academy of Orthopaedic Surgeons, 2012.

91. American Dental Association. Antibiotic prophylaxis: Total joint replacement. http://www.ada.org.2583.aspx#replace. Accessed 23 Sept 2013.

92. American Dental Association. Prophylaxis recommendations: Infective endocarditis (IE). http://www.ada.org/2583.aspx#endocarditis. Accessed 23 Sept 2013.

93. Meurman JH. Oral microbiota and cancer. J Oral Microbiol 2010;2:5195.

94. Cummins J, Tangney M. Bacteria and tumours: Causative agents or opportunistic inhabitants? Infect Agent Cancer 2013;8:11.

95. Mager DL. Bacteria and cancer: Cause, coincidence or cure? A review. J Transl Med 2006;4:14.

96. World Health Organization, International Agency for Research on Cancer (IARC), Working Group on the Evaluation of Carcinogenic Risks to Humans. Schistosomes, liver flukes and *Helicobacter pylori*. IARC Monographs on the Evaluation of Carcinogenic Risks to Humans. Lyon, France: IARC, 1994.

97. World Health Organization, International Agency for Research on Cancer (IARC), Working Group on the Evaluation of Carcinogenic Risks to Humans. Human papillomaviruses. IARC Monographs on the Evaluation of Carcinogenic Risks to Humans. Lyon, France: IARC, 1995.

98. World Health Organization, International Agency for Research on Cancer (IARC), Working Group on the Evaluation of Carcinogenic Risks to Humans. Epstein-Barr virus and Kaposi's sarcoma herpesvirus/human herpesvirus 8. IARC Monographs on the Evaluation of Carcinogenic Risks to Humans. Lyon, France: IARC, 1997.

99. Mravak-Stipetić M, Sabol I, Kranjciččić J, Knežević M, Grce M. Human papillomavirus in the lesions of the oral mucosa according to topography. PLoS One 2013;8:e69736.

100. Adamopoulou M, Vairaktaris E, Nkenke E, et al. Prevalence of human papillomavirus in saliva and cervix of sexually active women. Gynecol Oncol 2013;129:395–400.

101. World Health Organization/Institut Català d'Oncologia Information Centre on HPV and Cervical Cancer (HPV Information Centre). Human papillomavirus and related cancers: World, ed 3. Summary report update 22 Jun 2010. http://screening.iarc.fr/doc/Human%20Papillomavirus%20and%20Related%20Cancers.pdf. Accessed 23 Sept 2013.

102. Ylitalo N, Sørensen P, Josefsson AM, et al. Consistent high viral load of human papillomavirus 16 and risk of cervical carcinoma in situ: A nested case-control study. Lancet 2000;355:2194–2198.

103. Ribeiro KB, Levi JE, Pawlita M, et al. Low human papillomavirus prevalence in head and neck cancer: Results from two large case-control studies in high-incidence regions. Int J Epidemiol 2011;40:489–502.

104. Chaturvedi AK, Engels EA, Anderson WF, Gillison ML. Incidence trends for human papillomavirus–related and –unrelated oral squamous cell carcinomas in the United States. J Clin Oncol 2008;26:612–619.

105. Chocolatewala N, Chaturvedi P, Desale R. The role of bacteria in oral cancer. Indian J Med Paediatr Oncol 2010;31:126–131.

106. Katz J, Onate MD, Pauley KM, Bhattacharyya I, Cha S. Presence of *Porphyromonas gingivalis* in gingival squamous cell carcinoma. Int J Oral Sci 2011;3:209–215.

107. Dayama A, Srivastava V, Shukla M, Singh R, Pandey M. *Helicobacter pylori* and oral cancer: Possible association in a preliminary case control study. Asian Pac J Cancer Prev 2011;12:1333–1336.

108. Fernando N, Jayakumar G, Perera N, Amarasingha I, Meedin F, Holton J. Presence of *Helicobacter pylori* in betel chewers and non betel chewers with and without oral cancers. BMC Oral Health 2009;9:23.

109. Shimakage M, Horii K, Tempaku A, Kakudo K, Shirasaka T, Sasagawa T. Association of Epstein-Barr virus with oral cancers. Hum Pathol 2002;33:608–614.

110. Sand LP, Jalouli J, Larsson PA, Hirsch JM. Prevalence of Epstein-Barr virus in oral squamous cell carcinoma, oral lichen planus, and normal oral mucosa. Oral Surg Oral Med Oral Pathol Oral Radiol Endod 2002;93:586–592.

111. Gong HL, Shi Y, Zhou L, et al. The composition of microbiome in larynx and the throat biodiversity between laryngeal squamous cell carcinoma patients and control population. PLoS One 2013;8:e66476.

112. Akutsu Y, Matsubara H, Shuto K, et al. Pre-operative dental brushing can reduce the risk of postoperative pneumonia in esophageal cancer patients. Surgery 2010;147:497–502.

113. Marchesi JR, Dutilh BE, Hall N, et al. Towards the human colorectal cancer microbiome. PLoS One 2011;6:e20447.

114. Castellarin M, Warren RL, Freeman JD, et al. *Fusobacterium nucleatum* infection is prevalent in human colorectal carcinoma. Genome Res 2012;22:299–306.

115. Kostic AD, Chun E, Robertson L, et al. *Fusobacterium nucleatum* potentiates intestinal tumorigenesis and modulates the tumor-immune microenvironment. Cell Host Microbe 2013;14:207–215.

116. Rubinstein Mara R, Wang X, Liu W, Hao Y, Cai G, Han YW. *Fusobacterium nucleatum* promotes colorectal carcinogenesis by modulating E-cadherin/β-catenin signaling via its FadA adhesin. Cell Host Microbe 2013;14:195–206.

117. Strauss J, Kaplan GG, Beck PL, et al. Invasive potential of gut mucosa-derived *Fusobacterium nucleatum* positively correlates with IBD status of the host. Inflamm Bowel Dis 2011;17:1971–1978.

118. McCoy AN, Araújo-Pérez F, Azcárate-Peril A, Yeh JJ, Sandler RS, Keku TO. *Fusobacterium* is associated with colorectal adenomas. PLoS One 2013;8:e53653.

119. Wu Q, Yang ZP, Xu P, Gao LC, Fan DM. Association between *Helicobacter pylori* infection and the risk of colorectal neoplasia: A systematic review and meta-analysis. Colorectal Dis 2013;15:e352–e364.

120. Michaud DS, Joshipura K, Giovannucci E, Fuchs CS. A prospective study of periodontal disease and pancreatic cancer in US male health professionals. J Natl Cancer Inst 2007;99:171–175.

121. Michaud DS, Izard J, Wilhelm-Benartzi CS, et al. Plasma antibodies to oral bacteria and risk of pancreatic cancer in a large European prospective cohort study [epub ahead of print 18 Sept 2012]. Gut doi:10.1136/gutjnl-2012-303006.

122. Camargo MC, Koriyama C, Matsuo K, et al. Case-case comparison of smoking and alcohol risk associations with Epstein-Barr virus-positive gastric cancer [epub ahead of print 31 July 2013]. Int J Cancer doi: 10.1002/ijc.28402.

123. Salazar CR, Sun J, Li Y, et al. Association between selected oral pathogens and gastric precancerous lesions. PLoS One 2013;8:e51604.

124. Zhan P, Suo LJ, Qian Q, et al. *Chlamydia pneumoniae* infection and lung cancer risk: A meta-analysis. Eur J Cancer 2011;47:742–747.

125. Mäntylä P, Stenman M, Paldanius M, Saikku P, Sorsa T, Meurman JH. *Chlamydia pneumoniae* together with collagenase-2 (MMP-8) in periodontal lesions. Oral Dis 2004;10:32–35.

126. Hujoel PP, Drangsholt M, Spiekerman C, Weiss NS. An exploration of the periodontitis-cancer association. Ann Epidemiol 2003;13:312–316.

127. Giannobile WV, Kornman KS, Williams RC. Personalized medicine enters dentistry: What might this mean for clinical practice? J Am Dent Assoc 2013;144:874–876.

128. Razzouk S, Termechi O. Host genome, epigenome, and oral microbiome interactions: Toward personalized periodontal therapy. J Periodontol 2013;84:1266–1271.

The Mechanisms Behind Oral-Systemic Interactions

Marcelo O. Freire, DDS, PhD
Thomas E. Van Dyke, DDS, PhD

The localized inflammatory response to injury or infection is a spatially defined and temporally regulated condition that is self-limited. If the lesion does not resolve and becomes chronic, the acquired immune system is stimulated, including broad activation of cell-mediated immunity, lymphocytic pathways, and humoral immunity. The impact of the chronic persistent lesions or injury leads to systemic dysregulation of homeostasis, an extended response that goes beyond the confined localization of one tissue. The chronicity of the lesion alters molecular, cellular, and overall tissue responses in remote regions of the body, thus having a transient or permanent impact on overall health.

Oral conditions can significantly influence or be influenced by events locally and systemically. Periodontal diseases, periodontic-endodontic lesions, traumatic lesions, reactionary oral lesions (chronic irritation), premalignant lesions, oral cancer, and other conditions are very distinct in etiology and mechanism but have in common a programmed immune response that modulates disease progression, prognosis, and treatment. Periodontal tissues in particular have an anatomical and multitissue origin, are hypervascularized, and have a unique interface with microorganisms that are generally commensal, maintaining a controlled homeostatic response in health. Infectious and inflammatory diseases of the oral cavity, such as periodontitis, result from an imbalance of the commensal-host relationship in which there is excessive inflammation and overgrowth of commensal pathogens. It is now becoming clear that chronic oral infections and inflammation have a systemic impact. It is important to the fields of biology, medicine, and dentistry to understand the mechanisms of the intricate molecular interactions that underlie the relationship between oral conditions that arise locally and long-term systemic consequences.

Historically, descriptions of a localized response to injury and infection were recorded by the ancient Egyptian and Greek cultures. Hippocrates in the 5th century BCE introduced terms like *edema* that are still used to describe the local response in inflammation.[1] He also referred to inflammation as an early component of the healing process after tissue injury. Centuries later, the invention of the compound microscope by Janssen in the 1500s and the subsequent improvement of its optical resolution by Leeuwenhoek gave rise to the early descriptions of the tissue response to injury. Early concepts of inflammation were largely derived from intuition rather than careful scientific investigation. The controversial observations described by the ancient cultures provided the framework for critical experimentation in later centuries, when it became clear that it was necessary to elucidate the relationship between local responses and systemic health.

Still, until the middle of the 20th century, scientific and medical theory was based on observation and intuition rather than experimentation and application of the scientific method. An example is the concept that focal infection or injury is the basis of systemic disease. The focal infection theory was first introduced in 1891 by Miller, who proposed the relationship between oral and systemic infection in the book *The Human Mouth as a Focus of Infection*.[2] A prevailing theory of medicine around this time was that miasmas, or bad smells, caused disease, this in spite of Koch's discovery of the infectious nature of disease. Miller emphasized that oral microorganisms or their products caused the development of a variety of diseases in sites removed from the oral cavity, including arthritis, brain abscesses, pulmonary diseases, cardiovascular and gastric problems, and even stupidity.

The role of oral sepsis as a cause of systemic disease was described by William Hunter, a prominent British physician, who criticized dental restorations "built in, on, and around diseased teeth which form a veritable mausoleum of gold over a mass of sepsis to which there is no parallel in the whole realm of medicine."[3] In 1919, Rosenow published a series of animal experiments and human case reports supporting the concept of focal infection. He suggested cooperation between dentists and physicians to ensure that the focus of oral infection would be eliminated completely. It became common practice to extract all endodontically or periodontally involved teeth to eliminate any possible foci of infection, with the expectation that this would prevent or cure a plethora of local or systemic problems.[3]

The lack of scientific foundation eventually led to the disappearance of the concept of focal infection, because there was no clear basis for ascribing most systemic diseases to the presence of oral foci of infection. As a result, the focus of dental practice changed, and restorative dental procedures reemerged as the mainstay of most dental treatment plans. However, as a more scientific approach was applied to investigating clinical problems, it became clear that,

in fact, there are situations in which oral bacteria can affect distant structures, in particular the case of bacterial endocarditis in susceptible people.

Beginning in the late 1980s, a series of publications regarding the association between periodontitis and some systemic conditions, including coronary heart disease, stroke, and preterm birth and low birth weight, captured the attention of the dental profession. In some sense, this can be construed as a return to the theory of focal infection. However, the response of the dental and medical professions this time has been considerably more measured than in the early part of the 20th century. There is no suggestion that elimination of oral infection will cure cardiovascular disease (CVD). The relationship of oral disease to systemic disease has been investigated in terms of modifiable risk factors.

In recent years, important additions to the scientific literature recognize that inflammation is a hallmark response to bacteria or bacteremia that, as an evolutionary programmed reaction to injury and infection, is a major link between oral and systemic diseases.[4-6] The investigation of oral-systemic disease connections is a rapidly advancing area of research. Considering the existing data, it is important to reflect on all the possible relationships. Oral and systemic conditions may coexist but be disorders of different origin and have an intensifying effect on each other. Various infected or inflamed conditions of the oral cavity, including the periodontal diseases, can be associated with systemic diseases directly or indirectly, increase the risk for development of other diseases or vice versa, or in fact be causal. This chapter examines the mechanisms behind the link between oral and systemic diseases, emphasizing inflammation as the key to pathogenesis.

Inflammation

Innate immunity, characterized by the local inflammatory response, is the early host response to identify and eliminate infectious agents or damaged tissues. As an initial and protective response to challenges presented to host tissues, inflammation is characterized by vascular dilation, enhanced permeability of capillaries, increased blood flow, and leukocyte recruitment, which result in the five cardinal signs of inflammation: heat, redness, swelling, pain, and loss of function. Polymorphonuclear leukocytes (PMNs), or neutrophils (named for their staining characteristics with hematoxylin and eosin), are the first line of defense of the innate immune system. PMNs are professional phagocytes with potent oxidative and nonoxidative killing mechanisms to combat bacteria. PMN infiltration is followed by mononuclear cells, monocytes, and macrophages that enter the inflammatory site and clear cellular debris, bacteria, and apoptotic PMNs by phagocytosis without prolonging inflammation. The degree of inflammation activation is dependent on the nature of the inflammatory trigger, the response, its localization, and its persistence.[7]

The major sensors for the inflammatory response are innate immune cells that migrate to the injured site and resident stromal cells. Together, they trigger production of mediators that modulate the fate of inflammation. Neutrophils, macrophages, dendritic cells, and mast cells produce low–molecular weight proteins called *cytokines* that control initiation of inflammation, maintenance and regulation of its amplitude, and duration of the response. The regulation leading to the transcription of cytokine genes, their translation, and secretion of proinflammatory cytokines from a variety of cells is generally dependent on activation of transcription by nuclear factor κB (NFκB) nuclear protein. The NFκB-regulated pathways are activated by pattern-recognition receptors such as toll-like receptors (TLRs) that bind bacterial lipopolysaccharide (LPS) and other molecules.

Both inflammatory cytokines and chemoattractant cytokines, or chemokines, are produced for autocrine, endocrine, and paracrine functions.[4,8] The cytokines are low–molecular weight proteins that modulate inflammation positively or negatively. Cytokines are produced by resident cells, such as epithelial cells and fibroblasts, and phagocytes in the acute phase and early chronic phase of inflammation, as well as by immune cells in adaptive immunity.

After microbial recognition, cytokines of the innate response, including tumor necrosis factor α (TNF-α), interleukin (IL) 1β, and IL-6, are the first secreted and are signature innate cytokines. TNF-α is a pleotropic cytokine that has many functions, from signaling cell migration to tissue destruction. TNF-α upregulates the production of IL-1β and IL-6. TNF-α is also correlated with extracellular matrix degradation and bone resorption through actions promoting secretion of matrix metalloproteinases (MMPs) and receptor activator of NFκB ligand (RANKL) and coupled bone formation.[9]

Chemokines are cytokines with chemoattractant functions that induce cell migration to the site of infection or injury. Once blood leukocytes exit a blood vessel, they are attracted by functional gradients of chemotactic factors. Chemokines are synthesized by a variety of cells, including leukocytes and endothelial, epithelial, and stromal cells. Beyond their chemotactic role, chemokines function as messengers of distinct biologic processes, including cell proliferation, cell death, angiogenesis, and tumor metastasis. Bacterial peptides are also chemotactic for inflammatory cells.[10]

The innate immune recognition of different microorganisms is complex. Viral infections induce the production of interferons (IFN-α, IFN-β) and activation of cytotoxic lymphocytes (natural killer cells); bacterial pathogens are recognized by pattern-recognition receptors such as TLRs, which are expressed by tissue-resident macrophages and other host cells. Binding of TLRs induces the production of inflammatory cytokines, chemokines, and proinflammatory lipid mediators such as prostaglandins. These inflammatory mediators are the major players in establishing an effective inflammatory response and clearance of bacteria. Proinflammatory mediators, such as IL-1β, IL-6, TNF-α, and prostaglandin E_2 (PGE_2), are produced locally in inflamed tissues. Proinflammatory cytokines in circulation induce systemic actions, including leukocytosis and acute-phase proteins. Parasites, on the other hand, lead to the production of a different set of cytokines and cellular responses. These include IL-4, IL-5, and IL-13 by mast cells and basophils. With continued exposure, soluble antigens react with circulating specific antibody to form immune complexes that further amplify inflammation at sites of deposition.[5]

Locally produced lipid mediators, such as prostaglandins and leukotrienes, are proinflammatory signals and trigger the nervous system to promote fever and fatigue.[10] Prostaglandins and leukotrienes are derived from membrane lipids, particularly arachidonic acid. Arachidonic acid is metabolized by two major enzyme pathways, cyclooxygenases (COX) and lipoxygenases. COX-1 (constitutively expressed COX) and COX-2 (inducible COX) catalyze the conversion of arachidonic acid into prostaglandins, prostacyclins, and thromboxanes. Prostaglandins have 10 subclasses, of which D, E, F, G, H, and I are the most important in inflammation.

There are three major classes of lipoxygenase: 5, 12, and 15. Lipoxygenases catalyze the formation of hydroxyeicosatetraenoic acids (HETEs) from arachidonic acid, leading to the formation of leukotrienes. Excessive production of inflammatory mediators and/or an exacerbated sensing response to inflammatory triggers are correlated with progression from acute inflammation to chronic inflammation in many diseases.

Microorganisms that gain access to the blood are usually eliminated by the reticuloendothelial system within minutes (transient bacteremia) with no clinical symptoms. Local bacterial antigens that are systemically dispersed trigger significant systemic inflammation. Leukocytes, endothelial cells, and hepatocytes respond to bacteria and their virulence factors with secretion of proinflammatory immune mediators, called *acute-phase proteins*, such as C-reactive protein (CRP). Persistence of infection, with continuous exposure of the host to new antigens, results in the activation of humoral immunity and antibody production. Circulating specific antibodies form immune complexes with respective target antigens, which in turn activate the complement system and Fc receptors on phagocytes to amplify inflammation at sites of deposition. Likewise, proinflammatory mediators, such as IL-1β, IL-6, TNF-α, and PGE_2, produced locally in the inflamed tissues, may "spill" into the circulation and have systemic impact, such as induction of endothelial dysfunction.[9,11]

Although the inflammatory response is protective, failure to remove noxious materials produced by neutrophils via phagocytosis and failure of clearance of apoptotic inflammatory cells or delay of apoptosis characterize the chronic and pathologic lesion. The incomplete elimination of leukocytes from a lesion is observed in susceptible individuals; acute inflammation fails to resolve, and chronic disease and fibrosis develop. Accordingly, loss of resolution and failure to return tissue to homeostasis results in neutrophil-mediated destruction and chronic inflammation with accumulation of macrophages, which is a major cause of human inflammatory pathologies, cancers, type 2 diabetes, CVDs, and periodontal diseases.

The natural resolution of inflammation after an acute inflammatory response results from well-coordinated biochemical pathways that are activated late in the acute inflammatory response. The pathways are lipoxygenase pathways as well that involve the action of two different lipoxygenases on the same arachidonic acid molecule. The double substitution leads to the formation of lipoxins, a new series of eicosanoids that share the same backbone structure of the proinflammatory leukotrienes and HETEs but bind to distinct receptors. The active, receptor-mediated regulation halts neutrophil function, promotes neutrophil apoptosis, and promotes the nonphlogistic (noninflammatory) accumulation of macrophages that efficiently clear the lesion of remaining bacteria and apoptotic cells.

There are a number of resolution pathways, depending on the fatty acid substrate. Omega-3 fatty acids are metabolized by similar pathways to produce resolvins of the D and E series (from docosahexaenoic acid and eicosapentaenoic acid, respectively), protectins, and maresins. All of these factors drive resolution of inflammation through different receptors on inflammatory cells. It is now suggested that chronic inflammation results from a combination of excessive production of proinflammatory mediators and a failure of production of sufficient proresolution mediators (for review, see the article by Serhan et al[6]).

Periodontal Diseases

The local acute periodontal inflammatory response is a reaction to the local microbial biofilm. The commensal flora and inflammatory response evolved to maintain a relationship that leads to health, as observed in periodontal tissues and in other mucosal surfaces, including the oropharyngeal surface and the gut. Disturbance of homeostasis, characterized by increased inflammation and overgrowth of pathologic organisms, initiates chronic inflammation, which is followed by an acquired immune response that leads to tissue destruction or periodontitis.

Failure to remove both the trigger (pathogenic bacteria) and inflammatory cells, especially neutrophils, characterizes the chronic, pathologic lesion. The rapid and complete elimination of leukocytes from a lesion is the ideal outcome following an inflammatory event. In susceptible individuals, periodontal inflammation fails to resolve, and chronic inflammation becomes periodontal pathosis. Accordingly, inadequate resolution and failure to return tissue to homeostasis results initially in neutrophil-mediated destruction and chronic inflammation and later in a complex immune lesion characterized by destruction of extracellular matrix, bone, scarring, and loss of periodontal tissue function.[12,13]

The presence of bacterial plaque and gingivitis is prevalent in humans, affecting in excess of 90% of the adult dentate population. The same direct correlation cannot be said for periodontitis; despite abundant plaque deposits in most people, the prevalence of moderate periodontitis (attachment loss greater than 5 mm) is around 40% of the population.[14] However, this prevalence of periodontitis is not uniformly distributed across different races, ethnicities, and socioeconomic groups. This being the case, despite the universal presence of plaque, bacteria do not appear to be the major determinants of the progression of gingivitis to periodontitis. Although the popular dogma has been to accept that periodontitis arises from a specific subgingival infection, the concept that periodontitis arises when the periodontal tissues provide an adequate ecologic environment for opportunistic bacteria to flourish has been presented, for some time, by eminent oral microbiologists as an alternative mechanism.[15–17]

The host-parasite interaction is clearly responsible for the initiation of the gingivitis lesion, but what happens next is less clear. There is no definitive evidence that specific bacteria are responsible for the progression and manifestation of advanced periodontitis; a number of specific pathogens are *associated* with deep periodontal pockets. It can be argued that the specific bacteria are present as a result of the disease but do not cause the disease. This is no different than most mucosal biofilm pathoses, where the complicating issue, which remains unresolved, is "Which comes first—the host response or the change in the biofilm?"[18]

Several biologic pathways linking periodontal disease to induction of systemic inflammation have been identified.[17–19] In health, the sulcular epithelium and local innate immunity act as a natural barrier that prevents bacterial penetration. In gingival health, only a small number of bacteria, mostly facultative anaerobes, are found in the gingival crevice and bloodstream. However, in periodontal disease, inflamed tissue and ulcerated subgingival pocket epithelium are vulnerable to bacteria and provide bacteria a port of entry to the circulation.

Periodontal Inflammation in Oral Cancer

A higher incidence of cancer development is found in individuals with chronic inflammatory conditions; this insight has driven suggestions of possible linkage with periodontal inflammation.[20,21] Associations between periodontal disease and the risk for precancerous lesions and tumors have been shown, and a possible relationship between periodontal disease and oral neoplasm has been described; recent evidence from National Health and Nutrition Examination Survey (NHANES) III indicated that periodontitis was significantly related to the presence of tumors,[22] but stratified analysis found this association was only present in current smokers. A stronger association was found between periodontitis and human papillomavirus status in patients with oropharyngeal cancer.[23]

The risk of death from cancer is increased in patients with periodontitis. In a follow-up of subjects from NHANES I,[20,24] patients diagnosed with periodontitis had a 55% (95% confidence interval [CI]: 25% to 92%) increased risk of death from any cancer. There was a significantly increased risk for lung cancer; however, this was not evident in individuals who had never smoked.

The incidence of cancer was consistently increased in patients with periodontitis. A larger study with a 17.7-year follow-up identified 5,720 incident cancers in 48,375 men enrolled. Men who reported periodontal disease had a slightly increased total cancer incidence of 14% (95% CI: 7% to 22%), which remained significant when the analysis was limited to those who were never smokers.[25] There was a significantly increased risk of lung, kidney, pancreatic, and hematologic cancers after adjustment. Notably, risk for lung cancer was the only association when the number of teeth was used as the exposure.[25]

Similar genetic risk factors for periodontal disease and cancers were found in a prospective study in Sweden. The study identified more than 4,000 incident cancers after a median follow-up of 27 years.[26] At baseline, the participants were classified as having periodontal disease if they reported that at least half their teeth had loosened or fallen out on their own. Periodontal disease was associated with a 15% (95% CI: 1% to 32%) increased risk for all cancers. Periodontal disease was also associated with increased risk of colorectal, pancreatic, and prostate cancers.

In co-twin analyses, monozygotic twins with baseline periodontal disease showed a 50% increase in total cancer risk, but in dizygotic twins this association was markedly attenuated. Similar patterns emerged for digestive tract cancers, suggesting that shared genetic risk factors may partially explain associations between periodontal disease and cancers.[20,26]

Link Between Periodontal Disease and Systemic Conditions

Uncontrolled (chronic) inflammation is a hallmark of various human diseases, including periodontitis, diabetes, CVDs, and premature labor.[23–25] Despite advances in knowledge of causes and risk factors associated with chronic periodontitis, there are no signs of decline in prevalence. According to the US Centers for Disease Control, 647 million adults have periodontal disease as of 2012.[14] Periodontal diseases, including gingivitis and periodontitis, are leukocyte-driven inflammatory diseases characterized by soft tissue destruction and osteoclast-mediated bone loss. The etiology of periodontitis is recognized to be primarily bacterial but multifactorial, and a number of behavioral, environmental, microbial, systemic, and genetic risk factors influence host susceptibility and disease progression. The impact of a dysregulated inflammatory response has the potential for harm to the systemic health of individuals (Fig 5-1).

More than 100 years ago, the theory of focal infection revolutionized thinking regarding the relationship between an apparently local infection and its systemic actions.[27] The theory was eventually discredited because the treatments rendered were ill conceived and did far more harm than good. However, understanding of the observed associations between local infection and systemic disease has matured with the increased understanding of the role of inflammation in many systemic diseases, which was not appreciated until recently.

Periodontitis and diabetes

Among many diseases that impact the population globally, type 2 diabetes is a major public health problem. Worldwide, about 347 million adults suffer from type 2 diabetes.[28] According to the World Health Organization, the prevalence may double by the year 2030, and health care expenditures related to diabetes will increase significantly.[29]

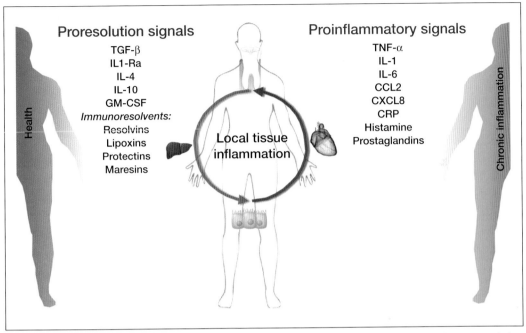

Fig 5-1 Local and systemic actions of tissue inflammation. Tissue-inflammatory processes link to systemic homeostasis. The nature of challenge and balance between the response from sensors and mediators leads to distinct fates of acute inflammation. Proinflammatory mediators such as IL-1, TNF-α, and others listed are important molecules that initiate the tissue response to injury and infection. The termination of acute processes is modulated by immunoresolvents and consequent upregulation of anti-inflammatory cytokines. An unresolved inflammatory process is the primary step leading to development of chronic inflammation and loss of local and systemic function. CCL2, chemokine (C-C motif) ligand 2; CXCL8, interleukin 8; TGF-β, transforming growth factor β; IL1-Ra, interleukin 1 receptor antagonist; GM-CSF, granulocyte-macrophage colony-stimulating factor.

Inflammatory diseases such as type 2 diabetes and chronic periodontal diseases have a reciprocal relationship. Among people diagnosed with type 2 diabetes, one-third present with severe periodontal disease, and adult diabetic patients with severe periodontitis have greater risk of poor glycemic control, increasing the risk of oral and systemic complications.[28] Hyperglycemia resulting from type 2 diabetes can impact PMNs and monocytes through various mechanisms, including the accumulation of advanced glycation end products that leads to an increase of extracellular production of superoxide by leukocytes and increased secretion of proinflammatory cytokines, such as IL-1β, insulinlike growth factor, TNF-α, and MMPs.[30]

Increased inflammation in periodontitis leads to prolonged activation of PMNs and monocytes, and ineffective clearance of bacteria and prolonged inflammation consequently aggravate systemic diabetes regulation. Systemic inflammation in type 2 diabetes, defined by increased circulating TNF-α, is associated with obesity and periodontitis and has been proposed as a mechanism for the connection between these conditions. A case-control study demonstrated that periodontitis is associated with elevated plasma triglycerides and total cholesterol.[31]

A relationship between inflammatory pathways and metabolic diseases, such as type 2 diabetes or insulin resistance, is one line of active investigation.[32] Attempts to understand the molecular pathways that regulate diabetes and insulin resistance require the study of adipose tissue. For example, adipose tissue is now recognized as a biologically active endocrine organ and not simply a site of inert lipid storage. Adipocytes, like any stromal cell, secrete cytokines, now collectively known as *adipokines*, into the circulation, including adiponectin, TNF-α, plasminogen activator inhibitor type 1, and resistin.[33]

The realization that adipocytes have a molecular influence on the entire system helps explain why obesity is frequently associated with inflammatory disease, type 2 diabetes, and atherosclerosis. Evidence suggests that inflammatory cells may be found within adipose tissue; perhaps the fat itself is actively involved in inflammatory processes, contributing to the release of proinflammatory mediators.

Fat tissue cytokine, adipokine, has many actions in sites away from its origin, including muscle, liver, and blood vessel walls, and is believed to play an important role in modulating glucose and lipid metabolism. Although adipose tissue may release a host of proinflammatory cells, adiponectin is of interest because it seems to be anti-inflammatory and, therefore, protective. For example, studies have shown that lower levels of plasma adiponectin are found in patients with both diabetes and coronary heart disease than in patients with diabetes without coronary heart disease, suggesting that adiponectin may be antiatherogenic.[18,31,33] Humans in insulin-resistant states also have lower levels of adiponectin; this was reversed by the administration of thiazolidinedione, an insulin-sensitizing compound.[30,31] There also seems to be a negative relationship between adiponectin and CRP, again suggesting that adiponectin has an anti-inflammatory role.

Diabetic patients have greater risk for developing chronic periodontitis, and those with elevated hemoglobin A_{1c} (HbA$_{1c}$) levels have a significantly higher prevalence of periodontitis and experience more tooth loss than do those with better metabolic control. Acute and chronic infections may adversely influence glycemic control.[28] Furthermore, it has been established that HbA$_{1c}$ is adversely affected by systemic inflammation.

It is now clear that a biologically plausible link between periodontitis and metabolic control has been determined. If effective treatment of periodontitis can modify glycemic control, as suggested in some studies,[28] then periodontal therapy may be an important contribution to a patient management program that incorporates lifestyle changes and medications.

Periodontal therapy has shown uniform outcomes across studies. While treated periodontal conditions have shown consistency in results, the effects of the therapy on diabetes are not clear. The standard treatment goal of periodontal therapy with regard to diabetes is to reduce HbA$_{1c}$ levels, because reductions in HbA$_{1c}$ have been shown to delay the development of diabetic complications. Although there have been efforts to reduce HbA$_{1c}$ levels through periodontal therapy, the ideal HbA1$_c$ level to be reached is not clear.[28,33–35] It is possible that periodontal therapy can improve HbA$_{1c}$ levels by 0.4% to 0.5%[35]; this systemic beneficial action of periodontal therapy demonstrates the importance of controlling local inflammatory conditions as part of diabetes management.

Periodontitis and cardiovascular disease

Severe periodontal disease affects 10% to 15% of the general population and has been linked to CVD in cross-sectional and cohort studies.[31,36,37] Studies report that elevated cell and cytokine-mediated markers of inflammation, including CRP, fibrinogen, and various cytokines, are associated with periodontal disease.[18,30] The same proinflammatory markers in periodontal disease have also been linked with atherothrombogenesis.[18,19,38] When the progression of periodontal disease is reduced, levels of inflammatory markers common to both diseases (ie, IL-6, TNF-α, and CRP) are decreased, which might in turn decrease the risk of vascular disease. It is still unknown whether inhibiting or reducing inflammation in general or CRP in particular will decrease the rate of vascular effects.[39]

In several atherosclerosis studies using animal models, periodontal disease was shown to be a contributing factor.[18,19,40] Activated immune cells in the atherogenic plaque produce pro-inflammatory cytokines (IFN, IL-1, and TNF-α), which induce the production of substantial amounts of IL-6. These cytokines are also produced in various tissues in response to infection and in the adipose tissue of patients with metabolic syndrome. IL-6 in turn stimulates the production of large amounts of acute-phase reactants, including CRP, serum amyloid A, and fibrinogen, especially in the liver.

Although cytokines at all steps have important biologic actions, their amplification at each step of the cascade makes the measurement of downstream mediators such as CRP particularly useful for clinical diagnosis. Increased high-sensitivity CRP plasma levels in patients with prehypertension or established hypertension may link these two conditions. Major depression, physical inactivity, family histories of CVD and periodontal disease, advancing age, and male sex are other risk factors for atherosclerotic CVD that are commonly found in patients with periodontitis and also may serve as confounders.[36]

Risk factors common to both CVD and periodontitis are thought to be related to increased systemic inflammation.[31] Diet, genetics, medications, and environmental factors influence the course of periodontal disease, and when periodontal disease is combined with these factors, they all influence cardiovascular health status. In CVD studies, periodontal disease was shown to be a contributing factor.[37,41]

Lipid of low-density lipoproteins is known to initiate and propagate an inflammatory response.[38] Once migration of leukocytes has occurred, monocytes differentiate into macrophages and proliferate. Fatty streaks develop; these consist of lipid-laden monocytes and macrophages as well as T lymphocytes, which eventually are joined by migrating smooth muscle cells. If the cascade of events goes unchecked, the fatty streaks develop into advanced lesions, whereby macrophages accumulate, a necrotic core is developed, and a fibrous cap is formed that blocks the lesion from the lumen.

This fibrous cap, which is characteristic of late-stage atherosclerosis, is of concern; rup-

ture of this fibrous cap is believed to underlie the vast majority of myocardial infarctions that may derive from these inflammatory processes. Cytokines such as INF-γ are involved in the destabilization of the plaque because they lead to a decrease in matrix synthesis as well as matrix degradation. In addition to these cytokines, MMP enzymes are involved in controlling degradation; macrophages express MMPs, further contributing to degradation.[31]

Periodontal inflammation causes a local and systemic cytokine response. As already mentioned, several studies have reported that elevated cell- and cytokine-mediated markers of inflammation are associated with periodontal disease.[36,37,40] Proinflammatory cytokines induce an acute-phase response in the liver characterized by elevated levels of CRP and fibrinogen, which in turn promote atherogenesis. In addition, gingival ulceration in periodontitis allows the migration of bacteria into the blood (bacteremia), which could provide a second inflammatory stimulus leading to atheroma formation.[42]

CVD, once characterized as a lipid disease because of the end-stage pathology, is now known to have a large inflammatory component. In recent years, epidemiologic studies have ascertained an association between CVD and other inflammatory diseases, in particular periodontal diseases.[4,36] Given the prolonged nature of the pathogenesis of CVD, it has been difficult to demonstrate cause and effect in this association. To that end, the relationship between CVD and periodontitis was investigated longitudinally in an animal model. New Zealand white rabbits were fed a 0.5% cholesterol diet for 13 weeks. This is known to cause atheromatous changes in the large arteries of the animals.[40] In the experiment, periodontitis was induced with a ligature and *Porphyromonas gingivalis* in half the animals, while the other half maintained a normal periodontium; all animals were fed the atherogenic diet.[40]

Using the size (area) of the atheromatous lesion as the primary outcome, the animals that had periodontitis exhibited twice the atheroma formation of the control animals.[40] These data provide direct longitudinal evidence that periodontal inflammation can impact the progression of CVD. Further investigation was unable to isolate bacteria from the arterial lesions; however, it was demonstrated that local inflammation was able to induce upregulation of the systemic inflammatory response, reflected by increased levels of circulating CRP and IL-1.[31,40] These data suggest that the impact of infection is not at the level of bacteremia and direct stimulation of arterial endothelium but rather the result of local inflammation inducing a systemic elevation of inflammation.[31]

Patients with periodontitis who have two or more known risk factors for atherosclerosis should be referred by the dental team for evaluation of atherosclerotic risk, which should include physical examination and annual measurement of blood pressure and blood lipid profile. Animal studies demonstrate that TLR receptor signaling influences the course of progression of the disease.[19]

Patients with periodontitis and abnormal serum lipid values, elevated levels of plasma CRP (as measured by the high-sensitivity CRP test), or both are recommended to follow a multifaceted lifestyle modification program to reduce risk of CVD. Cessation of cigarette smoking is recommended for all patients with periodontitis. Furthermore, all patients with periodontitis who have elevated blood pressure (greater than 140/90 mmHg) should be treated according to standard hypertension management protocols and should undertake lifestyle changes, including reduction of weight and dietary sodium intake, as appropriate.

Periodontal evaluation should be considered in patients with CVD who have signs or symptoms of gingival disease or unexplained tooth loss. Moreover, when periodontitis is newly diagnosed in patients with CVD, dentists and physicians should closely collaborate to optimize CVD risk reduction and periodontal care.[43]

Atherogenesis leading to atherosclerosis involves highly specific cellular and molecular responses that can be described as an inflammatory disease. Classic cardiovascular risk factors can be viewed as an injury or insult to which the body adapts, setting in motion a decades-long response. Regardless of the cause, the earliest changes in atherosclerosis occur in the endothelium. These lead to increased permeability

and adhesiveness, particularly of leukocytes, as well as increased procoagulation properties that result in activation of vasoactive molecules, cytokines, and growth factors.[9]

In the development of atherosclerosis, monocytes and T cells mediated by endothelial expression of adhesion molecules accumulate at the injury site. T cells are then activated, releasing mediators such as cytokines and chemokines. Chemokines, a class of cytokines that mediate chemoattraction (chemotaxis) between cells, attract leukocytes to the site. Through a cascade of signals, the process leading to entry of leukocytes into the endothelium involves the rolling, activation, and adherence of leukocytes. One particular adhesion molecule, vascular cell adhesion molecule 1, is of importance in the adherence process because it binds precisely with monocytes and T lymphocytes. Once adherent to the endothelium, monocytes transmigrate into the intima.[9]

During inflammation, there is a dramatic increase in chemokine secretion, resulting in selective recruitment of leukocytes to the injured tissue. Early proinflammatory cytokines, such as IL-1 and TNF-α, stimulate chemokine production. Another cytokine, IFN-γ, is secreted by T lymphocytes (specifically T-helper cell type 1); this induces chemokine production directly and by acting with IL-1 and TNF-α.

Two groups of chemokines associated with IFN-γ are CC and CXC. CC chemokines induce the migration of monocytes. For example, monocyte chemoattractant protein 1, a CC chemokine, seems to be responsible for migration of monocytes from the bloodstream into the surrounding tissue by binding to and activating CC chemokine receptors, in this case CC chemokine receptor 2. Depending on their structural characteristics, CXC chemokines can induce migration of neutrophils or attract lymphocytes. Research suggests that the differential expression of three IFN-γ–inducible CXC chemokines (IFN-inducible protein 10, monokine induced by IFN-γ, and IFN-inducible T-cell alpha chemoattractant) by atheroma-associated cells plays a role in the recruitment and retention of activated T lymphocytes within vascular wall lesions during atherogenesis.[16] This study also found increased expression of the receptor for these chemokines, CXC chemokine receptor 3, by T lymphocytes within human atherosclerotic lesions.

When the progression of periodontal disease is slowed, levels of inflammatory markers common to both diseases (ie, IL-6, TNF-α, and CRP) are decreased; this might in turn decrease the risk of vascular disease.[36] After researchers adjusted for risk factors, such as smoking, diabetes, alcohol intake, obesity, and blood pressure, subjects with periodontal disease had a 1.14- to 1.59-fold greater risk of developing CVD than did those without periodontal disease.[36,37,42]

Although inflammatory responses to injury and infection are essential to health, the response also causes problems when inflammatory processes are maladaptive, leading to chronic diseases such as diabetes and CVD. Innovative research is needed to elucidate the intricate pathways by which local chronic inflammation can impact large vessels.

Periodontitis and pregnancy

Periodontal diseases are inflammatory responses to infectious pathogens that, although distant from many organs, can also affect the fetoplacental unit.[44] In an attempt to contain or eliminate this infection, host cells activate a local inflammatory response against bacteria and their numerous virulence factors (eg, LPS). However, several studies report that inflammatory cytokines, periodontal bacteria, and/or their virulence factors may enter the blood circulation and disseminate throughout the body, triggering systemic inflammatory responses and/or ectopic infections.[36]

Not surprisingly, local inflammation is able to interfere with the homeostasis of normal pregnancy and labor. While a large number of epidemiologic studies have showed a positive association between periodontal disease and pathologic outcomes of pregnancy, the results presented have not always been confirmatory.[44]

In healthy pregnancy, the mother and the fetus exchange nutrients and waste through the umbilical cord that connects the placenta of the mother to the fetus. In amniotic fluid, levels of inflammatory mediators, including PGE_2, TNF-α,

and IL-1β, increase incrementally through pregnancy, reach a threshold, and promote uterine contraction, cervical dilation, and delivery.[45] It is of extreme importance that normal levels of inflammatory mediators as well as hormones be tightly regulated to maintain a normal course of pregnancy.[44]

Evidence suggests that periodontal pathogens interfere with homeostatic control of pregnancy. Through DNA identification and immunodetection, both P gingivalis and Aggregatibacter actinomycetemcomitans have been detected in biopsy specimens taken from placenta of women diagnosed with preeclampsia.[46] Most commonly, in amniotic fluids, Fusobacterium nucleatum was identified in patients suffering from premature labor or giving birth to babies with low birth weight.[47]

However, although there is clear evidence that bacterial presence in diverse tissues establishes pathologic conditions during pregnancy, the mechanisms by which the pathogens arise in the local tissues remain unclear.[44] Recent studies suggest that pathogens can gain access to the amniotic cavity by ascending from the vagina and the cervix, by hematogenous dissemination through the placenta, by accidental introduction at the time of invasive procedures (amniocentesis), and by retrograde spread through the fallopian tubes.[44,48] Besides the pathogens themselves, their virulent factors, including LPS, have been associated with triggering of the same type of pathologic actions to the maternal placenta and fetus.

Localized elevated levels of maternal IL-1β, IL-6, PGE_2, and TNF-α in the amniotic fluid have been associated with pregnancy alterations, including premature birth. Other biomarkers such as MMPs, estriol, elastase, protease, phospholipase, prolactin myeloperoxidase, and tissue inhibitor of MMP 1 (TIMP-1) have been evaluated[48] but with inconclusive results. CRP, an acute-phase molecule synthesized by the liver, activates systemic inflammation and proinflammatory cytokines; it is also associated with premature birth.[42] Other pregnancy complications have been associated with elevated levels of CRP, including intrauterine growth restriction and preeclampsia.[44]

Finally, a combination of local complications places the host at risk for poor pregnancy outcomes. For example, women with gestational diabetes mellitus have high risk to present elevated serum levels of CRP, IL-6, and TNF-α. Through inflammatory pathways, these cytokines interfere with insulin-signaling homeostasis. Therefore, carbohydrate metabolism, hormonal control, and inflammatory mediators together influence the fate of health during pregnancy and the outcome of labor.[44] For more information on periodontal infections and pregnancy outcomes, see chapter 10.

Resolution of Inflammation and the Periodontal Disease–Systemic Disease Link

It has become clear in recent years that periodontitis is an inflammatory disease that is initiated by the oral microbial biofilm.[15] This distinction implies that it is the host response to the biofilm that destroys the periodontium in the pathogenesis of the disease. As the understanding of pathways of inflammation has matured, a better understanding of the molecular basis of resolution of inflammation has emerged. Resolution of inflammation involves an active, agonist-mediated, well-orchestrated return of tissue homeostasis.[49] Table 5-1 details the actions of immunoresolvents in acute inflammatory disease models.

There is an important distinction between anti-inflammation and resolution: *Anti-inflammation* involves pharmacologic blocking of specific inflammatory pathways; *resolution* is mediated by physiologic pathways that restore homeostasis.[6] A growing body of research suggests that chronic inflammatory periodontal disease involves a failure of resolution pathways to restore homeostasis that leads to development of the chronic lesion.[6,11] Proof of concept studies in the 1980s demonstrated that pharmacologic anti-inflammatory measures prevented and slowed the progression of periodontal diseases in animals and man.[71] However, the side effect profile of such therapies precluded the use of nonsteroidal anti-inflammatory drugs or other enzyme inhibitors or receptor antagonists in periodontal therapy.[71]

The isolation and characterization of resolving agonist molecules, such as lipoxins, resolvins, protectins, and maresins, have opened a new area of research into the use of endogenous lipid mediators of resolution as potential therapeutic agents for inflammatory periodontitis. Work in animal models of periodontitis has revealed the potential of this therapeutic approach for prevention and treatment and forced reconsideration of the understanding of the pathogenesis of human periodontal diseases[73] (see Table 5-1; for review, see Freire and Van Dyke[72]).

The importance of agonists of resolution in eliminating inflammation has been confirmed in demonstrations of control of systemic inflammatory disease by exogenous addition of excess lipoxins or resolvins.[74] These findings are observed in concert with resolution of periodontitis in the same animal, suggesting that control of inflammation is central to the association between periodontitis and systemic disease. The report provided support and a rationale for the mechanism of the observed associations as well as a basis for the clinical concern that periodontitis increases the risk for a number of important systemic inflammatory diseases.[51,52]

Table 5-1	Animal studies of inflammatory disease, their immunoresolvents, and their actions	
Inflammatory disease/study model	**Immunoresolvent and its action**	**Study**
Periodontitis/rabbit	**Lipoxin A$_4$/ATL**	
	Prevents connective tissue and bone loss	Serhan et al[50]
	Accelerates healing of inflamed tissues	Serhan et al[50]
	Ceases infiltration of neutrophils	Serhan et al[50]
	Resolvin E1	
	Reduces bone loss	Hasturk et al[51]
	Regenerates lost soft tissue and bone tissue	Hasturk et al[52]
Peritonitis/mouse	**Lipoxin A$_4$/ATL**	
	Stops neutrophil recruitment	Bannenberg et al[53]
	Promotes lymphatic removal of phagocytes	Schwab et al[54]
	Resolvin E1	
	Decreases PMN infiltration	Arita et al[55]
	Regulates chemokine and cytokine production	Schwab et al[54]
	Promotes lymphatic removal of phagocytes	Bannenberg et al[53]
	Resolvin D1	
	Shortens resolution interval	Spite et al[56]
	Regulates microRNAs	Recchiuti et al[57]
	Reduces concentrations of LTB$_4$, PGD$_2$, PGF$_2$, and TXA$_2$ in exudates	Krishnamoorthy et al[58]
	Attenuates neutrophil recruitment	Norling et al[59]
	Lowers antibiotic requirement	Chiang et al[60]
	Increases animal survival	Chiang et al[60]
	Reduces bacterial titers	Chiang et al[60]
	Protectin D1	
	Promotes local clearance of apoptotic cells	Bannenberg et al[53]
	Regulates lymphatic removal of phagocytes	Ariel et al[61,62]
	Modulates T-cell migration	Schwab et al[54]
	Maresin-1	
	Blocks infiltration of PMNs into the peritoneum	Serhan et al[63]

(continued on next page)

Table 5-1 *(cont)*	Animal studies of inflammatory disease, their immunoresolvents, and their actions	
Inflammatory disease/study model	**Immunoresolvent and its action**	**Study**
Colitis/mouse	**Lipoxin A₄/ATL**	
	Reduces severe colitis	Aliberti et al[64]
	Attenuates gene expression of proinflammatory mediators	Gewirtz et al[65]
	Inhibits weight loss	Gewirtz et al[65]
	Reduces immune dysfunction	Wallace et al[66]
	Resolvin E1	
	Improves animal survival rate	Arita et al[55]
	Reduces weight loss	Arita et al[55]
	Promotes LPS detoxification	Campbell et al[67]
	Stops neutrophil recruitment	Ishida et al[68]
	AT-Resolvin D1	
	Reduces disease activity index	Bento et al[69]
	Attenuates gene expression of proinflammatory mediators	Bento et al[69]
	Attenuates neutrophil recruitment	Bento et al[69]
	Resolvin D2	
	Improves disease activity index	Bento et al[69]
	Reduces colonic PMN infiltration	Bento et al[69]
Retinopathy/mouse	**Resolvin E1/Resolvin D1/Protectin D1**	
	Protects against neovascularization	Connor et al[70]

ATL, aspirin-triggered 15-epi-lipoxin A₄; LTB₄, leukotriene B₄; PGD₂, prostaglandin D₂; PGF₂, prostaglandin F₂; TXA₂, thromboxane A₂. (Adapted from Freire and Van Dyke.[72])

Conclusion

The link between oral and systemic inflammatory processes and their consequences are directly related to the tissue response to challenge, usually microbial, and inflammation. The fate of this overall process is determined by the balance between mediators and sensors that amplify the inflammatory process and those that control the return to homeostasis. Diseases associated with uncontrolled acute inflammation are characterized by insufficient actions of resolution programs and inappropriate release and maintenance of high levels of toxic substances and proinflammatory mediators that may result in damage to host tissues and prolong the inflammatory response. In experimental animal models, compelling evidence demonstrates the actions of proresolution mediators in regulation of both local and systemic inflammatory responses, elucidating the role of endogenous mediators in systemic inflammatory processes and disease regulation.

A clearer picture is emerging of the central role of inflammation in the association between periodontitis and a number of systemic diseases and conditions. The target of periodontal therapy, whether it be control of the biofilm and/or control of the local inflammation, should be to control systemic inflammation associated with chronic systemic diseases.

References

1. Granger DN, Senchenkova E. Inflammation and the Microcirculation. San Rafael, CA: Morgan & Claypool Life Sciences, 2010.
2. Pallasch TJ, Wahl MJ. The focal infection theory: Appraisal and reappraisal. J Calif Dent Assoc 2000; 28:194–200.
3. Barnett ML. The oral-systemic disease connection. An update for the practicing dentist. J Am Dent Assoc 2006;137(suppl):5S–6S.
4. Van Dyke TE, Kornman KS. Inflammation and factors that may regulate inflammatory response. J Periodontol 2008;79(8 suppl):1503–1507.
5. Medzhitov R. Inflammation 2010: New adventures of an old flame. Cell 2010;140:771–776.
6. Serhan CN, Chiang N, Van Dyke TE. Resolving inflammation: Dual anti-inflammatory and pro-resolution lipid mediators. Nat Rev Immunol 2008;8:349–361.
7. Majno G, Joris I. Cells, Tissues, and Disease. Oxford: Oxford University, 2004.
8. Van Dyke TE. Cellular and molecular susceptibility determinants for periodontitis. Periodontol 2000 2007;45:10–13.
9. Van Dyke TE, van Winkelhoff AJ. Infection and inflammatory mechanisms. J Clin Periodontol 2013; 40(suppl 14):S1–S7.
10. Graves DT, Oates T, Garlet GP. Review of osteoimmunology and the host response in endodontic and periodontal lesions. J Oral Microbiol 2011;3:5304 doi:10.3402/jomv3i0.5304.
11. Fredman G, Oh SF, Ayilavarapu S, Hasturk H, Serhan CN, Van Dyke TE. Impaired phagocytosis in localized aggressive periodontitis: Rescue by Resolvin E1. PLoS One 2011;6:e24422.
12. Darveau RP. Periodontitis: A polymicrobial disruption of host homeostasis. Nat Rev Microbiol 2010; 8:481–490.
13. Eke PI, Thornton-Evans GO, Wei L, Borgnakke WS, Dye BA. Accuracy of NHANES periodontal examination protocols. J Dent Res 2010;89:1208–1213.
14. Eke PI, Dye BA, Wei L, et al. Prevalence of periodontitis in adults in the United States: 2009 and 2010. J Dent Res 2012;91:914–920.
15. Offenbacher S. Periodontal diseases: Pathogenesis. Ann Periodontol 1996;1:821–878.
16. Kornman KS, Van Dyke TE. Bringing light to the heat: "Inflammation and periodontal diseases: A reappraisal." J Periodontol 2008;79:1313.
17. Williams RC, Barnett AH, Claffey N, et al. The potential impact of periodontal disease on general health: A consensus view. Curr Med Res Opin 2008;24:1635–1643.
18. Reyes L, Herrera D, Kozarov E, Roldán S, Progulske-Fox A. Periodontal bacterial invasion and infection: Contribution to atherosclerotic pathology. J Clin Periodontol 2013;40(suppl 14):S30–S50.
19. Hayashi C, Papadopoulos G, Gudino CV, et al. Protective role for TLR4 signaling in atherosclerosis progression as revealed by infection with a common oral pathogen. J Immunol 2012;189:3681–3688.
20. Linden GJ, Herzberg MC, Working Group 4 of the Joint EFP/AAP Workshop. Periodontitis and systemic diseases: A record of discussions of Working Group 4 of the Joint EFP/AAP Workshop on Periodontitis and Systemic Diseases. J Clin Periodontol 2013;40(suppl 14):S20–S23.
21. Coussens LM, Werb Z. Inflammation and cancer. Nature 2002;420:860–867.
22. Tezal M, Grossi SG, Genco RJ. Is periodontitis associated with oral neoplasms? J Periodontol 2005; 76:406–410.
23. Tezal M, Scannapieco FA, Wactawski-Wende J, et al. Local inflammation and human papillomavirus status of head and neck cancers. Arch Otolaryngol Head Neck Surg 2012;138:669–675.
24. Hujoel PP, Drangsholt M, Spiekerman C, Weiss NS. An exploration of the periodontitis-cancer association. Ann Epidemiol 2003;13:312–316.
25. Michaud DS, Liu Y, Meyer M, Giovannucci E, Joshipura K. Periodontal disease, tooth loss, and cancer risk in male health professionals: A prospective cohort study. Lancet Oncol 2008;9:550–558.
26. Arora M, Weuve J, Fall K, Pedersen NL, Mucci LA. An exploration of shared genetic risk factors between periodontal disease and cancers: A prospective co-twin study. Am J Epidemiol 2010;171: 253–259.
27. Miller SU. Increased human body water loss at reduced ambient pressure. Aerosp Med 1962;33: 689–691.
28. Engebretson S, Kocher T. Evidence that periodontal treatment improves diabetes outcomes: A systematic review and meta-analysis. J Clin Periodontol 2013;40(suppl 14):S153–S163.
29. Zhang Y, Dall TM, Mann SE, et al. The economic costs of undiagnosed diabetes. Popul Health Manag 2009;12:95–101.
30. Taylor JJ, Preshaw PM, Lalla E. A review of the evidence for pathogenic mechanisms that may link periodontitis and diabetes. J Clin Periodontol 2013; 40(suppl 14):S113–S134.

31. Schenkein HA, Loos BG. Inflammatory mechanisms linking periodontal diseases to cardiovascular diseases. J Clin Periodontol 2013;40(suppl 14): S51–S69.

32. Chapple IL, Genco R, Working Group 2 of the Joint EFP/AAP Workshop. Diabetes and periodontal diseases: Consensus report of the Joint EFP/AAP Workshop on Periodontitis and Systemic Diseases. J Clin Periodontol 2013;40(suppl 14):S106–S112.

33. Bharti P, Katagiri S, Nitta H, et al. Periodontal treatment with topical antibiotics improves glycemic control in association with elevated serum adiponectin in patients with type 2 diabetes mellitus. Obes Res Clin Pract 2013;7:e129–e138.

34. Atouf F, Park CH, Pechhold K, Ta M, Choi Y, Lumelsky NL. No evidence for mouse pancreatic beta-cell epithelial-mesenchymal transition in vitro. Diabetes 2007;56:699–702.

35. Borgnakke WS, Ylöstalo PV, Taylor GW, Genco RJ. Effect of periodontal disease on diabetes: Systematic review of epidemiologic observational evidence. J Clin Periodontol 2013;40(suppl 14):S135–S152.

36. Genco RJ, Van Dyke TE. Prevention: Reducing the risk of CVD in patients with periodontitis. Nat Rev Cardiol 2010;7:479–480.

37. de Oliveira C, Watt R, Hamer M. Toothbrushing, inflammation, and risk of cardiovascular disease: Results from Scottish Health Survey. BMJ 2010; 340:c2451.

38. Cybulsky MI, Jongstra-Bilen J. Resident intimal dendritic cells and the initiation of atherosclerosis. Curr Opin Lipidol 2010;21:397–403.

39. Beck JD, Couper DJ, Falkner KL, et al. The Periodontitis and Vascular Events (PAVE) pilot study: Adverse events. J Periodontol 2008;79:90–96.

40. Jain A, Batista EL Jr, Serhan C, Stahl CL, Van Dyke TE. Role for periodontitis in the progression of lipid deposition in an animal model. Infect Immun 2003; 71:6012–6018.

41. Couper DJ, Beck JD, Falkner KL, et al. The Periodontitis and Vascular Events (PAVE) pilot study: Recruitment, retention, and community care controls. J Periodontol 2008;79:80–89.

42. Paraskevas S, Huizinga JD, Loos BG. A systematic review and meta-analyses on C-reactive protein in relation to periodontitis. J Clin Periodontol 2008;35: 277–290.

43. Devchand PR, Arita M, Hong S, et al. Human ALX receptor regulates neutrophil recruitment in transgenic mice: Roles in inflammation and host defense. FASEB J 2003;17:652–659.

44. Madianos PN, Bobetsis YA, Offenbacher S. Adverse pregnancy outcomes (APOs) and periodontal disease: Pathogenic mechanisms. J Clin Periodontol 2013;40(suppl 14):S170–S180.

45. Haram K, Mortensen JH, Wollen AL. Preterm delivery: An overview. Acta Obstet Gynecol Scand 2003;82:687–704.

46. Gonzales-Marin C, Spratt DA, Millar MR, Simmonds M, Kempley ST, Allaker RP. Levels of periodontal pathogens in neonatal gastric aspirates and possible maternal sites of origin. Mol Oral Microbiol 2011;26:277–290.

47. Han YW, Redline RW, Li M, Yin L, Hill GB, McCormick TS. Fusobacterium nucleatum induces premature and term stillbirths in pregnant mice: Implication of oral bacteria in preterm birth. Infect Immun 2004;72:2272–2279.

48. Gürsoy M, Könönen E, Gürsoy UK, Tervahartiala T, Pajukanta R, Sorsa T. Periodontal status and neutrophilic enzyme levels in gingival crevicular fluid during pregnancy and postpartum. J Periodontol 2010;81:1790–1796.

49. Van Dyke TE, Serhan CN. Resolution of inflammation: A new paradigm for the pathogenesis of periodontal diseases. J Dent Res 2003;82:82–90.

50. Serhan CN, Jain A, Marleau S, et al. Reduced inflammation and tissue damage in transgenic rabbits overexpressing 15-lipoxygenase and endogenous anti-inflammatory lipid mediators. J Immunol 2003; 171:6856–6865.

51. Hasturk H, Kantarci A, Ohira T, et al. RvE1 protects from local inflammation and osteoclast-mediated bone destruction in periodontitis. FASEB J 2006; 20:401–403.

52. Hasturk H, Kantarci A, Goguet-Surmenian E, et al. Resolvin E1 regulates inflammation at the cellular and tissue level and restores tissue homeostasis in vivo. J Immunol 2007;179:7021–7029.

53. Bannenberg GL, Chiang N, Ariel A, et al. Molecular circuits of resolution: Formation and actions of resolvins and protectins. J Immunol 2005;174:4345–4355.

54. Schwab JM, Chiang N, Arita M, Serhan CN. Resolvin E1 and protectin D1 activate inflammation-resolution programmes. Nature 2007;447:869–874.

55. Arita M, Yoshida M, Hong S, et al. Resolvin E1, an endogenous lipid mediator derived from omega-3 eicosapentaenoic acid, protects against 2,4,6-trinitrobenzene sulfonic acid-induced colitis. Proc Natl Acad Sci U S A 2005;102:7671–7676.

56. Spite M, Summers L, Porter TF, Srivastava S, Bhatnagar A, Serhan CN. Resolvin D1 controls inflammation initiated by glutathione-lipid conjugates formed during oxidative stress. Br J Pharmacol 2009;158:1062–1073.

57. Recchiuti A, Krishnamoorthy S, Fredman G, Chiang N, Serhan CN. MicroRNAs in resolution of acute inflammation: Identification of novel resolvin D1-miRNA circuits. FASEB J 2011;25:544–560.

58. Krishnamoorthy S, Recchiuti A, Chiang N, Fredman G, Serhan CN. Resolvin D1 receptor stereoselectivity and regulation of inflammation and proresolving microRNAs. Am J Pathol 2012;180:2018–2027.

59. Norling LV, Dalli J, Flower RJ, Serhan CN, Perretti M. Resolvin D1 limits polymorphonuclear leukocyte recruitment to inflammatory loci: Receptor-dependent actions. Arterioscler Thromb Vasc Biol 2012;32: 1970–1978.

60. Chiang N, Fredman G, Bäckhed F, et al. Infection regulates pro-resolving mediators that lower antibiotic requirements. Nature 2012;484:524–528.

61. Ariel A, Li PL, Wang W, et al. The docosatriene protectin D1 is produced by TH2 skewing and promotes human T cell apoptosis via lipid raft clustering. J Biol Chem 2005;280:43079–43086.

62. Ariel A, Fredman G, Sun YP, et al. Apoptotic neutrophils and T cells sequester chemokines during immune response resolution through modulation of CCR5 expression. Nat Immunol 2006;7:1209–1216.

63. Serhan CN, Yang R, Martinod K, et al. Maresins: Novel macrophage mediators with potent antiinflammatory and proresolving actions. J Exp Med 2009;206:15–23.

64. Aliberti J, Hieny S, Reis e Sousa C, Serhan CN, Sher A. Lipoxin-mediated inhibition of IL-12 production by DCs: A mechanism for regulation of microbial immunity. Nat Immunol 2002;3:76–82.

65. Gewirtz AT, Collier-Hyams LS, Young AN, et al. Lipoxin A4 analogs attenuate induction of intestinal epithelial proinflammatory gene expression and reduce the severity of dextran sodium sulfate-induced colitis. J Immunol 2002;168:5260–5267.

66. Wallace JL, Fiorucci S. A magic bullet for mucosal protection...and aspirin is the trigger! Trends Pharmacol Sci 2003;24:323–326.

67. Campbell EL, MacManus CF, Kominsky DJ, et al. Resolvin E1-induced intestinal alkaline phosphatase promotes resolution of inflammation through LPS detoxification. Proc Natl Acad Sci U S A 2010; 107:14298–14303.

68. Ishida T, Yoshida M, Arita M, et al. Resolvin E1, an endogenous lipid mediator derived from eicosapentaenoic acid, prevents dextran sulfate sodium-induced colitis. Inflamm Bowel Dis 2010;16:87–95.

69. Bento AF, Claudino RF, Dutra RC, Marcon R, Calixto JB. Omega-3 fatty acid-derived mediators 17(R)-hydroxy docosahexaenoic acid, aspirin-triggered resolvin D1 and resolvin D2 prevent experimental colitis in mice. J Immunol 2011;187:1957–1969.

70. Connor KM, SanGiovanni JP, Lofqvist C, et al. Increased dietary intake of omega-3-polyunsaturated fatty acids reduces pathological retinal angiogenesis. Nat Med 2007;13:868–873.

71. Howell TH. Blocking periodontal disease progression with anti-inflammatory agents. J Periodontol 1993;64(8 suppl):828–833.

72. Freire MO, Van Dyke TE. Natural resolution of inflammation. Periodontology 2000 2013;63:149–164.

73. Recchiuti A, Serhan CN. Pro-resolving lipid mediators (SPMs) and their actions in regulating miRNA in novel resolution circuits in inflammation. Front Immunol 2012;3:298.

74. Van Dyke TE. Inflammation and periodontal diseases: A reappraisal. J Periodontol 2008;79(8 suppl): 1501–1502.

Clinical Considerations:
What You Can Take Back to Your Practice

What is the effect of diabetes on oral health and glycemic control?

Diabetes, especially if poorly controlled, affects oral health by increasing the risk for periodontal disease and tooth loss. It can also lead to xerostomia and burning mouth syndrome. On the other hand, periodontitis can adversely affect glycemic control and increase the risk for complications such as cardiovascular disease and end-stage renal disease in patients with type 2 diabetes. Furthermore, loss of teeth resulting from periodontal disease can result in poor nutrition.

What is the biologic plausibility of the association between oral health and diabetes?

The bidirectional relationship between diabetes and periodontal disease is most likely related to the increased level of systemic inflammation each disease causes. This heightened systemic inflammation results in insulin resistance, poor glycemic control, and aggravated destruction of periodontal tissues.

Are oral infections independent risk factors for the development or progression of diabetes?

Emerging evidence suggests that oral infections, especially periodontal disease, are risk factors for initiation and progression of type 2 diabetes. However, this remains to be confirmed by further studies assessing if and to what extent prevention or treatment of periodontal disease will reduce the incidence or progression of diabetes and its complications.

Does the delivery of oral health care contribute to improvement of glycemic control?

There is evidence that periodontal treatment can reduce glycated hemoglobin when significant periodontal disease is present, in patients with poor glycemic control, and when adequate periodontal therapy has been carried out.

Is it safe to provide dental care to patients with diabetes?

It is safe and important to provide dental care to patients with diabetes since there is evidence that tooth loss can affect diet and result in nutritional inadequacies that can contribute to poor glycemic control.

What is the appropriate message to give to the public about the association between oral health and diabetes?

The message for the public is that diabetes, especially if poorly controlled, is an important risk factor for periodontal disease. Tooth loss is also increased twofold in patients with diabetes, and this loss often leads to poor nutrition, which can make dietary control of diabetes more difficult. People with diabetes can also suffer from xerostomia or burning mouth syndrome and are more susceptible to fungal infections.

6 | Oral Health and Diabetes

Robert J. Genco, DDS, PhD

Diabetes mellitus is a group of metabolic disorders characterized by hyperglycemia that results from defective insulin action or production. In the United States, 8.3% of the population had diabetes in 2010; of these, 18.8 million people were diagnosed and 7 million undiagnosed. Type 2 diabetes accounts for about 90% of these cases and type 1 for most of the other cases. Other types, such as gestational diabetes and maturity-onset diabetes of youth, are rare. The prevalence of diabetes in the United States is predicted to increase to 14% of the population by 2030.[1] An increase in the prevalence of diabetes is also predicted globally, with an increase to 70% of adults with diabetes in developing countries and 20% in developed countries by 2030.

Population growth, aging of the population, and urbanization that has resulted in changes in diet and exercise habits are likely to account for the increase in the worldwide numbers of individuals with diabetes by 2030. The proportion of type 1 diabetes varies geographically. However, in most countries, type 2 is the most prevalent form.

People with diabetes and chronically poor metabolic control suffer from death, heart disease, and stroke rates that are 2 to 4 times higher than those in individuals without diabetes.[2] Diabetes is the leading cause of new cases of blindness among adults and is the leading cause of kidney failure. About 60% to 70% of people with diabetes have mild to severe forms of nervous system damage, and more than 60% of nontraumatic lower limb amputations occur in people with diabetes. In the United States in 2012, the average medical expenditures among people with diabetes were 2.3 times higher than what would be expected in the absence of diabetes.[1]

Burden of Periodontal Disease

There is recent evidence for a high burden of periodontal disease among adults in the United States. More than 47% of adults in a 2009 to 2010 sample of adults older than 30 years of age were found to have periodontitis[3] (Fig 6-1). In this sample of adults included in the National Health and Nutrition Examination Survey (NHANES), the prevalence of periodontitis was highest in males, Mexican American individuals, and in persons at lower socioeconomic levels. In further analysis of the same 2009 to 2010 NHANES data, 60% of those with diabetes (defined as hemoglobin A_{1c} [HbA_{1c}] levels of 6.5%

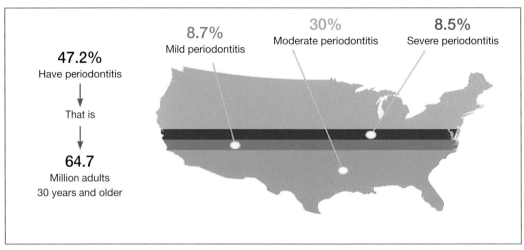

Fig 6-1 Rates of periodontitis among US adults. (Reprinted from Eke et al[3] with permission.)

or greater) were found to have moderate to severe periodontitis.

This high burden of periodontal disease is also seen globally.[4] For the global studies, the World Health Organization measured periodontal disease using a different index from that used in the US studies; however, a high prevalence of periodontal disease was observed in most countries surveyed. There were variations in prevalence among countries, and those variations were largely thought to be related to socioenvironmental conditions and behavioral risk factors. The variation and prevalence of periodontitis globally were also related to the general health status of the populations studied; higher levels of periodontitis were found among those with diabetes and those infected with human immunodeficiency virus.[4]

Unfortunately, there is a lack of awareness of the mutual relationship between diabetes and periodontitis, in spite of reports that a majority of adults with type 2 diabetes suffer from some form of periodontitis.[5] A considerable body of evidence shows a close bidirectional association between diabetes and periodontal disease.[6] The evidence for and implications of these associations are reviewed in this chapter.

Evidence for the Bidirectional Association Between Periodontal Disease and Diabetes

Epidemiologic studies

Diabetes and periodontal disease are complex chronic diseases that affect each other.[7,8] Diabetes, especially if poorly controlled, is a risk factor for periodontal disease. Both cross-sectional and longitudinal epidemiologic studies have consistently found greater prevalence and incidence of periodontal disease in patients with either type 1 or type 2 diabetes. The relationship is most pronounced in patients who do not have adequate glycemic control, as is the case for many other complications.[6] A meta-analysis of cross-sectional and longitudinal epidemiologic studies that evaluated the relationship between periodontal disease and diabetes found that greater probing depth and greater attachment loss were observed in individuals

Fig 6-2 Difference in rates of attachment loss among patients with or without type 2 diabetes. (Reprinted from Emrich et al[10] with permission.)

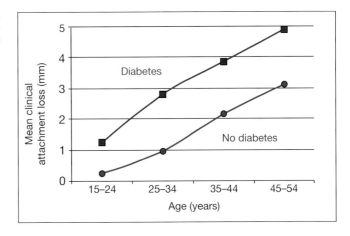

with type 2 diabetes than in comparable individuals without diabetes.[9] The prevalence, onset, and severity of periodontal disease have been documented by these studies. The greater severity and earlier onset of periodontal disease in patients with type 2 diabetes were confirmed in a study of the Native Americans of the Gila River Indian Community in Arizona[10] (Fig 6-2).

Several studies of large populations have shown that the prevalence and severity of periodontitis are also increased in individuals who are at high risk for diabetes, a condition that is sometimes called *prediabetes*. These individuals have elevated levels of blood glucose but not at the levels that would warrant diagnosis of diabetes.[11–13]

Mechanisms linking diabetes and periodontitis

Type 2 diabetes is characterized by a systemic inflammatory process that leads to insulin resistance and reduced pancreatic B-cell function and apoptosis, both of which cause increasing hyperglycemia. Periodontitis contributes to this systemic inflammation, which adversely affects glycemic control in patients suffering from both

diseases. The elevated systemic inflammation associated with periodontitis results mainly from the entry of periodontal organisms and their virulence factors into the systemic circulation. There is also strong evidence that advanced glycation endproducts resulting from hyperglycemia lead to activation of macrophages. Macrophages so activated then produce inflammatory cytokines and reactive oxygen species that increase the periodontal soft and hard tissue destruction found in patients with diabetes[14] (Fig 6-3).

The effects of diabetes on periodontitis and of periodontitis on diabetes are likely based on their both contributing to the hyperinflammatory state. These mechanisms help explain the bidirectional relationships between periodontitis and diabetes.[14] The evidence for the effect of periodontitis on diabetes suggests that periodontal disease not only contributes to worsened glycemic control but also is associated with increased mortality and morbidity from cardiovascular disease and diabetic nephropathy.[15] There is also emerging evidence of a role for periodontal disease in development of new cases of type 2 and possibly gestational diabetes mellitus.[15] Further studies are necessary to confirm and extend these later findings.

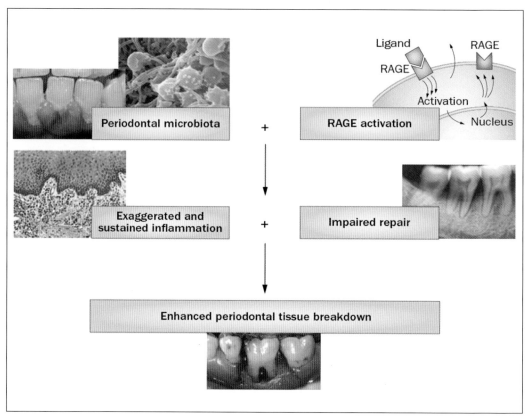

Fig 6-3 Relationship between systemic inflammation and periodontal breakdown. RAGE, receptor for advanced glycation endproducts.

Effects of periodontitis on glycemic control

There is evidence that periodontitis can adversely affect glycemic control in persons with diabetes, further supporting the bidirectional relationship of the two diseases. This evidence has been summarized in two systematic reviews.[8,15] Taylor et al,[16] in a longitudinal study, documented the adverse effects of periodontitis on glycemic control over time (Fig 6-4).

It is well known that acute and chronic infections adversely affect glycemic control in patients with diabetes.[17] Often glycemic control improves once such infections are resolved, so it is reasonable to predict that resolution of periodontal infections may improve glycemic control in patients with diabetes. A series of randomized controlled trials have addressed the question of whether, and to what extent, periodontal treatment improves glycemic control (Table 6-1). Several meta-analyses of intervention studies suggest that periodontal treatment results in a statistically significant reduction of HbA_{1c} level (a reduction of approximately 0.4% at 3 months) compared with no treatment for periodontal disease.[18–23] This is a clinical impact on diabetes management equivalent to adding a second agent to an antidiabetic drug treatment regimen.

Further studies are clearly needed in various patient groups, such as those who are resistant to antidiabetic drug therapy and lifestyle intervention and whose glycated hemoglobin levels remain elevated. In addition, optimal periodon-

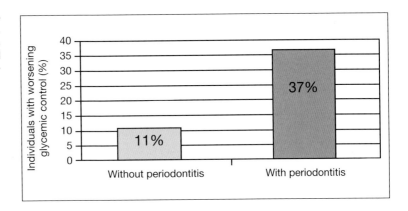

Fig 6-4 Results of a 2-year study indicating that periodontal disease affects glycemic control. (Reprinted from Taylor et al[16] with permission.)

Table 6-1	Effect of nonsurgical periodontal treatment on glycemic control in people with type 2 diabetes: All meta-analyses published as of May 2013					
Meta-analysis	No. of studies	No. of RCTs	Pooled no. of subjects	Change in HbA$_{1c}$ (%)	95% CI	P value
Janket et al[18]	4	1*	264	−0.7	−2.2, 0.9	NS
Darre et al[19]	9	9	485	−0.46†	0.11, 0.82	.01
Teeuw et al[20]	5	3*	180	−0.40†	−0.77, −0.04	.03
Simpson et al[21]	3	3	244	−0.40	−0.78, −0.01	.04
Sgolastra et al[22]	5	5	315	−0.65	−0.43, −0.88	< .05
Engebretson and Kocher[23]	9	9	775	−0.36	−0.54, −0.19	< .0001

RCTs, randomized controlled trials; CI, confidence interval; NS, not significant.
*Remaining (non-RCT) studies were clinical controlled trials.
†Standardized mean difference.

tal treatment aimed at reducing the periodontal pathogens is necessary to establish the extent to which these treatments help in restoring glycemic control. Most of these periodontal intervention studies were undertaken for 3 months, and longer studies are needed.

If the effects are reproducible and long term, periodontal therapy could be considered a part of the management of diabetes in view of its potential effect on glycemic control. This positive outcome would be above and beyond the beneficial effects of resolving periodontal infection to preserve the dentition, which in turn would lead to better nutrition, which would contribute indirectly to diabetes control, as discussed later in the chapter. Studies are also needed to determine if the prevention or treatment of periodontal disease and possibly other oral in-

fections can also reduce other complications of diabetes, including cardiovascular disease and nephropathy.

Guidelines for Dental Care of Patients with Diabetes

Diabetes mellitus is a common disorder among patients who are treated in dental practices. About 1 in 4 patients suffering from periodontitis also has diabetes mellitus. Periodontal disease adversely affects the metabolic control of diabetes patients. Furthermore, tooth loss from

Box 6-1	Guidelines for physicians and other medical professionals with regard to the oral health of patients with diabetes*

Because of the increased risk for development of periodontitis in patients with diabetes, the following recommendations are made:

- Patients with diabetes should be told that periodontal disease risk is increased by diabetes. They should also be told that if they suffer from periodontal disease their glycemic control may be more difficult and they are at higher risk for diabetic complications such as cardiovascular and kidney disease.
- As part of their initial evaluation, patients with type 1, type 2, or gestational diabetes should receive a thorough oral examination, which includes a comprehensive periodontal examination.
- For all patients who are newly diagnosed with type 1 or type 2 diabetes, subsequent periodontal examinations should occur (as directed by dental professionals) as part of their ongoing management of diabetes. Even if no periodontitis is diagnosed initially, annual periodontal review is recommended.
- Patients with diabetes presenting with any overt signs and symptoms of periodontitis, including loose teeth not associated with trauma, spacing or spreading of the teeth, gingival abscesses, and gingival suppuration, require prompt periodontal evaluation.
- Patients with diabetes who have extensive tooth loss should be encouraged to pursue dental rehabilitation to restore adequate mastication for proper nutrition.
- Oral health education should be provided to all patients with diabetes.
- Children and adolescents diagnosed with diabetes should be referred to a dental professional to receive annual oral screening for periodontal disease from the age of 6 to 7 years.
- Patients with diabetes should be advised that other oral conditions, such as dry mouth and burning mouth, may occur and, if so, they should seek advice from their dental practitioner. In addition, patients with diabetes are at increased risk of oral fungal infections and experience poorer wound healing than those who do not have diabetes.

*Reprinted from Chapple et al[8] with permission.

dental caries and periodontal disease can lead to poor nutrition, compromising dietary efforts at glycemic control and weight loss in patients with diabetes. Hence, excellent dental care aimed at maintaining a healthy dentition free of caries and periodontal disease is necessary for optimal care of patients with diabetes.

Medical history

A good medical history is especially important in patients with diabetes or individuals who are at risk for diabetes. Patients who have diabetes should be asked about the following:

- Duration of diabetes
- Type of diabetes
- Complications such as heart disease, kidney diseases, neuropathy, and others
- Recent glycemic control and/or HbA_{1c} levels
- Frequency of acute problems, especially hypoglycemic episodes
- Antidiabetic medications, including dosages and times of administration
- Concomitant medications, with an emphasis on those that may alter glucose control and those being used to prevent or manage complications of diabetes

Box 6-2	Guidelines for dental professionals with regard to the oral health of patients with diabetes*

- Patients with diabetes should be told that they are at increased risk for periodontitis. They should also be told that if they suffer from periodontal disease their glycemic control may be more difficult and they are at higher risk for other complications such as cardiovascular and kidney disease.
- Patients presenting with a diagnosis of type 1, type 2, or gestational diabetes should receive a thorough oral examination, which includes a comprehensive periodontal evaluation.
- If periodontitis is diagnosed, it should be properly managed. If no periodontitis is diagnosed initially, patients with diabetes should be placed on a preventive care regimen and monitored regularly for periodontal changes.
- Patients with diabetes who present with any acute oral or periodontal infections require prompt oral and periodontal care.
- Patients with diabetes who have extensive tooth loss should be encouraged to pursue dental rehabilitation to restore adequate mastication for proper nutrition.
- Oral health education should be provided to all patients with diabetes.
- Patients with diabetes should also be evaluated for other potential oral complications, including dry mouth, burning mouth, and candidal infections.
- An annual oral screening for early signs of periodontal involvement is recommended for children and adolescents diagnosed with diabetes, starting at the age of 6 years.
- Patients who present without a diagnosis of diabetes but who have obvious risk factors for type 2 diabetes and signs of periodontitis should be informed about their risk of having diabetes, assessed using a chairside HbA_{1c} test, and/or referred to a physician for appropriate diagnostic testing and follow-up care.

*Reprinted from Chapple et al[8] with permission.

Treatment planning modifications

Blood glucose monitoring should be considered before a dental procedure is started that may induce stress, bleeding, or pain. Patients with plasma glucose levels of less than 37 mg/dL should be given 15 g of oral carbohydrates before treatment. If the patient has chronically elevated blood glucose HbA_{1c} levels (>126 mg/dL), he or she should be referred to a physician for management to achieve adequate glycemic control. Adequate long-term glycemic control is crucial for maintenance of periodontal health and for proper healing after most oral procedures.

Appointments should be scheduled so that they do not coincide with peak insulin levels, because that is when patients are at increased risk of hypoglycemia. In general, morning appointments are best. Complications of diabetes, such as cardiovascular disease or renal disease, and the medications used to treat these complications must be considered in dental treatment planning.

Patients who are scheduled for major oral surgical procedures may require adjustments of their antidiabetic medication. These adjustments are best done in consultation with the physician who manages the patient's diabetes care.

Periodontal disease

Given the current evidence, the consensus of a group of clinical researchers is that it is appropriate to provide guidelines for periodontal care in patients with diabetes.[8] These guidelines for medical and dental professionals and recommendations for patients are reproduced in Boxes 6-1 to 6-4.

Box 6-3	Oral health recommendations for diabetic patients at the physician's office*

Why should I have my gums checked?

- If your physician has told you that you have diabetes, you should make an appointment with a dentist to have your mouth and gums checked.
- People with diabetes have a higher chance of getting gum disease.
- Gum disease can lead to tooth loss and may make your diabetes harder to control.

You may have gum disease if you have ever noticed:

- Red, bleeding, or swollen gums
- Pus from the gums
- Foul taste
- Longer-looking teeth
- Loose teeth
- Increasing spaces between your teeth
- Calculus (tartar) on your teeth

If you have noticed any of these problems, it is important to see a dentist as soon as possible.

Gum disease may be present and get worse without any symptoms that are apparent to you:

- Even if you do not think you have gum disease now, you should still get regular dental checkups as part of managing your diabetes.
- Your dentist will be able to pick up early signs of gum disease.

You need to clean your teeth and gums very carefully at home.

If you have diabetes, you may also suffer from dry mouth, burning mouth, yeast infections of the mouth, or poor healing of mouth wounds.

It is important to keep your mouth and your whole body as healthy as possible with regular dental and medical care.

*Reprinted from Chapple et al[8] with permission.

Tooth loss

Tooth loss, especially edentulism, can result in difficulty in chewing, which leads to poorer nutrition, and in poor esthetics and a negative social image.[24,25] Chronic periodontal disease and severe dental caries are the primary reasons for tooth loss in adults.[26] Factors such as low educational level, low socioeconomic status, greater age, poor access to care, lack of health insurance coverage, and a history of smoking are risk factors for tooth loss.

Because periodontal disease is associated with diabetes, it is important to consider whether diabetes is an underlying risk factor for tooth loss. Several studies of tooth loss in patients with diabetes have shown that there is a larger proportion of tooth loss, including edentulism, among individuals with diabetes. An analysis of the data from the 2003 to 2004 cycle of NHANES showed that the rate of edentulism

Box 6-4	Oral health recommendations for diabetic or prediabetic patients at the dental office*

People with diabetes have a higher chance of getting gum disease:

- If you have been told by your dentist that you have gum disease, you should follow up with necessary treatment as advised. This may require several appointments. Like diabetes, gum disease is a chronic condition and requires lifelong maintenance.
- You also need to clean your teeth and gums very carefully at home.
- If left untreated, gum disease may also make your diabetes harder to control.

Gum disease may be present and get worse without any symptoms that are apparent to you:

- If your dentist has told you that you do not have gum disease now, you should still get regular dental checkups as part of managing your diabetes.
- Your dentist will be able to pick up early signs of gum disease.

You may have gum disease if you ever notice:

- Red, bleeding, or swollen gums
- Pus from the gums
- Foul taste
- Longer-looking teeth
- Loose teeth
- Increasing spaces between your teeth
- Calculus (tartar) on your teeth

People with diabetes may also suffer from dry mouth, burning mouth, yeast infections of the mouth, or poor healing of mouth wounds.

If you have not been diagnosed with diabetes but your dentist identified some risk factors for diabetes, including signs of gum disease, it is important to get a medical checkup as advised:

- Your medical doctor can order blood tests to see if you have undiagnosed diabetes and can provide proper advice and care based on the results.
- Make an appointment to see your medical doctor as soon as possible.
- Remember to inform your dentist about the outcome of your visit to the medical doctor.

It is important to keep your mouth and your whole body as healthy as possible with regular dental and medical care.

*Reprinted from Chapple et al[8] with permission.

was 28% among those individuals aged 50 years or older with diabetes, while it was 14% in individuals of the same age group without diabetes.[27] Similarly, among individuals with at least some teeth, those with diabetes had a higher number of missing teeth than did adults without diabetes. This study carefully adjusted for other factors that also affected tooth loss, including age, race, level of education, and smoking.[27] Approximately 18% of cases of complete tooth loss in the United States are attributable to diabetes, which is of great concern in the management of patients with diabetes because tooth loss can affect diet.[27]

The association between tooth loss and reduced consumption of important dietary constituents, including fiber, fruits, and vegetables, has been reported.[28,29] In addition, a higher intake of saturated fatty acids is associated with tooth loss, which may help explain the association between edentulism and chronic heart disease.[30] It is also reasonable to assume that the reduced consumption of dietary fiber and fruits and vegetables accounts in part for the association between edentulism/tooth loss and diabetes.

A review of the overall health and food habits among older adults in Japan also sheds light on the relationship between tooth loss and diet.[31] A program has been in existence since 1991 to increase the number of individuals who reach the age of 80 years with 20 teeth (the "80/20" program). The percentage of 80/20 achievers increased from 10.9% in 1993 to 24.1% in 2005. Those who had retained 20 teeth at age 80 years consumed fewer total calories and lower levels of carbohydrates.[31] The change in the diet likely resulted in part from greater retention of teeth, and this is likely to be associated with better overall health.

A study of largely African American and American Indian older adult populations showed that those participants with fewer than 10 teeth consumed less fruit, meat, beans, and oils. They also derived more energy from solid fat, alcohol, and added sugar than did individuals with 11 or more teeth. Nutritional intervention for older individuals should certainly consider the effects of tooth loss on dietary patterns, especially in patients with diabetes.[32]

It is likely that the impact of periodontal disease on diabetes is in part related to increased levels of systemic inflammation and in part indirectly related to the altered diet associated with tooth loss. Both factors serve to worsen diabetes and its complications. Hence, early diagnosis, prevention, and effective treatment of periodontal disease have great potential to lessen the onset, progression, and complications of diabetes.

Other oral manifestations

There are other oral manifestations of diabetes that may impact dental care. Decreased salivary secretion and increased levels of cariogenic organisms, including *Streptococcus mutans* and *Lactobacillus*, may predispose patients, especially those with type 1 diabetes, to dental caries.[33] In addition, there are reports of oral mucosal disease in patients in diabetic popula-

tions. These include a greater predominance of fissured tongue and oral candidiasis.[34,35]

Complaints of xerostomia may be the result of thirst, which is common in patients with diabetes. Xerostomia also may result from sensory nerve dysfunction as a neurologic complication of diabetes. Xerostomia also may be caused by medications taken by patients with diabetes. If medications are determined to be the cause of the xerostomia, the clinician should consider altering the dose or changing the medication in consultation with the physician, which may provide relief for the patient. If this is not feasible, patients may benefit from the use of sugar-free gum or candy. They also may benefit from the use of non–alcohol-containing mouthrinses or saliva substitutes.

Diabetic neuropathy may manifest in the oral cavity as symptoms of burning mouth. The treatment protocols for xerostomia are also effective for burning mouth.

Neuropathy can also result in taste impairment in patients with diabetes.[36] This dysfunction can seriously affect the patient's ability to maintain a proper diet, which is central to glycemic control. The management of diabetic neuropathy may improve taste sensation; however, often such treatment is not effective. In any case, patients with altered taste sensation should be made aware that this is an unpleasant side effect of diabetes and that they should make efforts to consume a diet recommended to maintain healthy blood sugar levels as well as to control their weight while coping with the altered taste sensation.

Management of acute complications

Acute complications of diabetes may occur in the dental office, hypoglycemia being the most common. Ketoacidosis, especially in patients with type 1 diabetes, and hyperglycemic hyperosmolar syndrome may also occur.[36]

Hypoglycemia

Hypoglycemia, or a low level of blood glucose, is more likely to occur in patients with type 1 di-

Box 6-5	Management of hypoglycemia in the dental office[37]

- Give the patient 15 to 20 g of carbohydrates by mouth if possible (eg, 4 to 6 oz of fruit juice, 3 to 4 tsp sugar, or several pieces of hard candy).
- If the patient is not able to take food by mouth and an intravenous line is in place, administer 30 to 40 mL of 50% dextran (D50) or 1 mg of glucagon.
- If an intravenous line is not in place, administer 1 mg of glucagon subcutaneously or intramuscularly.
- The patient's plasma glucose should be checked in about 15 minutes; if the level is not near normal and the patient is still symptomatic, repeat the oral sugar dosage.
- If hypoglycemia persists or if the patient exhibits more severe symptoms of hypoglycemia, seek emergency medical care, because hypoglycemia can lead to seizures and death.

abetes who maintain tight glycemic control but may also occur in patients with type 2 diabetes. Hypoglycemia often results from insulin excess under normal circumstances. As blood glucose levels fall, insulin production decreases, and glucagon is then secreted from the pancreas, resulting in release of stored glucose from the liver. In addition, epinephrine is released, leading to a rise in blood glucose levels. If this normal physiologic response is dysfunctional, hypoglycemia may result. Epinephrine may also lead to many of the signs and symptoms of hypoglycemia, including shakiness, diaphoresis, and tachycardia.

The early symptoms and signs of hypoglycemia include confusion, agitation, anxiety, shakiness, and tremors. If hypoglycemia is not treated, more serious signs and symptoms, such as diaphoresis, dizziness, and tachycardia, may occur. This can lead to loss of consciousness and seizures and eventually death. Because severe hypoglycemia can be life-threatening, it should be treated promptly.

The risk factors for hypoglycemia include skipping or delaying of meals, too much insulin medication, an increase in exercise without adjustment of antidiabetic medication, excessive alcohol consumption, a past history of hypoglycemia, and long-term good glycemic control.

If a patient shows signs of hypoglycemia, the staff should follow the management protocol described in Box 6-5.

Ketoacidosis and hyperglycemic hyperosmolar syndrome

Ketoacidosis is a serious complication of diabetes that occurs when the body produces high levels of blood acids called *ketones,* which happens when the body cannot produce enough insulin. The symptoms often develop over 24 hours and include excessive thirst, frequent urination, nausea and vomiting, abdominal pain, fatigue, shortness of breath, fruit-scented breath, and confusion. High blood sugar levels and high urinary ketone levels are often found.

Hyperglycemic hyperosmolar syndrome involves extremely high blood sugar levels (without ketones) and dehydration. It is a complication of type 2 diabetes. Symptoms include confusion, increased thirst, lethargy, fever, nausea, weakness, and perhaps convulsions.

Both ketoacidosis and hyperglycemic hyperosmolar syndrome are less common than hypoglycemia, but they can occur in dental offices. Ketoacidosis is seen in patients with type 1 diabetes and is reversed with insulin therapy. Hyperglycemia most often reverses as the blood sugar level returns to normal or near-normal levels. Severe symptoms of both conditions can be serious and should be handled as a medical emergency.

Medical Management of Diabetes Mellitus

To provide optimal care for their patients with diabetes, dental practitioners must be familiar with the principles and implications of the medical management of the disease. Treatment of diabetes involves lifestyle changes and medications that help reduce hyperglycemia. It also includes preventive and treatment interventions to manage complications such as retinopathy, cardiovascular and cerebrovascular diseases, nephropathy, and neuropathy as well as other complications such as periodontitis. Proper diet, exercise, and good oral hygiene are lifestyle changes that are essential.[37]

Lifestyle changes

Diet is a pivotal intervention with the goals of improving glycemic control, reducing weight, and achieving lipid control.[38] Dietary carbohydrate control is especially important; this includes restrictions on the intake of refined carbohydrates and an emphasis on overall carbohydrate consumption that consists mostly of whole grains, fruit, vegetables, and low-fat milk.[39] Fat intake is limited to 30% of the total caloric intake and proteins to 10% to 20% of total caloric intake. Alcohol should be consumed with food and limited to one drink per day for women and two per day for men.[40,41]

Exercise is another essential component of diabetes control. In addition to weight loss, exercise is associated with a decrease in hyperglycemia as well as increased insulin sensitivity in patients with diabetes.[42] In addition, exercise may control hypertension and improve lipid profiles and thereby reduce the risk of the cardiovascular and cerebrovascular complications common in patients with diabetes.

Lifestyle changes have been shown in several studies to delay, and perhaps prevent, the onset of diabetes in individuals who exhibit impaired fasting glucose (prediabetic subjects) and obesity. In one study, lifestyle changes, including loss of 7% to 10% of body weight and an average of 5 sessions of 30 minutes each per week of moderate exercise, resulted in a 58% reduction in the incidence of development of type 2 diabetes over 3 years, compared with a placebo control group in which extensive lifestyle changes were not implemented.[43]

Of course, careful medical evaluation should be undertaken for diabetic complications that may alter the exercise regimen. Patients should check their blood glucose levels before beginning exercise and after exercise if any of the signs or symptoms of hypoglycemia occur.

Antidiabetic medications

Several studies have shown that pharmacologic intervention for glucose control may reduce the risk of complications associated with diabetes over 10 or more years. The Diabetes Control and Complications Trial carried out in the United States in patients with type 1 diabetes showed that maintaining near-normal plasma glucose levels reduced the risk of microvascular complications, including retinopathy, neuropathy, and nephropathy.[44] Similar delays in the onset and progression of microvascular complications are likely in patients with type 2 diabetes who maintain good blood glucose control.[45]

In a second large study, the United Kingdom Prospective Diabetes Study, patients with type 2 diabetes were prescribed an intensive lifestyle regimen.[46] A control group was compared to an intensive therapy group, which was prescribed sulfonylureas or insulin with an aim to achieving a fasting plasma glucose level of 108 mg/dL. During a median follow-up time of 10 years, a mean HbA_{1c} level of 7.0% was achieved by the intensive treatment group, while the control group exhibited a mean HbA_{1c} level of 7.9%. This resulted in a 25% risk reduction for combined eye, kidney, and nerve complications in the intensive control group. Interestingly, there was little or no effect on macrovascular endpoints, including cardiovascular disease.

These studies point to the importance of glycemic control in preventing microvascular complications; however, it is not yet clear to what extent glycemic control alone will result in a reduction in the risk of cardiovascular complications. It appears that a reduction of other cardiovascular risk factors, including dyslipidemia and hypertension, as well as glycemic control is needed to reduce the risk of cardiovascular disease in patients with type 2 diabetes.

It is important to understand that antidiabetic medications can lead to side effects, including hypoglycemia.

Insulin

Insulin therapy is used by all patients with type 1 diabetes. It is also used by many individuals with type 2 diabetes, especially when diet and oral medication are inadequate to obtain glycemic control. Insulin preparations differ markedly in their onset, peak time of action, and effective duration. It is important for the dentist to know the peak insulin action time for the insulin preparation that the patient is using, because this period is when the risk for hypoglycemia is highest. Insulin analogs, especially those that are very long-acting such as insulin glargine, are associated with lower risk for hypoglycemia.

Oral antidiabetic agents

Oral antidiabetic agents also vary in their risk of inducing hypoglycemia. The sulfonylureas have high (glyburide or glipizide) to moderate (glimepiride) risk. Other antidiabetic medications have low risk, including acarbose and miglitol. Others pose very low risk; these include metformin, rosiglitazone, and pioglitazone. Some of the more recently approved antidiabetic agents, such as pramlintide and exenatide, have hypoglycemia as a side effect when they are added to sulfonylureas.

Effect on dental care

Effective management of diabetes and complications of diabetes is a dynamic field, changing with the introduction of new antidiabetic medications, insulin pumps, and pancreas transplants, as well as introduction of glucose monitoring and self-monitoring procedures. Effective management includes dietary and exercise regimens, which require compliance by the patient.

Management of dental patients with diabetes requires the dental practitioner to understand each patient's diabetes-management regimen, the success or shortcomings of treatment, and the long-term prognosis for the patient. The dental professional can also assist the medical team in comanaging patients who have both dental diseases and diabetes. It is not known to what extent management of glycemic control will result in control of periodontal disease, but the strong correlation between uncontrolled hyperglycemia and periodontal disease suggests that management of hyperglycemia will likely result in less risk of periodontal disease. What is known is that healing is better in patients who have good glycemic control; hence, the response to dental therapy, especially surgical therapy, is likely to be better in patients with good glycemic control.

Screening for Diabetes in the Dental Office

Knowledge of the diabetic status of dental patients, especially those with periodontal disease and other oral manifestations of diabetes, is important for their oral as well as overall care. Uncontrolled diabetes is associated with increased progression of periodontal disease.[6] Early diagnosis of diabetes and stabilization of glycemic control can reduce the risk of complications. Furthermore, early detection of prediabetes and intensive lifestyle changes can reduce the incidence of type 2 diabetes. Therefore, early diagnosis of diabetes and identification of patients at high risk for diabetes (ie, those with prediabetes) are important for the overall management of diabetes and especially important for patients who are also seeking dental care, including periodontal treatment and dental implants.

The dental office is an underutilized point of contact with the health care system. Recently, the dental office has been proposed as a site for screening for undiagnosed diabetes and prediabetes, because 60% or more of the US population had seen a dentist in the previous 2 years.[47] In a dental clinic population, prediabetes was predicted in more than 90% of patients having 4 or more missing teeth, periodontal probing depths of 5 mm or more at about 25% of sites, and a capillary blood HbA_{1c} level of 5.7% or greater.[48]

In a recent field trial, diabetes screening was carried out for 1,022 dental patients aged 45 years and older.[49] The patients were eligible for the study if they had no knowledge of their diabetes status; more than 40% of the 1,022 dental patients had a capillary blood HbA_{1c} level equal to or greater than 5.7%. HbA_{1c} levels of 5.7% to 6.4% are defined by the American Diabetes Association as high risk for diabetes or prediabetes, and a level of 6.5% or higher is a diagnostic criterion for diabetes. Hence, in this study, any patient with a screening HbA_{1c} level equal to or greater than 5.7% was referred to a physician for evaluation. Of the patients referred and for whom a diagnosis was returned to the dental office, 12% had diabetes, and 23% were at high risk for diabetes (prediabetes). This study had a reasonably high yield; that is, 15% of the 1,022 screened patients had either prediabetes or diabetes. None of these dental patients admitted knowledge of having diabetes or being at high risk for diabetes prior to this screening. The potential is for detection of diabetes or prediabetes in 1 of 8 dental patients over the age of 45 years who are unaware of their diabetes status.

Barriers to full implementation of HbA_{1c} screening for prediabetes and diabetes in dental practices include cost, lack of insurance reimbursement, and, perhaps most important, patient compliance with the referral to seek a medical diagnosis. Many of these barriers can likely be overcome in the future. Capillary blood screening for HbA_{1c} is a feasible, accurate method of screening for diabetes and prediabetes in a dental practice. The yield could be improved by triaging patients based on prior existing periodontal disease, missing teeth, and their risk profile for diabetes.

Diabetes screening at clinical sites such as dental offices and pharmacies could be of great service, because at present 26% of individuals with diabetes are unaware of their condition.[1] Furthermore, a large percentage of individuals with prediabetes are unaware of their high risk for development of diabetes. As was already mentioned, early treatment of diabetes can lead to better glycemic control with fewer medications and fewer complications. In addition, intensive lifestyle modifications in patients with prediabetes can prevent the onset of diabetes at least over a 3-year period.[43] This is one of the few chronic diseases for which a safe and effective regimen has been developed to prevent its onset.

Of course, patients often do not comply with intensive lifestyle changes such as dietary changes or exercise regimens on a long-term basis. Dental professionals can help patients to comply with these regimens, because dentists often see these patients regularly; the dental team can reinforce the need for intensive lifestyle modification to sustain diabetes prevention or management.

A clinical pathway program has been developed to share medical and dental information to provide optimal care for patients with diabetes who seek periodontal care.[50] By linking patients' medical and dental records, this team has shown that coordinated treatment planning can be carried out by physicians and dentists and that outcomes are improved when treatment is coordinated for those patients with both diabetes and dental disease.

In another study, medical conditions associated with dental conditions, including periodontitis, were discovered using linked electronic medical records.[51] In this study, the shared electronic health records of 2,475 patients who were undergoing dental treatment in a dental school and medical treatment in the same university hospital were assessed. Diabetes mellitus types 1 and 2, hypertension, hypercholesterolemia, hyperlipidemia, and conditions related to adverse pregnancy were associated with periodontitis. For effective comanagement of patients who attend both dental school clinics and their related medical colleges for treatment, it is important that specific patients who suffer from these dental and medical conditions be identified. This would allow treatment plans and management to be coordinated to promote better overall health in patients.

Many risk factors, including smoking and obesity, are common to periodontal disease and other chronic diseases, including cardiovascular disease and cancer as well as diabetes. Modification of these common risk factors by both the dental and medical teams, working in a coordinated fashion, has great potential to provide major benefits to society in reducing the morbidity and mortality associated with these prevalent chronic diseases as well as the risk for periodontal disease.

In the chronic care model, collaboration by physicians, dentists, and other health care professionals can be carried out to achieve better clinical outcomes for patients. These practice models offer great potential benefit. Effective patient communication and patient cooperation are essential for success, and these can be enhanced by new practice models.[52,53] Interprofessional patient management may be most optimally carried out in a chronic care model or in a medical home model, but with some effort it is also likely to be successful in more traditional practice settings.

The health benefits and actual costs associated with dental office screening for and interprofessional management of diabetes need to be rigorously evaluated by well-designed randomized field clinical trials under actual practice conditions.

plications of diabetes, such as xerostomia and tooth loss. Dentists should be aware of any antidiabetic medications patients are taking and ensure that glycemic control is adequate before undertaking any procedures. Dentists must be aware of the signs and symptoms of acute complications of diabetes, such as hypoglycemia, diabetic ketoacidosis, and hyperglycemic hyperosmolar syndrome, and how to manage these conditions.

Likewise, dental patients who have periodontal disease and exhibit additional risk factors for diabetes, such as obesity, should be made aware of the relationship between these two diseases and referred to their physician for assessment of their diabetic status.

Early identification and early treatment of diabetes and prediabetes have many benefits for the patient in terms of improved health and reduced risk of complications. It appears that involvement of the dental profession in early screening could have a beneficial effect. Furthermore, the use of common electronic health records, coordinated treatment planning, and common risk factor management among dentists, physicians, pharmacists, nurses, and other health care professionals is likely to improve outcomes and the overall health of patients with diabetes and periodontitis as well as reduce overall patient care cases.

Conclusion

Diabetes and periodontitis are two common, serious conditions that have a bidirectional association. The prevalence and incidence of periodontal disease are greater in patients with type 1 or type 2 diabetes. Furthermore, periodontitis can adversely affect glycemic control in patients with diabetes. The reciprocal effects of diabetes on periodontitis and of periodontitis on diabetes are likely based on their both contributing to a hyperinflammatory state.

Dental management of patients with diabetes requires extra caution and, when possible, coordination of care with their physician. Such patients should be routinely assessed for periodontal involvement as well as other oral com-

References

1. American Diabetes Association. National Diabetes Fact Sheet. http://www.diabetes.org/in-my-community /local-offices/miami-florida/assets/files/ada-fact -sheet-2011-one-pager.pdf. Accessed January 2011.
2. DeFronzo RA, Ferrannini E. Insulin resistance. A multifaceted syndrome responsible for NIDDM, obesity, hypertension, dyslipidemia and atherosclerotic cardiovascular disease. Diabetes Care 1991; 14:173–194.
3. Eke PI, Dye BA, Wei L, Thornton-Evans GO, Genco RJ. Prevalence of periodontitis in adults in the United States: 2009 and 2010. J Dent Res 2012;91: 914–920.
4. Petersen PE, Ogawa H. The global burden of periodontal disease: towards integration with chronic disease prevention and control. Periodontol 2000 2012;60:15–39.

5. Weinspach K, Staufenbiel I, Memenga-Nicksch S, Ernst S, Geurtsen W, Gunay H. Level of information about the relationship between diabetes mellitus and periodontitis—Results from a nationwide diabetes information program. Eur J Med Res 2013; 18:6.

6. Genco RJ, Borgnakke WS. Risk factors for periodontal disease. Periodontology 2000 2012;61:1–37.

7. Grossi S, Genco RJ. Periodontal disease and diabetes mellitus: A two-way relationship. Ann Periodontol 1998;3:51–61.

8. Chapple ILC, Genco R, Working Group 2 of the Joint EFP/AAP Workshop. Diabetes and periodontal diseases: Consensus report of the Joint EFP/AAP Workshop on Periodontitis and Systemic Diseases. J Clin Periodontol 2013;40(suppl 14):S106–S112.

9. Chavarry NG, Vettore MV, Sansone C, Sheiham A. The relationship between diabetes mellitus and destructive periodontal disease. Oral Health Prev Dent 2009;7:107–127.

10. Emrich LJ, Shlossman M, Genco RJ. Periodontal disease in non-insulin dependent diabetes mellitus. J Periodontol 1991;62:123–130.

11. Losche W, Karapetow F, Pohl A, Pohl C, Kocher T. Plasma lipid and blood glucose levels in patients with destructive periodontal disease. J Clin Periodontol 2000;27:537–541.

12. Zadik Y, Bechor R, Galor S, Levin L. Periodontal disease might be associated even with impaired fasting glucose. Br Dent J 2010;208:E20.

13. Lalla E, Kunzel C, Burkett S, Cheng B, Lamster IB. Identification of unrecognized diabetes and pre-diabetes in a dental setting. J Dent Res 2011;90:855–860.

14. Taylor JJ, Preshaw PM, Lalla E. A review of the evidence for pathogenic mechanisms that may link periodontitis and diabetes. J Periodontol 2013;84(4 suppl):S113–S134.

15. Borgnakke WS, Ylostalo PV, Taylor GW, Genco RJ. Effect of periodontal disease on diabetes: Systematic review of epidemiologic observational evidence. J Periodontol 2013;84(4 suppl):S135–S152.

16. Taylor GW, Burt BA, Becker MP, et al. Severe periodontitis and risk for poor glycemic control in subjects with non-insulin-dependent diabetes mellitus. J Periodontol 1996;67(suppl):1085–1093.

17. Sammalkorpi K. Glucose intolerance in acute infections. J Intern Med 1989;225:15–19.

18. Janket SJ, Wightman A, Baird AE, Van Dyke TE, Jones JA. Does periodontal treatment improve glycemic control in diabetic patients? A meta-analysis of intervention studies. J Dent Res 2005;84:1154–1159.

19. Darre L, Vergnes JN, Gourdy P, Sixou M. Efficacy of periodontal treatment on glycaemic control in diabetic patients: A meta-analysis of interventional studies. Diabetes Metab 2008;34:497–506.

20. Teeuw WJ, Gerdes VE, Loos BG. Effect of periodontal treatment on glycemic control of diabetic patients: A systematic review and meta-analysis. Diabetes Care 2010;33:421–427.

21. Simpson TC, Needleman I, Wild SH, Moles DR, Mills EJ. Treatment of periodontal disease for glycaemic control in people with diabetes. Cochrane Database Syst Rev 2010;(5):CD004714.

22. Sgolastra F, Severino M, Pietropaoli D, Gatto R, Monaco A. Effectiveness of periodontal treatment to improve metabolic control in patients with chronic periodontitis and type 2 diabetes: A meta-analysis of randomized clinical trials. J Periodontol 2013;84:958–973.

23. Engebretson S, Kocher T. Evidence that periodontal treatment improves diabetes outcomes: A systematic review and meta-analysis. J Periodontol 2013;84(4 suppl):S153–S163.

24. Beltran-Aguilar ED, Barker LK, Canto MT, et al. Centers for Disease Control and Prevention. Surveillance for dental caries, dental sealants, tooth retention, edentulism, and enamel fluorosis: United States, 1988–1994 and 1999–2002. MMWR Surveill Summ 2005;54(3):1–43.

25. Sheiham A, Cushing AM, Maizels J. The social impact of dental disease. In: Slade GD (ed). Measuring Oral Health and Quality of Life. Chapel Hill, NC: Department of Dental Ecology, School of Dentistry, University of North Carolina, 1997:47–56.

26. Thorstensson H, Johansson B. Why do some people lose teeth across their lifespan whereas others retain a functional dentition into very old age? Gerodontology 2010;27:19–25.

27. Patel MH, Kumar JV, Moss ME. Diabetes and tooth loss. An analysis of data from the National Health and Nutrition Examination Survey, 2003–2004. J Am Dent Assoc 2013;144:478–485.

28. Felton DA. Edentulism and co-morbid factors. J Prosthodont 2009;18:88–96.

29. Sheiman A, Steele JG, Marcenes W, et al. The relationship among dental status, nutrient intake, and nutritional status in older people. J Dent Res 2001;80:408–413.

30. Elter JR, Champagne CM, Offenbacher S, Beck JD. Relationship of periodontal disease and tooth loss to prevalence of coronary heart disease. J Periodontol 2004;75:782–790.

31. Yamanaka K, Nakagaki H, Morita I, Suzaki H, Hashimoto M, Sakai T. Comparison of the health condition between the 8020 achievers and the 8020 non-achievers. Int Dent J 2008;58:146–150.

32. Savoca MR, Arcury TA, Leng X, et al. Severe tooth loss in older adults as a key indicator of compromised dietary quality. Public Health Nutr 2010; 13:466–474.

33. Karajalainen KM, Knuuttila ML, Kaar ML. Salivary factors in children and adolescents with insulin-dependent diabetes mellitus. Pediatr Dent 1996;18: 306–311.

34. Guggenheimer J, Moore PA, Rossie K, et al. Insulin-dependent diabetes mellitus and oral soft tissue pathologies. 1. Prevalence and characteristics of non-candidal lesions. Oral Surg Oral Med Oral Pathol Oral Radiol Endod 2000;89:563–539.

35. Guggenheimer J, Moore PA, Rossie K, et al. Insulin-dependent diabetes mellitus and oral soft tissue pathologies. 2. Prevalence and characteristics of Candida and candidal lesions. Oral Surg Oral Med Oral Pathol Oral Radiol Endod 2000;89:570–576.

36. Mealey BL. Diabetes mellitus. In: Greenberg MS, Glick M (eds). Burket's Oral Medicine: Diagnosis and Treatment, ed 10. Hamilton, ON: Decker, 2003: 563–577.

37. Kidambi S, Patel S. Diabetes mellitus: A medical overview. In: Genco RJ, Willams RC (eds). Periodontal Disease and Overall Health: A Clinician's Guide. Yardley, PA: Professional Audience Communications, 2010:55–82. http://www.colgateprofessional.com/LeadershipUS/ProfessionalEducation/Articles/Resources/pdf/OSCD.pdf. Accessed 3 September 2013.

38. Fernandez-Real JM, Ricart W. Insulin resistance and chronic cardiovascular inflammatory syndrome. Endocr Rev 2003;24:278–301.

39. Sheard NF, Clark NG, Brand-Miller JC, et al. Dietary carbohydrate (amount and type) in the prevention and management of diabetes: A statement by the American Diabetes Association. Diabetes Care 2004;27:2266–2271.

40. Franz MJ, Bantle JP, Beebe JP, et al. Evidence-based nutrition principles and recommendations for the treatment and prevention of diabetes and related complications. Diabetes Care 2003;26(suppl 1): S51–S61.

41. Franz MJ, Bantle JP, Beebe JP, et al. Nutrition principles and recommendations in diabetes. Diabetes Care 2004;27(suppl 1):S36–S46.

42. Eriksonn J, Taimola S, Eriksson K, Parviainen S, Peltonen J, Kujula U. Resistance training in the treatment of non-insulin dependent diabetes mellitus. Int J Sports Med 1997;18:242–246.

43. Knowler WC, Barrett-Connor E, Fowler SE, et al. Reduction in the incidence of type 2 diabetes with lifestyle intervention or metformin. N Engl J Med 2002;346:393–403.

44. Diabetes Control and Complications Trial Research Group. The effect of intensive treatment of diabetes on the development and progression of long-term complications in insulin-dependent diabetes mellitus. N Engl J Med 1993;329:977–986.

45. Ohkubo Y, Kishikawa H, Araki E, et al. Intensive insulin therapy prevents the progression of diabetic microvascular complications in Japanese patients with non-insulin-dependent diabetes mellitus: A randomized prospective 6-year study. Diabetes Res Clin Pract 1995;28:103–117.

46. U.K. Prospective Diabetes Study (UKPDS) Group. Intensive blood-glucose control with sulphonylureas or insulin compared with conventional treatment and risk of complications in patients with type 2 diabetes (UKPDS 33). Lancet 1998;352:837–853.

47. Strauss SM, Tuthill J, Singh G, et al. A novel intra-oral diabetes screening approach in periodontal patients: Results of a pilot study. J Periodontol 2012;83:699–706.

48. Lalla E, Kunzel C, Burkett S, Cheng B, Lamster IB. Identification of unrecognized diabetes and prediabetes in dental setting. J Dent Res 2011;90:855–860.

49. Genco RJ, Schifferle RE, Dunford RG, Falkner KL, Hsu WC, Balukjian J. Screening for diabetes mellitus in dental practices: A field trial. J Am Dent Assoc [in press].

50. Ota M, Seshima F, Okubo N, et al. A collaborative approach to care for patients with periodontitis and diabetes. Bull Tokyo Dent Coll 2013;54:51–57.

51. Boland MR, Hripcsak G, Albers DJ, et al. Discovering medical conditions associated with periodontitis using linked electronic health records. J Clin Periodontol 2013;40:474–482.

52. Bojadzievski T, Gabbay RA. Patient-centered medical home and diabetes. Diabetes Care 2011;34: 1047–1053.

53. Stellefson M, Dipnarine K, Stopka C. The chronic care model and diabetes management in US primary care settings: A systematic review. Prev Chronic Dis 2013;10:E26.

Clinical Considerations:
What You Can Take Back to Your Practice

What is the effect of oral health on cardiovascular disease?

Epidemiologic studies show strong associations between poor oral health and cardiovascular disease. This association may differ among different populations and age groups.

Are oral infections independent risk factors for the development of cardiovascular disease?

Epidemiologic studies demonstrate strong associations between oral infections and cardiovascular disease and events. The effect is of clinical significance and is independent of other known risk factors. However, we cannot yet claim that oral infections are causes for the development or progression of cardiovascular events.

What is the biologic plausibility of the association between oral health and cardiovascular disease?

Oral microbes colonize atherosclerotic plaque via bacteremia, and they may contribute to the eventual destabilization of the plaque. They may also lead to myocardial infarction or ischemic stroke. Also, oral microbes contribute to the cumulative burden of systemic inflammatory responses that may lead to atherosclerosis.

Does the delivery of oral health care contribute to improvement of cardiovascular disease outcomes?

Well-designed intervention studies demonstrate improvement in several established biomarkers for cardiovascular disease. However, there are no studies showing improved clinical signs or symptoms.

Is it safe to provide dental care to patients with cardiovascular disease?

From the perspective of disseminating oral bacteria, the transient bacteremia caused by infrequent dental procedures represents much less hazard than everyday activities such as toothbrushing and flossing or mastication of hard food items. Provision of dental care to patients at risk for ischemic events should be done after consultation with the attending physician/cardiologist.

What is the appropriate message to give to the public about the association between oral health and cardiovascular disease?

Gum disease and heart disease may go together, but scientists cannot yet prove that one leads to the other. The association may be due to unhealthy lifestyles (eg, smoking, poor nutrition, sedentary lifestyle). Adopting healthy lifestyles in the context of oral health prevention or treatment may bring benefits to atherosclerosis onset and development. Microbes that usually live in the mouth enter the bloodstream, especially in the presence of gum disease. Therefore, it is important for clinicians to emphasize to their patients that health of the mouth is part of overall health and well-being.

The Cardiovascular System and Oral Infections

7

Maurizio S. Tonetti, DMD, PhD, MMSc
Filippo Graziani, DDS, MClinDent, PhD

The hypothesis that oral infections may contribute to atherosclerosis was formulated in the mid-1980s by a group of Finnish cardiologists.[1] It is relevant to attempt an understanding of the rationale for this line of research. Groundbreaking epidemiologic studies had identified the "classic" risk factors for atherosclerosis, but cardiologists were faced with the clinical dilemma that only 1 in 2 heart attacks could be explained by the classic set of risk factors: hypertension, dyslipidemia, diabetes, and smoking. Research was needed to identify mechanisms that explained a significant portion of the burden of disease and, more importantly, to find ways to prevent it. An interesting hypothesis that chronic infection (and later chronic inflammation) may contribute to the atherosclerotic process was formulated. In this broader context, and given the obvious high prevalence of chronic oral infections, early associations were sought between the presence of oral infections and cardiovascular events: Subjects with acute cardiovascular events seemed to have poorer oral health than control subjects. The field was born.

At the turn of the 21st century, an impressive collection of scientific evidence stood in support of the hypothesis that chronic infections were among the major contributors to atherosclerosis and its sequelae. The validity of this hypothesis was confirmed by studies indicating that individuals exposed to chronic infections have 2 to 3 times greater odds of having carotid atherosclerosis.[2] Chronic obstructive pulmonary disease with infectious exacerbations, chronic bronchitis, chronic sinusitis, and chronic or recurrent urinary tract infections—as well as an amorphous group of "other" infections—were all associated with higher odds of carotid atherosclerosis. Pathogens sustaining these chronic infections were considered either to have a direct effect on the vasculature or to act as a source of systemic inflammation that in turn would trigger the atherosclerotic process. Indeed, epidemiologic studies linking systemic inflammation, atherosclerosis, and cardiovascular events have shown consistent associations between levels of systemic inflammatory markers and increases in carotid intima-media thickness, myocardial infarction, and nonhemorrhagic stroke.

The infection hypothesis was tested with clinical randomized controlled trials (RCTs) aimed at preventing cardiovascular events with the use of long-acting broad-spectrum antibiotics such as azithromycin. Early reports showed encouraging results, but later full-scale studies and meta-analyses showed no preventive effect from antibiotic treatment.[3] The infection hypothesis had failed to provide a tangible benefit.

Table 7-1	Estimated difference in serum CRP concentration between individuals with periodontitis and individuals without periodontitis*[†]			
Study or subcategory	**n**	**Periodontitis CRP mean (SD)**	**n**	**Control CRP mean (SD)**
Bizzarro et al[7] SeP	38	3.10 (4.40)	39	1.90 (2.00)
Bizzarro et al[7] MoP	53	3.10 (3.30)	39	1.90 (2.00)
Salzberg et al[8] GaP	93	3.72 (2.88)	91	1.54 (2.95)
Salzberg et al[8] LaP	97	2.57 (2.95)	91	1.54 (2.95)
Havemose-Poulsen et al[9] GaP	27	5.00 (2.70)	25	3.00 (2.00)
Havemose-Poulsen et al[9] LaP	18	5.00 (5.40)	25	3.00 (2.00)
Joshipura et al[10]	91	2.20 (2.25)	377	1.80 (3.00)
Buhlin et al[11]	50	3.28 (4.64)	46	1.74 (1.68)
Amar et al[12]	17	2.30 (2.30)	21	1.00 (1.00)
Craig et al[13]	44	5.78 (1.07)	25	2.46 (1.44)
Noack et al[14]	50	4.06 (5.55)	65	1.70 (1.91)
Loos et al[15]	107	2.64 (3.48)	43	1.21 (1.34)
Fredriksson et al[16]	17	2.62 (2.90)	17	0.87 (1.73)
Total (95% CI)	**702**		**904**	

Test for heterogeneity: $Chi^2 = 51.41$; $df = 12$ ($P < .00001$), $I^2 = 76.7\%$. *(continued on next page)*
Test for overall effect: $Z = 5.42$ ($P < .00001$).
*Reprinted from Paraskevas et al[6] with permission.
[†]Case-control studies.
WMD, weighted mean difference; SD, standard deviation; CI, confidence interval; df, degrees of freedom; SeP, severe periodontitis; MoP, moderate periodontitis; GaP, generalized aggressive periodontitis; LaP, localized aggressive periodontitis.

From the moment the systematic review showed that there was no benefit in using systemic antibiotics to eliminate obscure infections to prevent cardiovascular events, the hypothesis that oral infections could contribute to the overall atherosclerotic burden was seen with less favor. Supporters of the link between oral infection and atherosclerosis pointed out that azithromycin or other systemic antibiotics would fail to act specifically against biofilm-centered infections, such as periodontitis.[4] Indeed, the periodontal literature has shown only marginal effects from the use of systemic antibiotics in the absence of mechanical root instrumentation (biofilm dispersion).[5]

This is at least part of the reason why many researchers active in this field stress that periodontitis is a source of chronic, nonresolving inflammation and frequently play down the fact that periodontitis is a biofilm-centered infection:

Cardiologists these days are much less excited about infection than about inflammation as a mechanism leading to atherosclerosis.

From an oral health standpoint, the hypothesis of a relationship between oral health and systemic diseases fits very well with the key developments of our understanding of periodontitis established in the late 1980s to mid-1990s: the existence of a systemic predisposition to periodontitis and in general the existence of a relationship between local periodontal disease and systemic inflammatory and immune challenges. Indeed, both epidemiologic research pointing to the existence of high-risk groups and pathophysiologic research pointing to the existence of biochemical changes that would prime healthy sites in diseased subjects toward susceptibility to periodontitis seem to be consistent with the notion that the periodontal disease process does not remain localized to the

WMD (random) 95% CI	Weight (%)	WMD (random) [95% CI]
	6.40	1.20 [–0.33, 2.73]
	8.11	1.20 [0.11, 2.29]
	9.10	2.18 [1.34, 3.02]
	9.10	1.03 [0.19, 1.87]
	7.33	2.00 [0.71, 3.29]
	3.53	2.00 [–0.61, 4.61]
	10.16	0.40 [–0.15, 0.95]
	6.98	1.54 [0.17, 2.91]
	7.77	1.30 [0.13, 2.47]
	9.84	3.32 [2.67, 3.97]
	6.14	2.36 [0.75, 3.97]
	9.38	1.43 [0.66, 2.20]
	6.15	1.75 [0.14, 3.36]
	100.00	1.65 [1.05, 2.24]

-4   -2   0   2   4

oral cavity and that the organism as a whole senses what is going on in the periodontium. A critical piece of evidence in this regard was the publication of a systematic review and meta-analysis of the systemic inflammatory changes associated with periodontitis.[6] In case-control studies, individuals with periodontitis showed 1.65-mg/L higher concentrations of C-reactive protein (CRP) than did unaffected subjects[7–16] (Table 7-1). This finding was significant in several ways. First, it established that periodontitis is sensed by the innate acute-phase response system and leads to a chronic systemic inflammatory status. Second, the size of the elevation in CRP was remarkable: CRP is an excellent predictor of cardiovascular outcomes, and cardiovascular risk has been predicted based on serum CRP concentrations. An increase of the magnitude observed for periodontitis is sufficient to shift an otherwise healthy subject to a high-risk category. These data support the hypothesis that periodontitis—as a chronic inflammatory condition driven by a biofilm-centered infection—contributes to the systemic inflammatory load of a subject.

Mechanisms

Over the last two decades, a wealth of mechanistic data has explored potential mechanisms at the basis of the biologic plausibility of the association between periodontitis and atherosclerosis. Mainly two types of mechanisms are involved: (1) Bacteria from periodontal disease may enter the circulation[17] and contribute directly to the development of atherogenesis (or thrombosis) and/or (2) systemic inflammation, resulting from periodontitis, can contribute to atherosclerotic cardiovascular disease (ACVD). These data have been reviewed in depth by the recent European Federation of Periodontology/American Academy of Periodontology (EFP/AAP) workshop.[18,19]

There are some biologic suggestions of a potential role of periodontal pathogens on the formation of atherosclerotic plaque. Oral and systemic inoculation of *Porphyromonas gingivalis* in apolipoprotein E–deficient (ie, more susceptible to atherosclerosis) animal models has shown that together with infection of periodontal tissues, which was measured as alveolar bone loss, a systemic response toward *P gingivalis* was mounted.[20,21] Higher aortic expression of vascular cell adhesion molecule 1 and tissue factor was also noted in the *P gingivalis*–inoculated animals.[20] Moreover, atherosclerotic lesions of the proximal aortas and aortic trees were more advanced and occurred earlier in *P gingivalis*–challenged animals.[21] Conversely, atherosclerotic lesions did not appear in the control animals despite their higher susceptibility.

The following findings provide further evidence of the association between periodontal pathogens and atherosclerosis:

- *The DNA of periopathogens has been localized within atherosclerotic plaque.* Assessment of 50 human endoarterectomy specimens showed that in at least 44% of the specimens, the DNA of some target periopathogens, including *Tanerella forsythia*, *P gingivalis*, and *Actinobacillus actinomycetemcomitans*, was present.[22] Further studies confirmed these findings.[23,24]
- *Periopathogens are able to invade endothelial cells.* *P gingivalis* has shown the capability to invade several cell lines, and the majority of *P gingivalis* strains may invade vascular tissues.[25]
- *Periopathogens may trigger platelet aggregation on their membrane.* Platelet aggregation is characteristic of atheromas. It has been shown that *P gingivalis* may facilitate platelet aggregation through its fimbriae and may determine a potent platelet aggregation–inducing activity through its vesicles (membrane evaginations projecting to the outer environment).[26]
- *P gingivalis accelerates the transition of macrophages to foam cells.* An important feature in the development of early atherosclerotic lesions is cholesterol uptake into macrophages to form foam cells. Murine macrophages could be stimulated by *P gingivalis* to accumulate low-density lipoproteins to form foam cells.[27]
- *Periopathogens have been linked to an increased host inflammatory reaction.* Systemic inflammation is closely linked to the onset of atherosclerosis.[28] Subjects affected by periodontal disease develop an intense local production of proinflammatory cytokines that may enter the bloodstream, as shown by the high levels of inflammatory biomarkers in both gingival tissues and serum.[29,30] This triggers a systemic acute-phase inflammatory response, characterized by increased levels of acute-phase proteins such as CRP and by vascular dysfunction.[10,31,32]

The association between periodontal pathogens and atherosclerosis is therefore biologically plausible, and thus emphasis has been generally given to the strength and the consistency of the findings. In summary, a plausible biologic mechanism would suggest that bacteria or their toxic byproducts may easily gain access to the circulatory system. Indeed, episodes of bacteremia have been detected after normal activity such as chewing or toothbrushing. Similar to bacterial dissemination, excessive local production of proinflammatory cytokines may obtain access to the bloodstream and trigger a systemic acute-phase response. Thus, when compared with matched periodontal healthy subjects, periodontal subjects show higher levels of CRP and interleukin 6 (IL-6); a lower number of erythrocytes; lower hemoglobin concentrations; higher values of haptoglobin; moderate leukocytosis; and increased cholesterol, low-density lipoprotein, and glucose levels.[33] These differences were also significant when the analyses accounted for a series of possible confounding factors (age, sex, smoking, socioeconomic status, diabetes, body mass index, and alcohol use).

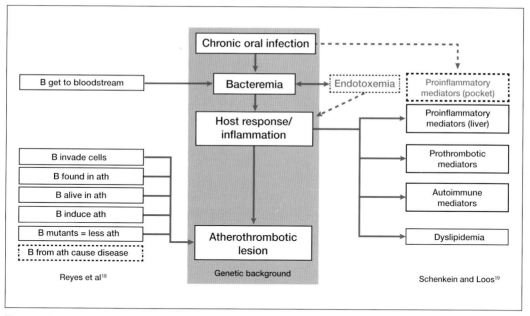

Fig 7-1 Biologically plausible mechanisms linking periodontitis and atherothrombogenesis. ath, atheroma; B, bacteria. Dotted boxes indicate limited or no evidence. (Reprinted from Tonetti et al[34] with permission.)

The two hypotheses (bacteremia and chronic inflammation) have been recently reviewed at the Joint EFP/AAP Workshop on Periodontitis and Systemic Diseases.[34] Significant evidence was identified for both hypotheses, and the current understanding of the mechanisms is described in Fig 7-1.

The consensus deliberations on the specific position papers highlighted the fact that, at present, it is impossible to recognize the relative contribution of a direct bacterial effect—mediated by translocation and metastatic effect of bacteria or bacterial components—and the effect of spillover of inflammatory mediators produced locally in the inflamed periodontal tissues on the vascular endothelium. While it is indeed recognized that the two hypotheses would over-lap and that bacteremia will ultimately cause inflammation, a better understanding of the relative contribution of the two hypotheses may help us to design better preventive or therapeutic approaches.

A critical assessment of the mechanistic evidence highlights that, while each piece of evidence taken individually is moderately interesting, the consistency of the data across in vitro, ex vivo, and experimental research with a variety of animal models provides high levels of confidence regarding the existence of potential mechanisms. Their relevance and actual clinical importance must be assessed by different types of studies: analytical epidemiology and intervention trials.

| Box 7-1 | Conclusions about epidemiologic evidence derived from the Joint EFP/ AAP Workshop on Periodontitis and Systemic Diseases[34] |

- *Risk:* The outcome in all studies in the systematic review[37] indicated that the occurrence of periodontitis was prior to an incident cardiovascular event of ACVD. This higher level of evidence of association allows for statements of risk to be made.
- *Definitions of periodontitis:* "Periodontitis measured using clinical attachment loss/periodontal probing depth and/or radiographic assessment of bone loss has been associated with increased risk for various measures of ACVD independent of established cardiovascular risk factors." Periodontitis was not measured by self-reporting, interview, or simplified partial-mouth recordings.
- *Strength of association:* "Statistically significant excess risk for ACVD in individuals with periodontitis was reported to be independent of established cardiovascular risk factors." The amount of excess risk adjusted for other ACVD risk factors, however, varied by type of cardiovascular outcome and by age and sex. The risk was found to be greater for cerebrovascular disease than for coronary heart disease and greater in males and in younger individuals. No excess risk was reported between measures of periodontitis and incident coronary heart disease in individuals over 65 years, which supports previous findings that established individual ACVD risk factors are weaker in older adults. This was an important point during the workshop discussions: The presence of a degree of specificity in the association was thought to be an element that would strengthen the case for a true relationship. In addition, the workshop consensus was that there is insufficient evidence to indicate whether or not periodontitis is associated with the incidence of secondary cardiovascular events (a second ACVD event after the original event). It was recognized that this finding has implications

for future clinical trials and that, under ideal circumstances, more epidemiologic evidence would be needed for the planning of such intervention trials. Indeed, in the planning of intervention trials it is important to have a relationship between the outcome and the exposure (primary or secondary cardiovascular event and periodontitis).
- *Potential relevance:* "Even low to moderate excess risk reported in studies is enough to be important from a public health perspective because of the high prevalence of periodontitis." Essentially, given the high burden of periodontitis (and potentially gingivitis) in the population, even a moderate measure of risk may be relevant for a population, because periodontitis is both preventable and treatable, and thus a large number of cases of ACVD may be prevented by improving the oral health of the population.
- *Confounding:* Given the fact that chronic inflammatory diseases like cardiovascular disease and periodontitis share several risk factors (such as smoking, diabetes, obesity, and nutrition), there is concern that the purported association can be explained at least in part by such exposures. Indeed, the recent workshop concluded: "There are many potentially important confounders of the association between periodontitis and ACVD risk, including co-morbidities such as diabetes and lifestyle factors such as smoking. However, established cardiovascular risk factors do not completely explain the excess cardiovascular risk in subjects with periodontitis." In all of the studies reviewed, smoking status was controlled for, and in many studies excess risk was demonstrated in subjects who had never smoked. Excess risk for periodontitis was also demonstrated in studies that controlled for diabetes. However, excess risk could be associated with un-

Box 7-1 (cont) Conclusions about epidemiologic evidence derived from the Joint EFP/AAP Workshop on Periodontitis and Systemic Diseases[34]

known confounders. The ENCODE project, a deep sequencing project to identify all functional elements of the genome, recently found that common genetically determined pathways underpin various complex inflammatory diseases. Therefore, such genetic determinants could be confounding factors. In support of this last statement, a recent report has identified a common susceptibility locus for both cardiovascular disease and periodontitis on chromosome 9p21.3, in the long noncoding RNA ANRIL locus.[38,39] While all studies in the systematic review had to control for at least age and sex, and while smoking was "controlled" for in the analyses, the potential for residual confounding in the explanation of the association remains significant and is the result of the design of these epidemiologic studies.

Epidemiology

Early studies reported associations between various definitions of periodontitis and atherosclerotic vascular diseases.[35] The majority of the early studies were cross-sectional, and thus the validity of their results was hampered by the potential of reverse causality bias (cardiovascular diseases opening a window of susceptibility to periodontitis rather than the opposite) as well as by the use of vastly different definitions of disease, ranging from self-reporting to telephone interview, to different protocols for partial-mouth examinations. Furthermore, these studies did not appropriately correct for confounding factors: Periodontitis and ACVD share a variety of risk factors. Common risk factors (indicators) include cigarette smoking, obesity, male sex, stress, depression, physical inactivity, and a low-quality diet. Critics have pointed out these limitations and the need for better data analysis.

Nonetheless, the majority of the early epidemiologic studies have indicated an increase in risk. A meta-analysis acknowledging wide variations in study design and disease definition estimated that the adjusted additional risk was about 15% higher for cerebrovascular outcomes and about 13% higher for cardiovascular outcomes.[36]

In the recent EFP/AAP workshop, emphasis was placed on incident risk estimated in longitudinal studies in which the periodontal status had to be determined before the observation period.[37] This study design addresses the reverse causality bias. The workshop position paper included 12 studies (6 studies on coronary heart disease, 3 studies on cerebrovascular disease, 2 studies on both coronary heart and cerebrovascular disease mortality, and 1 study on peripheral arterial disease).[34] All but one study reported positive associations between various periodontal disease measures and the incidence of ACVD, at least in specific subgroups. The association was stronger in younger adults, and there was no evidence for an association between periodontitis and incident coronary heart disease in subjects older than 65 years; in this respect, it must be emphasized that, in most epidemiologic studies of ACVD, single risk factors are significant in younger subjects. Only one study evaluated the association between periodontitis and a second cardiovascular event. While heterogeneity in study outcomes and design prevented a meta-analysis, the data seemed remarkably consistent; indeed, participants in the workshop believed that several aspects of the epidemiologic evidence warranted discussion and were sufficient to permit conclusions to be made (Box 7-1).

Although it is well recognized that the epidemiologic evidence of an association between periodontitis and ACVD has increased in strength and overall quality, the majority of the large longitudinal studies were designed for different purposes, and the periodontal component was an additional element; hence, the study design may be at risk of bias. Considerable debate is taking place in the scientific community about whether a better understanding of the association between periodontitis and ACVD requires a specifically designed epidemiologic study or it would be a better use of the scarce available resources to simply focus on the needed intervention studies to establish causality. This is a reflection of a broader unresolved debate on causality, risk, and prevention between epidemiologists and clinical investigators.

Intervention Trials

Results from definitive clinical trials are considered the ultimate element of proof in establishing the nature of the relationship between periodontitis and ACVD. The logical framework is that, if the elimination or attenuation of the cause is randomized through treatment of periodontitis (or its prevention at the population level), an attenuation of the effect (the ACVD outcome under study) should be observed. The design of such trials, however, is an exceedingly complex exercise: It requires a good understanding of the most likely mechanism(s) to be targeted by the intervention, the identification of a population that is at risk and amenable to receive treatment, and the availability of an ethically appropriate control treatment.

Delivery of treatment

Surprisingly little attention has been paid in recent years to identifying the best possible periodontal intervention to achieve a general health benefit. The assumption that the best possible periodontal outcome (minimal gingival inflammation and shallow pockets in the whole of the dentition) represents the best candidate treatment is both rational and reasonable but far from having been proven. As yet, only one series of studies aimed at assessing the optimal benefit in terms of systemic inflammatory markers has been performed, by D'Aiuto et al, between 2002 and 2005.[33,40,41] These studies explored different regimens of root instrumentation and the adjunctive benefit of local delivery of minocycline (with an important anti-inflammatory effect). These studies identified several important aspects in terms of differential efficacy, adverse events, and timing of the effect of treatment.

Efficacy

Better efficacy was observed for both periodontal and systemic inflammatory outcomes after an intensive treatment regimen consisting of complete-mouth mechanical instrumentation, extraction of teeth with hopeless prognosis, local application of minocycline microspheres in all sites with probing depths greater than 4 mm, and oral hygiene instructions delivered over 24 to 36 hours.[33] Efficacy in terms of local periodontal parameters paralleled changes in systemic inflammatory parameters. Some studies have employed periodontal treatment regimens that included periodontal surgery to achieve optimal control of periodontitis.[42]

Some large studies conducted in the US have shown limited changes in the periodontal outcomes and have been associated with no change in the systemic parameter under investigation. The limited results obtained with periodontal therapy have been questioned and have highlighted that no systemic benefit should be expected in the absence of an effective delivery of the intervention. Current consensus among experts seems to be to specify therapeutic targets that must be achieved in terms of reducing gingival inflammation and probing depths rather than to specify a given regimen.

Adverse events

The studies by D'Aiuto et al[41,43,44] demonstrated that shortly after the delivery of periodontal treatment, subjects presented with a systemic inflammatory response that included an increase in acute-phase response (CRP, serum amyloid A, coagulation, and neutropenia) and an increase in markers of endothelial cell damage (E-selectin, von Willebrand factor, D-dimers, and flow-mediated dilation of the brachial artery). These adverse events are not unexpected, because mechanical instrumentation induces significant bacteremia and endotoxemia that are likely to cause the observed changes. The intensity of the observed changes, however, was surprising, because for several parameters, changes represented a 10-fold increase from baseline levels. These changes persisted for a period of up to 1 week.

Follow-up studies to assess the relative intensity of systemic inflammatory changes after subgingival debridement or periodontal flap surgery indicated that the greatest inflammatory response was observed immediately after complete-mouth subgingival debridement and that, surprisingly, surgical trauma seemed to have a smaller impact.[45] Minassian et al[46] explored the relevance of this systemic inflammatory response with its underlying bacteremia and trauma. They looked at a large insurance claim database to examine the incidence rate of cardiovascular events with regard to their relationship to dental appointments in which invasive dental procedures were performed. After invasive dental treatment, there was a small but measurable increase in the risk of having a cardiovascular event. The increased risk persisted for up to 3 months after the dental appointment.

Timing of treatment

Studies that have followed the time course of systemic responses after local periodontal therapy show a biphasic response characterized by an early worsening of both biochemical parameters (CRP and inflammation[44]) and functional parameters (flow-mediated dilation[47]). This biphasic response raises important issues related to the timing of outcome assessment: For several biochemical parameters, it seems important to allow healing of the early acute-phase response before assessing the potential benefit of treatment. Repeated episodes of treatment (either nonsurgical or surgical) complicate timing of sampling and outcome assessment.

Recognition of the complexity of the systemic treatment effects and the fact that periodontal therapy initially may bring a small added risk, rather than a benefit, in terms of cardiovascular events raises important ethical issues in the design of the proper intervention trials, specifically in terms of the target population.

Population at risk

Two types of population (and two types of intervention trial) have been considered: (1) Individuals who are free from significant identified systemic comorbidities (and at relatively low risk of presenting cardiovascular events) and (2) individuals who have already suffered from a cardiovascular event (and are at a much higher risk of having new events).

In the systemically healthy population, the experimental rationale for treating periodontitis would be to interfere with the process of atherogenesis and therefore to do a primary prevention trial. In such a population, the adverse events of periodontal therapy are probably less relevant in the sense that a healthy individual could tolerate well the increased burden associated with periodontal therapy. This is the optimal population in which to show prevention or delay of the atherosclerotic process assessed by measuring a variety of so-called surrogate cardiovascular outcomes (arterial elasticity, hypertension, intima-media thickness, etc). However, the problem is that these surrogate outcomes bear relatively little weight in the decision-making process to identify aspects to target with prevention: Stronger evidence based on true cardiovascular events is favored in the cardiology community. The challenges of running a trial aimed at preventing true cardiovascular events in an otherwise healthy population are formidable: The low rate of expected events will require either a very large sample size or a very long follow-up period. Not unexpectedly, trials in systemically healthy individuals with periodontitis have focused on surrogate markers.

Running an intervention trial in a population at increased risk (ie, with a previous experience of a cardiovascular or cerebrovascular event) poses great challenges as well. First, these individuals are normally medicated to lower the risk of a second event: Many of the drug molecules may interfere with multiple aspects of the mechanisms at the basis of a relationship between periodontitis and atherosclerosis. Second, the available periodontal intervention may represent a small but concrete short-term risk of a secondary event.[46] The advantages of performing a trial in this type of population are associated with the higher incidence of events in these populations; individuals have reached an overall burden of atherosclerotic diseases that make them at risk for a second event. Therefore, it is possible to decrease the sample size and/or the time of follow-up.

The periodontitis and vascular events (PAVE) study represents a feasibility study for such a secondary prevention trial.[48] The trial was remarkable because it was possible to recruit a population among individuals who had recently suffered from a primary cardiovascular event. It also showed the challenge related to the delivery of treatment: The experimental group showed moderate periodontal improvements, while the control group (left in the intention of the study investigators to community care, expected to be mainly supragingival cleaning with a hygienist) received a considerable level of periodontal treatment.[48]

Control intervention

Identification of an ethically acceptable control periodontal treatment seems to be a key aspect in the design of a definitive trial. The background of the ethical discussion is represented by the current standard of periodontal care available to the population. Depending on the different health care systems and the existence of a waiting time to receive treatment and/or the availability of specialist care, two options have been considered. The first option consists of delaying periodontal treatment until the end of a relatively short follow-up period of the trial and delivery of a standardized placebo treatment (eg, supragingival cleaning and oral hygiene instructions) within the trial. The second consists of leaving the control group to community care.

Both options have limitations and advantages and disadvantages. Delayed treatment seems ethically possible only if the duration of follow-up is adequately short (probably in the range of 6 to 12 months); it also requires adequate safety monitoring to ensure the institution of standard-of-care treatment if periodontitis progresses. The biggest advantage of such an approach is that it will maximize the difference in local periodontal parameters—and, it is hoped, systemic inflammatory burden—between the test and the control groups.

Community care is probably one of the few options for studies of longer duration. Its experimental appeal is based on the assumption that community periodontal therapy on one hand represents the current standard of treatment but on the other hand falls short of the optimal level of care that can be delivered by highly specialized teams in the context of the trial. The experience with the PAVE study shows that, at least in some countries like the United States, the periodontal-systemic link has received such a level of professional and media attention that subjects randomized to community care will endeavor to receive the best level of care that they can access.[49] Indeed, the ethics associated with the control group represent the biggest challenge in running a trial in a society with optimal access to periodontal care.

Results of intervention trials

Several RCTs have been performed to date to assess the role of periodontal intervention on systemic parameters. These trials were recently systematically reviewed and summarized by D'Aiuto et al[50] in the context of the Joint EFP/AAP Workshop on Periodontitis and Systemic Diseases. It should be emphasized that all these studies are pilot studies; therefore, even the results of meta-analyses must be interpreted with caution (and not as the best available level of evidence). In evidence-based medicine, results of a meta-analysis of small pilot studies are usually considered evidence to proceed with a properly sized, definitive multicenter trial.

D'Aiuto et al[50] analyzed RCTs reporting the benefit of periodontal therapy on two types of outcomes: (1) ACVD biomarkers such as lipids, white blood cell counts, CRP, acute-phase reactants (other than CRP), cytokines, hemostatic factors, matrix metalloproteinases, and oxidative stress; and (2) surrogate ACVD outcomes such as blood pressure and endothelial function. In their analysis, the quality of the available evidence was graded according to the classification scheme of the US Preventive Services Task Force.[51] After retrieval of data, the strength of the available evidence for each biomarker and surrogate outcome was assessed based on the following scale[52,53]:

1. *Strong evidence* (multiple relevant, high-quality RCTs)
2. *Moderate evidence* (one relevant, high-quality RCT and one or more relevant, low-quality RCTs)
3. *Limited evidence* (one relevant, high-quality RCT or multiple relevant, low-quality RCTs)
4. *No evidence* (only one relevant, low-quality study, no relevant RCTs, or contradictory outcomes)

In their analyses, D'Aiuto et al[50] identified that a moderate level of evidence to draw initial conclusions was available for four outcomes: lipids, CRP, IL-6, and endothelial function. The initial data available pointed to a beneficial effect of periodontal therapy on CRP, IL-6, and endothelial function, while the moderate level of evidence available did not support evidence of an effect of periodontal therapy on lipids. For all other biomarkers and functional parameters examined, evidence was too limited to allow even a preliminary conclusion to be drawn.

The results of this systematic review and meta-analysis were remarkable in several ways but mostly for the fact that evidence failed to support a potential beneficial effect of periodontal therapy via a change in lipids. At the present stage of knowledge, therefore, the mechanism that seems to be potentially involved is the inflammatory one, measured by CRP, IL-6, and endothelial function. The workshop recognized the importance of specificity in terms of pathway because it was felt that specificity adds credibility to the findings.[34]

At present, data indicate that periodontal treatment leads to an improvement in serum CRP levels in otherwise healthy subjects. For this specific parameter, D'Aiuto et al[50] referred the reader to a previously published high-quality systematic review and meta-analysis by Paraskevas et al.[6] In that study, the size of the reported benefit was a decrease of 0.5 mg/L (95% confidence interval of 0.1 to 0.9) in serum high-sensitivity CRP (Table 7-2). For comparison, such an improvement would be sufficient to lower the CRP-associated risk of future cardiovascular events and is in the range of CRP improvement that can be obtained with pharmacologic treatment with statins. It should be emphasized that the trials included in the systematic review and meta-analysis by Paraskevas et al[6] reported on systemically healthy individuals with severe, generalized periodontitis. It is at present unclear if a periodontal intervention could decrease CRP in subjects with cardiovascular disease or other comorbidities.

The data on endothelial function reviewed by D'Aiuto et al[50] were also of interest. The endothelium is a key regulator of blood vessel biology because it affects coagulation, inflammation, and growth and remodeling of blood vessel walls. The impairment of endothelial function and integrity, called *endothelial dysfunction,* occurs in the early stages of atherosclerosis and its progression.[55,56] Endothelial dysfunction is considered a long-term predictor of ACVD events.[57] It is frequently measured as flow-mediated dilation of the brachial artery using a noninvasive ultrasound technique.[58]

An early case-control study showed that subjects with severe periodontitis had lower values of flow-mediated dilation than did healthy controls.[12] The systematic review by D'Aiuto et al[50] identified seven intervention trials describing the effects of periodontal therapy on endothelial dysfunction. The majority of the trials reported an improvement of endothelial function after periodontal therapy.[42,47,54,59–62]

Of the RCTs, the largest was performed by Tonetti et al,[47] who randomized 121 healthy individuals suffering from severe generalized periodontitis to either a cycle of supragingival mechanical scaling and polishing (control) or

Table 7-2	Effect of periodontal therapy on serum CRP concentrations*			
Study or subcategory	n	Diff Exp Tx mean (SD)	n	Diff Control Tx mean (SD)
D'Aiuto et al[33]	20	0.40 (1.01)	24	−0.10 (1.65)
D'Aiuto et al[33]	21	0.00 (2.25)	24	−0.10 (1.65)
Seinost et al[54]	31	0.60 (1.38)	31	0.00 (0.80)
Total (95% CI)	72		79	

Test for heterogeneity: $Chi^2 = 0.57$, $df = 2$ ($P = .75$), $I^2 = 0\%$.
Test for overall effect: $Z = 2.32$ ($P = .02$).
*Reprinted from Paraskevas et al[6] with permission.
Exp, experimental group; Tx, treatment; WMD, weighted mean difference; SD, standard deviation; CI, confidence interval; df, degrees of freedom.

(continued on next page)

an intensive treatment regimen consisting of complete-mouth scaling and root planing, extraction of hopeless teeth, and local delivery of minocycline microspheres in all pockets. Six months after therapy, the intensive treatment regimen led to an improvement in endothelial function of 2.0% (95% confidence interval of 1.2 to 2.8; $P < .001$) over the control treatment (Fig 7-2). The observed improvement in endothelial function was directly associated with the obtained improvements in periodontal parameters.

Higashi et al[60,61] extended these results of an improvement of endothelial function to individuals suffering from hypertension and ACVD. These trials are significant because they seem to suggest that periodontal treatment may reverse the early stages of atherosclerosis, even in subjects with established cardiovascular disease.

With regard to trials on the effect of periodontal therapy on true cardiovascular outcomes (myocardial infarction, stroke, angina, or intima-media thickness at the carotid bifurcation), recent systematic reviews did not retrieve data with the exception of reports from small pilot trials.[50,63] One clinical study reported on the effects of periodontal therapy on carotid intima-media thickness over a 12-month period in 35 otherwise healthy subjects.[64] While the study did not have an RCT design, and thus the strength of the conclusions is limited, of interest was the broad set of biomarkers that was assessed during the trial, which showed both a chronologic and quantitative parallel to measures of carotid intima-media thickness.

	WMD (random) 95% CI		Weight (%)	WMD (random) [95% CI]
			28.84	0.50 [−0.29, 1.29]
			13.38	0.10 [−1.07, 1.27]
			57.78	0.60 [0.04, 1.16]
			100.00	0.50 [0.08, 0.93]

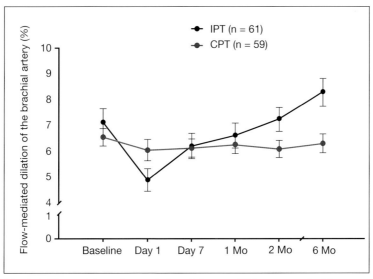

Fig 7-2 Effect of intensive periodontal therapy (IPT) compared with supra-gingival debridement (community periodontal treatment [CPT]) on endothelial dysfunction. The vertical axis depicts the percentage of flow-mediated dilation of the brachial artery. (Reprinted from Tonetti et al[47] with permission.)

Conclusion

The participants of the recent EFP/AAP workshop believed that, in the light of the present incomplete evidence, the following conclusions should be drawn[34]:

- There is consistent and strong epidemiologic evidence that periodontitis imparts an increased risk for future ACVD.
- The impact of periodontitis on ACVD is biologically plausible: Translocated circulating oral microbiota may directly or indirectly induce systemic inflammation that impacts the pathogenesis of atherothrombogenesis.
- While in vitro, animal, and clinical studies do support the existence of the interaction and biologic mechanism, intervention trials to date are not adequate to draw further conclusions.

The workshop consensus was that the following recommendations can be made to oral health practitioners[34]:

- Practitioners should be aware of the emerging and strengthening evidence that periodontitis is a risk factor for development of ACVD and should advise patients of the risk.
- The rationale for prevention, diagnosis, and treatment of periodontitis remains the preservation of the dentition and avoidance of the crippling effects of periodontitis-induced alveolar bone loss and tooth loss.
- Based on the weight of the evidence, periodontitis patients with other risk factors for ACVD, such as hypertension, obesity, and smoking, who have not seen a physician within the last year should be referred for a physical.
- Modifiable lifestyle-associated risk factors for periodontitis (and ACVD) should be addressed in the dental office and in the context of comprehensive periodontal therapy (eg, smoking cessation programs and advice on lifestyle modifications such as diet and exercise). This goal may be better achieved in collaboration with appropriate specialists and may bring health gains beyond the oral cavity.
- Treatment of periodontitis in patients with a history of cardiovascular events should follow American Heart Association guidelines for elective procedures.

Besides these consensus conclusions, it seems important to recognize that the challenges of having sufficient evidence to draw firmer conclusions are formidable and that both dental and medical practitioners as well as their patients will have to deal with the present incomplete picture for years to come. At present, there seem to be some firm points: The association between periodontal disease and atherosclerosis seems to be consistent. It is unclear, however, if the link can be explained fully by modifiable risk factors shared between periodontitis and cardiovascular diseases.

Because risk factor modification is now a well-recognized component of periodontal therapy, a pragmatic approach will likely see periodontists and other oral health care professionals treat periodontitis and address the risk factors as part of the periodontal therapy. This may bring general health benefits because of the control of the shared risk factors and—perhaps—because of the control of the systemic inflammatory burden contributed by periodontitis. Conversely, and this is the important implicit point made by the recent American Heart Association statement that critically evaluated the evidence of a relationship between periodontitis and cardiovascular disease,[64] it is wise for periodontists and oral health care professionals to avoid making claims that periodontal therapy improves cardiovascular health. Such assertions are premature and may confuse patients with cardiovascular disease, who belong under the care of their physician or cardiologist in a medical practice.

References

1. Mattila KJ, Nieminen MS, Valtonen VV, et al. Association between dental health and acute myocardial infarction. BMJ 1989;298:779–781.

2. Kiechl S, Egger G, Mayr M, et al. Chronic infections and the risk of carotid atherosclerosis: Prospective results from a large population study. Circulation 2001;103:1064–1070.

3. Andraws R, Berger JS, Brown DL. Effects of antibiotic therapy on outcomes of patients with coronary artery disease: A meta-analysis of randomized controlled trials. JAMA 2005;293:2641–2647.

4. Paju S, Pussinen PJ, Sinisalo J, et al. Clarithromycin reduces recurrent cardiovascular events in subjects without periodontitis. Atherosclerosis 2006;188: 412–419.

5. López NJ, Socransky SS, Da Silva I, Japlit MR, Haffajee AD. Effects of metronidazole plus amoxicillin as the only therapy on the microbiological and clinical parameters of untreated chronic periodontitis. J Clin Periodontol 2006;33:648–660.

6. Paraskevas S, Huizinga JD, Loos BG. A systematic review and meta-analyses on C-reactive protein in relation to periodontitis. J Clin Periodontol 2008; 35:277–290.

7. Bizzarro S, Van der Velden U, Ten Heggeler JM, et al. Periodontitis is characterized by elevated PAI-1 activity. J Clin Periodontol 2007;34:574–580.

8. Salzberg TN, Overstreet BT, Rogers JD, Califano JV, Best AM, Schenkein HA. C-reactive protein levels in patients with aggressive periodontitis. J Periodontol 2006;77:933–939.

9. Havemose-Poulsen A, Westergaard J, Stoltze K, et al. Periodontal and hematological characteristics associated with aggressive periodontitis, juvenile idiopathic arthritis, and rheumatoid arthritis. J Periodontol 2006;77:280–288.

10. Joshipura KJ, Wand HC, Merchant AT, Rimm EB. Periodontal disease and biomarkers related to cardiovascular disease. J Dent Res 2004;83:151–155.

11. Buhlin K, Gustafsson A, Pockley AG, Frostegård J, Klinge B. Risk factors for cardiovascular disease in patients with periodontitis. Eur Heart J 2003;24: 2099–2107.

12. Amar S, Gokce N, Morgan S, Loukideli M, Van Dyke TE, Vita JA. Periodontal disease is associated with brachial artery endothelial dysfunction and systemic inflammation. Arterioscler Thromb Vasc Biol 2003;23:1245–1249.

13. Craig RG, Yip JK, So MK, Boylan RJ, Socransky SS, Haffajee AD. Relationship of destructive periodontal disease to the acute-phase response. J Periodontol 2003;74:1007–1016.

14. Noack B, Genco RJ, Trevisan M, Grossi S, Zambon JJ, De Nardin E. Periodontal infections contribute to elevated systemic C-reactive protein level. J Periodontol 2001;72:1221–1227.

15. Loos BG, Craandijk J, Hoek FJ, Wertheim-van Dillen PM, Van der Velden U. Elevation of systemic markers related to cardiovascular diseases in the peripheral blood of periodontitis patients. J Periodontol 2000;71:1528–1534.

16. Fredriksson M, Gustafsson A, Asman B, Bergström K. Hyper-reactive peripheral neutrophils in adult periodontitis: Generation of chemiluminescence and intracellular hydrogen peroxide after in vitro priming and FcγR-stimulation. J Clin Periodontol 1998;25:394–398.

17. Tómas I, Diz P, Tobías A, Scully C, Donos N. Periodontal health status and bacteraemia from daily oral activities: Systematic review/meta-analysis. J Clin Periodontol 2012;39:213–228.

18. Reyes L, Kozarov E, Herrera D, Roldan S, Progulske-Fox A. Periodontal bacterial invasion and infection: Contribution to cardiovascular disease. J Clin Periodontol 2013;40(suppl 14):30–50.

19. Schenkein HA, Loos BG. Inflammatory mechanisms linking periodontal diseases to cardiovascular diseases. J Clin Periodontol 2013;40(suppl 14): 51–69.

20. Lalla E, Lamster IB, Hofmann MA, et al. Oral infection with a periodontal pathogen accelerates early atherosclerosis in apolipoprotein E-null mice. Arterioscler Thromb Vasc Biol 2003;23:1405–1411.

21. Li L, Messas E, Batista EL Jr, Levine RA, Amar S. *Porphyromonas gingivalis* infection accelerates the progression of atherosclerosis in a heterozygous apolipoprotein E-deficient murine model. Circulation 2002;105:861–867.

22. Haraszthy VI, Zambon JJ, Trevisan M, Zeid M, Genco RJ. Identification of periodontal pathogens in atheromatous plaques. J Periodontol 2000;71: 1554–1560.

23. Fiehn NE, Larsen T, Christiansen N, Holmstrup P, Schroeder TV. Identification of periodontal pathogens in atherosclerotic vessels. J Periodontol 2005; 76:731–736.

24. Aimetti M, Romano F, Nessi F. Microbiologic analysis of periodontal pockets and carotid atheromatous plaques in advanced chronic periodontitis patients. J Periodontol 2007;78:1718–1723.

25. Dorn BR, Burks JN, Seifert KN, Progulske-Fox A. Invasion of endothelial and epithelial cells by strains of *Porphyromonas gingivalis*. FEMS Microbiol Lett 2000;187:139–144.

26. Sharma A, Novak EK, Sojar HT, Swank RT, Kuramitsu HK, Genco RJ. *Porphyromonas gingivalis* platelet aggregation activity: Outer membrane vesicles are potent activators of murine platelets. Oral Microbiol Immunol 2000;15:393–396.

27. Kuramitsu HK, Qi M, Kang IC, Chen W. Role for periodontal bacteria in cardiovascular diseases. Ann Periodontol 2001;6:41–47.

28. Ridker PM. Intrinsic fibrinolytic capacity and systemic inflammation: Novel risk factors for arterial thrombotic disease. Haemostasis 1997;27(suppl 1):2–11.

29. Hutter JW, van der Velden U, Varoufaki A, Huffels RA, Hoek FJ, Loos BG. Lower numbers of erythrocytes and lower levels of hemoglobin in periodontitis patients compared to control subjects. J Clin Periodontol 2001;28:930–936.

30. Offenbacher S, Farr DH, Goodson JM. Measurement of prostaglandin E in crevicular fluid. J Clin Periodontol 1981;8:359–367.

31. Slade GD, Offenbacher S, Beck JD, Heiss G, Pankow JS. Acute-phase inflammatory response to periodontal disease in the US population. J Dent Res 2000;79:49–57.

32. Wu T, Trevisan M, Genco RJ, Falkner KL, Dorn JP, Sempos CT. Examination of the relation between periodontal health status and cardiovascular risk factors: Serum total and high density lipoprotein cholesterol, C-reactive protein, and plasma fibrinogen. Am J Epidemiol 2000;151:273–282.

33. D'Aiuto F, Parkar M, Nibali L, Suvan J, Lessem J, Tonetti MS. Periodontal infections cause changes in traditional and novel cardiovascular risk factors: Results from a randomized controlled clinical trial. Am Heart J 2006;151:977–984.

34. Tonetti MS, Van Dyke TE, Working Group 1 of the Joint EFP/AAP Workshop. Periodontitis and atherosclerotic cardiovascular disease: Consensus report of the Joint EFP/AAP Workshop on Periodontitis and Systemic Diseases. J Clin Periodontol 2013;40(suppl 14):S24–S29.

35. Beck JD, Offenbacher S. Relationships among clinical measures of periodontal disease and their associations with systemic markers. Ann Periodontol 2002;7:79–89.

36. Khader YS, Albashaireh ZS, Alomari MA. Periodontal diseases and the risk of coronary heart and cerebrovascular diseases: A meta-analysis. J Periodontol 2004;75:1046–1053.

37. Dietrich T, Sharma P, Walter C, Weston P, Beck J. The epidemiological evidence behind the association between periodontitis and incident atherosclerotic cardiovascular disease. J Clin Periodontol 2013;40(suppl 14):70–84.

38. Schaefer AS, Richter GM, Groessner-Schreiber B, et al. Identification of a shared genetic susceptibility locus for coronary heart disease and periodontitis. PLoS Genet 2009;5(2):e1000378.

39. Bochenek G, Häsler R, El Mokhtari NE, et al. The large non-coding RNA ANRIL, which is associated with atherosclerosis, periodontitis and several forms of cancer, regulates ADIPOR1, VAMP3 and C11ORF10. Hum Mol Genet 2013;22:4516–4527.

40. D'Aiuto F, Nibali L, Parkar M, Suvan J, Tonetti MS. Short-term effects of intensive periodontal therapy on serum inflammatory markers and cholesterol. J Dent Res 2005;84:269–273.

41. D'Aiuto F, Parkar M, Andreou G, et al. Periodontitis and systemic inflammation: Control of the local infection is associated with a reduction in serum inflammatory markers. J Dent Res 2004;83:156–160.

42. Elter JR, Hinderliter AL, Offenbacher S, et al. The effects of periodontal therapy on vascular endothelial function: A pilot trial. Am Heart J 2006;151:47. e1–47.e6.

43. D'Aiuto F, Nibali L, Mohamed-Ali V, Vallance P, Tonetti MS. Periodontal therapy: A novel non-drug-induced experimental model to study human inflammation. J Periodontal Res 2004;39:294–299.

44. D'Aiuto F, Parkar M, Tonetti MS. Acute effects of periodontal therapy on bio-markers of vascular health. J Clin Periodontol 2007;34:124–129.

45. Graziani F, Cei S, Tonetti M, et al. Systemic inflammation following non-surgical and surgical periodontal therapy. J Clin Periodontol 2010;37:848–854.

46. Minassian C, D'Aiuto F, Hingorani AD, Smeeth L. Invasive dental treatment and risk for vascular events: A self-controlled case series. Ann Intern Med 2010;153:499–506.

47. Tonetti MS, D'Aiuto F, Nibali L, et al. Treatment of periodontitis and endothelial function. N Engl J Med 2007;356:911–920.

48. Beck JD, Couper DJ, Falkner KL, et al. The periodontitis and vascular events (PAVE) pilot study: Adverse events. J Periodontol 2008;79:90–96.

49. Couper DJ, Beck JD, Falkner KL, et al. The periodontitis and vascular events (PAVE) pilot study: Recruitment, retention, and community care controls. J Periodontol 2008;79:80–89.

50. D'Aiuto F, Orlandi M, Gunsolley JC. Evidence that periodontal treatment improves biomarkers and CVD outcomes. J Clin Periodontol 2013;40(suppl 14):85–105.

51. US Preventive Services Task Force. Guide to Clinical Preventive Services: Report of the US Preventive Services Task Force, ed 2. Washington, DC: US Dept of Health and Human Services, 1996.

52. van Tulder MW, Tuut M, Pennick V, Bombardier C, Assendelft WJ. Quality of primary care guidelines for acute low back pain. Spine (Phila Pa 1976) 2004;29:E357–E362.

53. West S, King V, Carey TS, et al. Systems to rate the strength of scientific evidence. Evid Rep Technol Assess (Summ) 2002;(47):1–11.

54. Seinost G, Wimmer G, Skerget M, et al. Periodontal treatment improves endothelial dysfunction in patients with severe periodontitis. Am Heart J 2005;149:1050–1054.

55. Ross R. The pathogenesis of atherosclerosis: A perspective for the 1990s. Nature 1993;362:801–809.

56. Gimbrone MA Jr, Cybulsky MI, Kume N, Collins T, Resnick N. Vascular endothelium. An integrator of pathophysiological stimuli in atherogenesis. Ann N Y Acad Sci 1995;748:122–131.

57. Schachinger V, Britten MB, Zeiher AM. Prognostic impact of coronary vasodilator dysfunction on adverse long-term outcome of coronary heart disease. Circulation 2000;101:1899–1906.

58. Charakida M, Masi S, Luscher TF, Kastelein JJ, Deanfield JE. Assessment of atherosclerosis: The role of flow-mediated dilatation. Eur Heart J 2010; 31:2854–2861.

59. Blum A, Kryuger K, Mashiach EM, et al. Periodontal care may improve endothelial function. Eur J Intern Med 2007;18:295–298.

60. Higashi Y, Goto C, Hidaka T, et al. Oral infection-inflammatory pathway, periodontitis, is a risk factor for endothelial dysfunction in patients with coronary artery disease. Atherosclerosis 2009;206:604–610.

61. Higashi Y, Goto C, Jitsuiki D, et al. Periodontal infection is associated with endothelial dysfunction in healthy subjects and hypertensive patients. Hypertension 2008;51:446–453.

62. Mercanoglu F, Oflaz H, Oz O, et al. Endothelial dysfunction in patients with chronic periodontitis and its improvement after initial periodontal therapy. J Periodontol 2004;75:1694–1700.

63. Lockhart PB, Bolger AF, Papapanou PN, et al. Periodontal disease and atherosclerotic vascular disease: Does the evidence support an independent association? A scientific statement from the American Heart Association. Circulation 2012;125:2520–2544.

64. Piconi S, Trabattoni D, Luraghi C, et al. Treatment of periodontal disease results in improvements in endothelial dysfunction and reduction of the carotid intima-media thickness. FASEB J 2009;23:1196–1204.

Clinical Considerations:
What You Can Take Back to Your Practice

What is the effect of obesity on oral health?

Obesity contributes to the systemic inflammatory burden and has been shown to be a risk factor for periodontal disease. If obesity is associated with excessive caloric intake, and fermentable carbohydrates are a large part of the diet, this may lead to an increase in dental caries. Obesity has also been associated with altered (early) tooth eruption.

Are oral infections independent risk factors for the development of obesity?

Though not fully addressed in the literature, it is not biologically plausible that oral infections directly increase the risk of obesity.

What is the biologic plausibility of the association between oral health and obesity?

Obesity is an inflammatory condition. Adipose tissue contains both adipocytes and increased numbers of macrophages, which produce inflammatory mediators that contribute to the systemic inflammatory burden and can exacerbate the local inflammatory response in the periodontal tissues. Further, obesity is an important risk factor for type 2 diabetes mellitus, which is a recognized risk factor for periodontitis.

Does the delivery of oral health care contribute to reduced obesity?

Provisions of dental services, either preventive or therapeutic (treatment of dental caries or periodontal disease) do not contribute directly to reducing obesity. However, treatment of dental disease, elimination of pain, and establishment of a functional dentition can improve mastication and allow patients to eat a range of foods without the need to limit the diet to softer, carbohydrate-rich foods. In the larger context, oral health care providers can deliver a healthy lifestyle message to dental patients, including the need to eat a healthy diet, exercise, and control weight.

Is it safe to provide dental care to obese patients?

Being overweight or obese is associated with a number of important comorbidities (ie, hypertension, cardiovascular disease). In the absence of these comorbidities, it is safe to provide dental services to overweight and obese patients.

What is the appropriate message to give to the public about the association between oral health and obesity?

The relationship between oral health and obesity is complex. Obesity can affect periodontal health, and a healthy mouth will allow mastication of a full range of foods and thereby a healthy diet. An important message that can be delivered by oral health care providers is that living a healthy lifestyle, including not smoking, exercising, controlling weight, and maintaining oral health, will decrease the risk of many chronic diseases.

8 Obesity: The Oral-Systemic Connection

Ira B. Lamster, DDS, MMSc
Ilene Fennoy, MD, MPH
Mary Tavares, DMD, MPH

Obesity is one of the world's most serious public health problems, affecting both developing and developed countries. The prevalence has dramatically increased in the last few decades, reaching epidemic proportions. According to the World Health Organization (WHO), *overweight* and *obesity* can be defined as an abnormal or excessive level of fat accumulation that may impair health.[1] Like many chronic diseases, obesity has significant associated morbidity, mortality, and economic impact and is largely preventable.[2] Obesity-associated health problems include type 2 diabetes mellitus, hypertension, cardiovascular diseases, and certain malignancies.[3] The morbidity and mortality associated with these disorders take a devastating toll on affected individuals and are linked to poor quality of life and a reduced life span. The economic burden on society is also enormous; the cost in the United States was estimated in 2008 to be US$147 billion.[4]

Because obesity has such a negative impact on individual health as well as on society, oral health care professionals must consider a role in obesity management for their patients. This chapter discusses obesity and its effects on systemic and oral health, focusing on the relationship between obesity and specific oral diseases and disorders.

Assessment of Obesity

Quantitative assessment of body fat is important for clinical research and practice. Body Mass Index (BMI) is the most common measure used for these purposes. It is a useful but imperfect measure to classify individuals into categories based on height and weight. BMI is calculated by dividing weight in kilograms by height in meters squared (Box 8-1). When inches and pounds are used, a conversion factor of 703 is used. In epidemiologic studies, obesity is often defined with BMI as a single measure that can be compared across studies and populations, and BMI has been demonstrated to predict development of disease (morbidity) and mortality.[5] According to the WHO criteria, *overweight* is defined as a BMI greater than or equal to 25 kg/m^2, while *obesity* is defined as a BMI greater than or equal to 30 kg/m^2. These values are scaled the same for all ages and both sexes.[1,3]

Age- and sex-specific BMI percentiles are used to classify children and adolescents age 2 to 20 years into weight status categories. These factors must be considered because in children, unlike adults, the amount of body fat differs between boys and girls and changes with age.[6] Typically, a standard BMI calculation

---

Box 8-1   Calculation of BMI

Weight in pounds ÷ height in inches ÷ height in inches × 703

For example, a person who is 6 ft tall and weighs 230 lb would have a BMI of:
230 ÷ 72 ÷ 72 × 703 = 31.2

In this case, the person would be classified as obese.

Table 8-1   Weight status categories for children (BMI percentile) and adults (BMI)

Weight status category	BMI percentile range	BMI
Underweight	Less than the 5th percentile	< 18.5
Healthy weight	5th percentile to less than the 85th percentile	18.5–24.9
Overweight	85th percentile to less than the 95th percentile	25.0–29.9
Obese	Equal to or greater than the 95th percentile	≥ 30.0

is plotted against age on a sex-specific BMI-for-age growth chart.[7] BMI-for-age weight status categories and the corresponding percentiles are shown in Table 8-1.

BMI is useful because it allows the establishment of population guidelines and accounts for individuals who are of different heights. Although BMI is simple and easy to calculate, it is an indirect measure of body fat and does not allow for consideration of body frame or for differences in body mass composition (fat versus muscle). These limitations make BMI a less reliable measure of body fat for the elderly and some ethnic groups[5] and also must be viewed in relation to other important health variables such as hypertension and lack of physical activity. It also does not consider distribution of body fat. Specifically, abdominal fat is related to the risk for developing obesity-associated diseases.[8]

Waist circumference and waist-to-hip ratio are other indirect measures of body fat, particularly for abdominal adiposity. Although the actual measurements can be difficult to standardize, they have been validated by computed tomographic measurement of body fat. Waist circumference is a key element in the definition of metabolic syndrome.[9] Skinfold thickness measured with calipers can also be an indirect gauge of body fat. While simple to use and a good predictor of total and regional fat distribution, this measure is also difficult to standardize for research purposes. There are no established data to support the use of skinfold thickness to predict morbidity and mortality.[5]

Measurement of body fat can be made more accurately with technology such as underwater weighing (densitometry), isotope dilution (hydrometry), computed axial tomography, magnetic resonance imaging, and dual-energy x-ray absorptiometry (DEXA).[5] However, their cost, complexity, and lack of portability make these methods impractical for epidemiologic studies or routine clinical examinations.

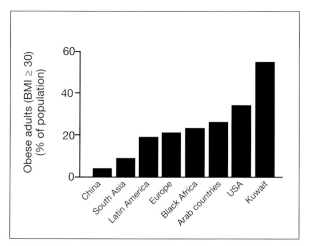

Fig 8-1 Rates of adult obesity (BMI ≥ 30) throughout the world. (Reprinted from Tavares et al[10] with permission.)

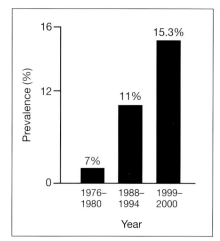

Fig 8-2 Prevalence of type 2 diabetes in children age 6 to 16 years in the United States. (Reprinted from Tavares et al[10] with permission.)

Prevalence of Obesity

International trends

The WHO estimated in 2008 that 35% of the world's adults aged 20 years and older were overweight and that 11%, more than 200 million men and nearly 300 million women, were obese.[1] It concluded that more than 1 in 10 of the global adult population is considered obese, and this trend has escalated in the past decade. The same report states that 65% of the world's population lives in countries where obesity causes more deaths than underweight conditions.[1] Figure 8-1 displays adult obesity (BMI ≥ 30) prevalence for selected countries around the world.[10–12] Rates are rising rapidly, particularly in African regions, Arab countries, and in the United States.[1]

The prevalence of global childhood overweight and obesity increased from 4.2% in 1990 to 6.7% in 2010. This trend is expected to climb to 9.1% (approximately 60 million children) by 2020.[13] The increasing trend toward earlier and higher rates of obesity among children is underscored by the 2010 WHO report that approximately 43 million of the world's children younger than the age of 5 years were overweight.[1]

Worldwide, the prevalence of overweight and obesity in developed countries is nearly double that of developing countries. Paradoxically, the vast majority of affected children (35 million) live in developing countries.[1] In absolute numbers, Asia has the highest number of overweight and obese children; more than half of affected children from developing countries live in this region.[13]

An ominous global trend is the decreasing age of onset for type 2 diabetes mellitus. The prevalence of children aged 6 to 11 years with type 2 diabetes has doubled in the past 20 years[10,14] (Fig 8-2).

National trends

Data taken from the 2009 to 2010 National Health and Nutrition Examination Survey (NHANES) revealed that more than one-third of adults in the United States were obese; there were no significant differences between the sexes. Individuals 60 years or older were more likely to be obese than younger adults.[15] If the current trends continue, it is predicted that about 3 of 4 Americans will be overweight or obese by 2020.[16]

Obesity rates are not evenly distributed among the states. In 2011, the adult obesity rate exceeded 30% in 12 states, primarily situated in the southeastern United States; an additional 27 states had adult obesity rates greater than 25%. If this current trajectory continues, the Robert Wood Johnson Foundation estimates that, by 2030, at least 44% of adults in every state will be obese.[17]

As of 2010, 18% of children aged 6 to 11 years and 18.4% of adolescents aged 12 to 19 years were considered obese in the United States. This represents an overall 54.5% increase in children and a 63.6% increase in adolescents in this category since 2000.[18,19] Within the adolescent demographic, 13.9% meet the adult classification of obesity.[19] This presents an ominous forecast, because obese adolescents have a 16 times greater risk of becoming obese adults than do adolescents who are not obese.[20] Furthermore, a child who was overweight at any one point during the elementary school years is 25 times more likely to be overweight at age 12 years than a child who was never previously overweight.[21]

In 2009 to 2010, there appeared to be a possible slowing of the upward trend in obesity. There was no change in the overall prevalence of childhood obesity when compared with 2007 to 2008. However, significant differences in prevalence of obesity by race and ethnicity were found. In 2009 to 2010, 21.2% of Hispanic children and adolescents and 24.3% of non-Hispanic black children and adolescents were obese, while the prevalence was 14.0% in non-Hispanic white children and adolescents.[22] Generally, in the United States, obesity and overweight conditions disproportionately affect Hispanic, African American, multiracial, and low-income populations.[23]

Causes of Obesity

Obesity is mainly attributed to the systemic energy imbalance created by excessive caloric intake and inadequate levels of energy utilization (ie, a lack of physical activity). Therefore, diet and activity play a significant role in this condition, but they are modulated by other risk factors for obesity. These include socioeconomic status, minority status, geographic location, access to education, cultural beliefs, and genetic influences.[24] An ever-growing body of literature points to additional factors, including sleep patterns and other factors, which start as early as the prenatal period.

Prenatal and postnatal factors

Several studies point to a strong correlation between maternal status and infant weight. One study of sibling births found a consistent association between maternal weight gain during pregnancy and infant birth weight.[25] When compared with infants born of women who gained only 18 to 22 lb during pregnancy, the infants of women who gained 53 lb or more were twice as likely to weigh more than 8.8 lb at birth.

Prenatal factors appear to influence weight beyond infancy. Three-year-old children whose mothers had gained what was defined as "excessive" weight during pregnancy were more than 4 times at risk of being overweight compared with the children of mothers who gained "inadequate" weight.[26] These findings question the categorization of maternal weight gain, because women who gained "adequate" weight had a higher chance of having an overweight 3-year-old than did the mothers who gained "inadequate" weight.

Gestational diabetes is an additional factor in child obesity. The risk of being overweight at ages 5 to 7 years was greater in children whose mothers had untreated gestational diabetes than in children whose mothers did not experience gestational diabetes.[27] Women who received treatment for gestational diabetes had a lower risk of having overweight children.

Prenatal risk factors for obesity may extend beyond maternal weight gain. A meta-analysis of 14 studies demonstrated evidence that women who smoked during pregnancy were more likely to have children who were obese at ages 3 to 7 years than were women who did not smoke.[28] Two of the studies within the meta-analysis found the same results after tracking children to age 14 years and into young adulthood.

Diet

Since the 1970s, American diets have shifted toward processed foods, greater use of edible oils, and the increased popularity of sugar-sweetened beverages. Further, the advent of new technologies has resulted in a markedly more sedentary lifestyle.[24] While conventional wisdom says that the quantity of calories individuals eat and drink would have an impact on their weight, a growing body of research indicates that the quality and pattern of food consumption are also important. Certain foods and patterns are protective against chronic diseases and help with weight control, while others, particularly highly processed foods and sugary drinks, increase disease risk and weight gain.

Large prospective studies have found that a low-fat diet is not necessarily associated with weight loss. In the United States, the percentage of fat calories consumed has decreased while obesity rates have increased,[29,30] and consumption of a low-fat diet has not necessarily improved chronic disease outcomes.[31] Part of the reason for these findings is that easily digestible refined carbohydrates have replaced fats, leading to weight gain and an increased risk of disease. In one large study of lifestyle change, increasing the intake of French fries, potato chips, sugared drinks, and refined grains (white flour and rice) resulted in significant weight gain over time.[32] These food items have a high glycemic index and glycemic load, causing rapid increases in blood sugar and insulin. The resulting sensation of hunger results in increased food consumption and eventual weight gain, leading to higher risks of diabetes and heart disease.[33,34]

The type of fat consumed is more important than the quantity with respect to cardiovascular health, and the same may hold true for weight control.[35,36] The Nurses' Health Study, which followed 42,000 middle-aged and older women for 8 years, found that increased consumption of trans fats and saturated fats was correlated with weight gain, but increased consumption of healthy monounsaturated and polyunsaturated fats was not.[37]

Sugar-sweetened beverages

In the United States, sugared beverages made up about 4% of daily calorie intake in the 1970s but represented about 9% of calories by 2001.[38] Data from the National Center for Health Statistics for 2005 to 2008 found that half of Americans consume some type of sugary drink on any given day.[39] Of these, 25% consume at least 200 calories from sugared drinks, and 5% consume at least 567 calories, which is equivalent to drinking four cans of soda.

Multiple systematic reviews and meta-analyses have found associations between the intake of sugary drinks, particularly soft drinks, and increased body weight and BMI in adults and children.[40,41] An intervention that nearly completely eliminated sugared beverage intake in a diverse group of adolescents resulted in a beneficial effect on body weight and provided support for the American Academy of Pediatrics guidelines limiting sugar-sweetened beverage consumption.[42]

Meal patterns

Eating patterns have changed in the past 40 years. Portion sizes of food eaten at home and away from home have increased for adults and children, as has consumption of fast food.[43] By 2006, American children were getting a larger percentage of their calories from fast food than from school food.[44] Additionally, meal frequency and snacking have increased over the past 30 years. Children get a quarter of their daily calories from between-meal foods, primarily sweet and salty snacks and sugary drinks.[24]

Physical activity

Children and adults are less active today than they were in the past. Technologic advancements and social changes have decreased the amount of physical activity that was once required for work, home life, and transportation. Although participation in leisure activities such as sports and exercise has increased slightly, these pursuits account for only a fraction of daily physical activity.[45–48]

Physical inactivity plays a significant role in weight gain and is an additional contributor to obesity. The Women's Health Study, which followed 34,000 women for 13 years, found that women who were normal weight at the study's start needed the equivalent of 1 hour a day of moderate-to-vigorous physical activity to maintain a steady weight.[49] In the Nurses' Health Study II, women gained, on average, about 20 lb over the 16 years of the study.[50,51] However, those who increased their physical activity by 30 minutes per day gained less weight than did women whose activity levels remained constant.

Physical activity has the effect of increasing total energy expenditure, which can result in energy balance or weight loss as long as additional food is not eaten to compensate for expended calories. It decreases body fat overall and around the waist, preventing abdominal obesity that is linked with chronic diseases. Additional benefits of physical activity include reduced depression and anxiety.[52,53]

Pathophysiology

Obesity and inflammation

Adipose tissue is no longer considered a simple storage organ but a vibrant, active tissue involved in physiologic and immune regulation.[54] It is composed of multiple cell types that can be categorized (1) by function—white fat used primarily as a storage organ for fuel reserves versus brown fat used for heat generation; (2) by location—subcutaneous versus visceral fat;

and (3) by cell type—non–fat cells including fibroblasts, endothelial cells, and macrophages, which make up 50% of the resident cells versus adipocytes.[55] Excessive adipose tissue, particularly visceral adiposity, is associated with increased cardiovascular risk, type 2 diabetes, and periodontal disease, all having an inflammatory component.[56–58] Indeed, excessive adiposity or obesity is itself recognized as an inflammatory condition[59] characterized by macrophage recruitment,[60] increased production of tumor necrosis factor α (TNF-α),[61] elevated C-reactive protein (CRP)[62] and interleukin 6 (IL-6),[63] and a range of other cytokines and inflammatory molecules (Fig 8-3).

Macrophage infiltration represents one of the key elements in the inflammation associated with obesity.[56,60] Stromal vasculature cells of visceral adipose tissue yielded increased macrophage messenger RNA transcripts that correlated with increased body mass in mice with both genetic and diet-induced obesity.[60] Furthermore, both adipocyte size and BMI were predictors of the numbers of macrophages in various fat depots of the animals.[60]

Macrophages are of two types: proinflammatory (M1, classic activation) or anti-inflammatory (M2, alternative activation).[64] Interferon γ, cytokine secretion, IL-12, bacterial lipolysaccharides, and T-cell activation are all mediators of the classic activation pathway, while immunosuppression of T-cell immune reactions through mediators such as IL-10, IL-13, and IL-4 are characteristic of the alternative pathway.[64] Obesity alters the distribution of the type of macrophages toward an increase in the proinflammatory M1 macrophages.[65] These proinflammatory macrophages overexpress genes for factors involved in macrophage migration and phagocytosis, such as IL-6 and chemokine receptor type 2.[66] The contribution by nonadipocyte cells, particularly macrophages, was greater than that of adipocytes for a variety of these inflammatory mediators, including cathepsin S, macrophage migratory inhibiting factor (MIF), and IL-1β receptor antagonist.[67] Thus, macrophages in adipose tissue are a major contributor to the inflammatory response observed in obesity.

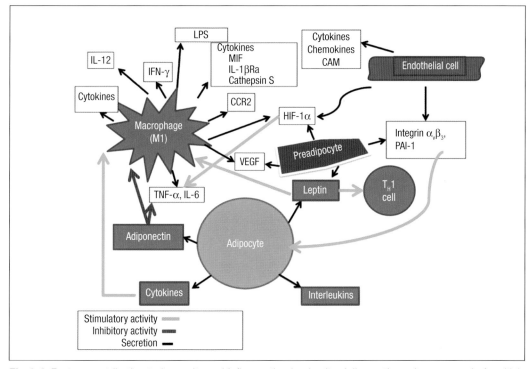

Fig 8-3 Factors contributing to immunity and inflammation in obesity. Adipose tissue is composed of multiple cells. The adipocyte, the characteristic cell of adipose tissue, secretes adipokines, cytokines, and interleukins, all of which play either stimulatory or inhibitory roles in the inflammatory process, including altering macrophage migration and T-helper cell (T$_H$1) distribution toward a more inflammatory pattern. Other cellular components of adipose tissue, including the macrophage, endothelial cell, and preadipocyte, all of which secrete cytokines as well as other products such as HIF-1α, affect proliferation of different cells, including immune cell function. LPS, lipopolysaccharides; IFN-γ, interferon γ; MIF, macrophage migration inhibiting factor; IL-1βRa, interleukin 1β receptor antagonist; CCR2, chemokine receptor 2; CAM, cell adhesion molecules; HIF-1α, hypoxia inducibile factor 1α; PAI-1, plasminogen activator inhibitor 1; VEGF, vascular endothelial growth factor.

Adipocytes secrete proteins, referred to as *adipokines*. These adipokines include leptin and adiponectin as well as interleukins and cytokines, all of which have effects on the immune system.[68] Leptin, a 16-kDa protein, primarily secreted by white adipose tissue and sharing structural homology with cytokines, is secreted in proportion to adipose tissue mass[69] and nutritional status.[70] It is considered to be a signal of energy sufficiency.[68] However, leptin also acts as a cytokine and has been shown to regulate T-cell production of additional cytokines such as stimulation of the T$_H$1 cell type, with its proinflammatory cytokine production, versus the T$_H$2 cell type, with its immunoregulatory cytokine production.[71–73] As a cytokine, leptin activates

phagocytosis by macrophages/monocytes, chemotaxis of neutrophils, and release of oxygen radicals by the leukocytes.[74,75] Adipocyte-derived leptin directly and indirectly stimulates immune responses, augmenting the effects of the non–fat cell component of adipose tissue.

In contrast, adiponectin exhibits dual roles with respect to inflammation. In patients with autoimmune disorders, adiponectin levels increase both locally and systemically in the presence of inflammation.[76] Serum levels are elevated in both systemic lupus erythematosus and rheumatoid arthritis.[77] In patients with rheumatoid arthritis, adiponectin binds to AdipoR receptors on chrondrocytes in a dose-dependent manner and increases messenger RNA expression of matrix metalloproteinases associated with increased destruction of collagen.[78] Both IL-6 and pro–matrix metalloproteinase 1, the principal mediators of inflammation in rheumatoid arthritis, are upregulated by adiponectin.[79] Increased levels of adiponectin have also been found in synovial fluid from subjects with osteoarthritis and rheumatoid arthritis.[80]

The anti-inflammatory activity of adiponectin has been well documented in obese individuals and individuals with metabolic disorders and is negatively correlated with weight gain and obesity.[81–83] Adiponectin modulates insulin sensitivity[84] and vascular reactivity.[85] In addition, adiponectin inhibits colony-forming units of macrophages and granulocytes and suppresses mature macrophage functions.[86]

A reciprocal relationship exists between TNF-α and IL-6 and adiponectin: Production of both TNF-α and IL-6 is inhibited by adiponectin,[87,88] while TNF-α and IL-6 inhibit adiponectin gene expression and secretion.[89] Low adiponectin levels in obese persons are associated with insulin resistance,[90,91] which is at least in part regulated by TNF-α[61,92] and IL-6.[93]

Binding of adiponectin to its receptor activates 5'-AMP-activated protein kinase (AMPK), increases peroxisome proliferator activator receptor alpha ligand activity, and inhibits nuclear factor κB signaling.[88,94,95] Adiponectin regulates endothelial nitric oxide synthase (eNOS) through the promotion of eNOS phosphorylation by an AMPK signaling mechanism.[96] Endothelial nitric oxide plays a protective function, promoting vasodilatation and inhibiting platelet aggregation.[97] In addition, adiponectin inhibits reactive oxygen species, limiting endothelial cell proliferation.[98] The low adiponectin levels in obese individuals therefore support the inflammatory state through loss of suppression of TNF-α and IL-6 and downregulation of anti-inflammatory pathways.[76]

Obesity and angiogenesis

Endothelial cells contribute to the inflammatory process by coordinating the recruitment of leukocytes into the adipose mass.[99] Activation of endothelial cells results in the production of cell adhesion molecules (CAMs), chemokines, cytokines, and ectoenzymes. These mediators guide leukocytes into underlying tissues through a series of steps involving (1) tethering and rolling by adhesion molecules such as selectin; (2) firm adhesion and activation by chemoattractants on the endothelium and adhesion molecules such as integrins on the leukocytes or CAMs on the endothelium; and (3) movement of leukocytes through cell-cell endothelial junctions involving molecules such as platelet endothelial CAMs.[99,100] Cytokines associated with inflammation, such as IL-6 and TNF-α, induce endothelial activation.[101] As a result, the endothelial cell can function as a regulator of the movement of leukocytes into the underlying tissues.

In addition, substances secreted by microvascular endothelial cells have been shown to promote proliferation of preadipocytes, supporting a role of the endothelium as a contributor to fat mass expansion.[102,103] Integrin $\alpha_v\beta_3$ and plasminogen activator inhibitor 1, produced by both endothelial cells and preadipocytes, have been identified as key substances in the coordinated development of both endothelial cells and adipose tissue at the same site,[104] while peroxisome proliferator activator receptor gamma, involved in adipocyte differentiation, has been shown to interfere with both adipose tissue development and angiogenesis if overexpressed.[105] Furthermore, blocking of angiogenesis by use of vascular endothelial growth factor receptor 2–blocking antibody resulted in a similar failure of both angiogenesis and adipose tissue development,[105] as did the use of a variety of other angiogenesis inhibitors.[106] Adipogenesis is therefore dependent on angiogenesis.

Hypoxia is considered a key initiator of the endothelial activation associated with expanding fat tissue.[107] As the fat mass expands with increasing recruitment of leukocytes, the local oxygen supply is inadequate to meet the demand, causing relative hypoxia. Adipose tissue in obese mice has been demonstrated to be in a hypoxic state compared with that of lean mice.[108,109] Hypoxia-inducible factor 1 (HIF-1), a transcription factor, is activated under low oxygen conditions and binds to multiple genes in the *cis*-acting hypoxic response, which is responsible for glucose metabolism and angiogenesis as well as inflammation, cellular stress, extracellular matrix remodeling, and apoptosis.[110] Furthermore, an increase in HIF-1α transcription factor along with an increase in secretion of leptin and vascular endothelial growth factor occurs when human preadipocytes are exposed to hypoxic conditions.[111]

Macrophages in the non–fat cell compartment of adipose tissue also demonstrate gene expression for HIF-1α.[109,112] Under hypoxic conditions, gene expression by macrophages for TNF-α, IL-6, IL-1, migratory inhibiting factor, and vascular endothelial growth factor are increased.[109] With both macrophages and preadipocytes providing evidence of increased cytokine production in the hypoxic state, it is likely that hypoxia underlies the inflammatory state associated with obesity. Therefore, expanding adipose tissue, which contains adipocytes, macrophages, and stromal vascular cells, promotes chronic inflammation through the secretion of inflammatory mediators.

Consequences of Obesity

Morbidity and mortality

Worldwide, being overweight or obese is the fifth leading risk factor for death. In 2013, the WHO estimated that 2.8 million adults die each year as a result of being overweight or obese. Furthermore, these conditions contribute to 44% of the diabetes burden, 23% of the ischemic heart disease burden, and between 7% and 41% of certain cancers.[1] Using the WHO metric of disability-adjusted life years, which measures lost years of healthy life, 2.3% of global disability-adjusted life years (approximately 35.8 million) are caused by overweight or obesity.[113] An analysis of 57 prospective studies reported that a BMI greater than 30 was associated with a life expectancy reduction of 2 to 4 years as compared with adults of healthy weight. Severe obesity (BMI > 40) was associated with a decrease of 8 to 10 years of life expectancy, which is similar to the effects of smoking.[114]

From the clinical perspective, obesity increases the risk of type 2 diabetes, sleep apnea, orthopedic complications, periodontal disease,[115] high plasma lipid levels, hypertension, and other cardiovascular risk factors.[116,117] Epidemiologic studies have shown that obesity is also associated with increased risk of cancers of the colon, endometrium, postmenopausal breast, kidney, esophagus, pancreas, gallbladder, and liver as well as some hematologic malignancies.[118,119] Overweight and obese children who continue in that state into adulthood have increased risks of developing diabetes and cardiovascular disease. However, these risks can be attenuated if the children become nonobese adults.[120] Maternal obesity may affect children before birth, linking obesity and diabetes with autism spectrum disorder and developmental delays.[121]

Psychosocially, obesity can have a long-term negative impact, leaving individuals vulnerable to the development of depression, anxiety, social isolation, discrimination, a lower quality of life, and stigmatization.[122] Weight-related stigmatization affects adults and children, taking the form of teasing, bullying, harassment, and hostility.[123] Obesity has also been associated with unemployment, absenteeism, and the potential for lower wages in comparison to nonobese employees.[124]

Medical costs

According to the US Centers for Disease Control, in 2008 roughly US$147 billion (9.1% of all medical spending) was devoted to obesity-related conditions. On average, the cost of health care for an obese individual exceeds that for a normal-weight person by US$1,429 per year.[3]

Obesity imposes a significant economic burden on both public and private payers. In an analysis of 2006 medical expenditures, researchers reported that the portions of total expenditures attributable to obesity included 8.5% of Medicare spending, 11.8% of Medicaid spending, and 12.9% of private payer

Box 8-2	Criteria for diagnosis of metabolic syndrome (any three or more)

- Hypertension (130/85 mm Hg or higher)
- Elevated fasting plasma glucose (100 mg/dL or higher)
- Waist circumference of 40 inches or more for men and 35 inches or more for women
- High-density lipoprotein cholesterol of less than 40 mg/dL for men and less than 50 mg/dL for women
- Elevated triglycerides (150 mg/dL or higher)

spending. The per capita percentage increase in annual costs attributable to obesity was estimated to be 36% for Medicare (US$1,723 in additional spending per beneficiary), 47% for Medicaid (US$1,021), and 58% for private payers (US$1,140).[4] Among adolescents, the total excess cost related to the prevalence of overweight and obesity in 2008 was estimated to be US$254 billion, comprising US$208 billion in lost productivity and US$46 billion in direct medical costs, as well as 1.5 million life-years lost prematurely.[125]

Total medical costs related to obesity are projected to double every decade to account for 16% to 18% of total US health care expenditures by 2030.[126] At this alarming rate, it is crucial for all health care providers to spread the message about the serious risks of obesity and how it can be prevented with proper diet and lifestyle modifications.

Metabolic syndrome

Metabolic syndrome is a cluster of risk factors that increase the chance of macrovascular disease (including myocardial infarction and stroke) and type 2 diabetes mellitus. The syndrome is intimately related to obesity, specifically midbody weight gain, and insulin resistance. Specific criteria have been developed to identify metabolic syndrome, which is diagnosed if an individual exhibits at least three of the criteria[127] (Box 8-2).

Obesity and the Oral Cavity

The current interest in the relationship of body weight and obesity to oral diseases partially derives from the recognized association between diabetes and obesity and the importance of the relationship between diabetes and oral health (reviewed in chapter 6). The mechanism that is believed to account for the relationship between diabetes and periodontitis is enhanced local and systemic inflammation, and the role of adipocyte- and macrophage-associated production of inflammatory mediators is an important part of that relationship. In addition, weight gain is often related to food intake, and the intake of fermentable carbohydrates can have an effect on the dentition and other tissues in the oral cavity. Finally, overweight and obesity are associated with sleep apnea, and dental professionals are expanding their role in treating this disorder.

Being overweight or obese has also been associated with an increased risk of oral/dental disease. These associations require dental professionals to be vigilant, treat disorders when they are detected, and develop a preventive regimen to reduce the chance of future complications. Further, oral health care professionals must consider their role in obesity management for their patients. Dentists are well versed in delivering a nutrition message related to carbohydrate intake, and this new responsibility could improve both the oral health and general health of patients treated in dental offices.

Table 8-2	Association between periodontitis and the conditions of overweight and obesity*		
Study	N	OR (95% CI)	% Weight
Buhlin et al[131]	96	4.54 (1.59, 13.00)	9.58
Genco et al[132]	12,367	1.48 (1.13, 1.93)	21.18
Nishida et al[133]	372	3.17 (1.79, 5.61)	16.31
Saito et al[134]	584	4.30 (2.10, 8.90)	13.87
Kushiyama et al[135]	1,070	1.09 (0.77, 1.53)	20.09
Han et al[136] (males)	96	2.50 (0.85, 7.38)	9.27
Han et al[136] (females)	102	1.47 (0.52, 4.16)	9.70
Overall (I^2 = 73%, P < .001)		2.13 (1.40, 3.26)	100.00

Odds ratio — 0.25 0.5 1 2 4 8 16

*Reprinted from Suvan et al[130] with permission.
Note: Weights are from random effects analysis.

Periodontal disease

In light of the contribution of obesity to the total inflammatory burden and the importance of the inflammatory response to the progression of periodontitis, the relationship of obesity to periodontitis has been examined. There is evidence from an animal model that obesity can affect the severity of periodontal destruction.[128] Using Wistar rats, researchers established two groups of animals. One group was fed a regular diet and the other a diet high in calories. After 90 days, silk ligatures were placed in the crevice around a maxillary second molar; all animals were killed 30 days later. More weight gain was observed in the animals fed the high-calorie diet. Greater alveolar bone loss was observed on the palatal aspect of animals in the obese group.

The same model has been studied without the use of silk ligatures to induce periodontal destruction. A similar pattern of periodontal destruction was observed in the later study: The obese animals demonstrated significantly greater bone loss on palatal surfaces.[129]

The association between clinical periodontal disease and obesity has been the subject of systematic reviews and meta-analyses. Chaffee and Weston[58] examined 554 citations, and 70

studies met their specific entry criteria, which included publication in English or Spanish, inclusion of a control or comparable group, and a defined relationship between periodontitis and obesity. An emphasis was placed on reporting of periodontitis by accepted clinical parameters and not other variables such as level of oral hygiene or the number of missing teeth.

The 70 studies represented 57 separate study populations. Of these, 28 studies contributed to the calculation of the odds ratio (OR) of the association between periodontal disease and obesity, which was 1.35 (95% confidence interval [CI]: 1.23 to 1.47). There were stronger associations for younger versus older adults, women, and those that did not smoke. Because most of the studies were cross-sectional, it could not be determined if obesity contributed to periodontal disease or vice versa.

A subsequent systematic review and meta-analysis[130] included 33 studies in the systematic review and 19 in the meta-analysis. There was a statistically significant association between periodontitis and obesity (OR = 1.81; CI = 1.42 to 2.30), between periodontitis and being overweight (OR = 1.27; CI = 1.06 to 1.151), and between periodontitis and the combined overweight and obese weight categories (OR = 2.13; CI = 1.40 to 3.26; Table 8-2). Again, cause and effect could not be assessed because of the cross-sectional nature of most of the studies.

Commenting on the biologic plausibility of this association, two explanations were proposed.[130] The first is an exaggerated inflammatory response. Adipocytes and other cell types in fat tissue produce a range of proinflammatory cytokines, and the concentration of acute-phase proteins and the number of circulating leukocytes are elevated in obese individuals.[137] This could enhance the inflammatory response in the local periodontal tissues. In support of this concept, elevated levels of TNF-α in gingival crevicular fluid (GCF) from obese patients have been reported.[138]

The other proposed mechanism is related to reduced sensitivity to insulin, which is important to the linkage between obesity and the development of type 2 diabetes mellitus. Related to circulating levels of proinflammatory cytokines, the result would be elevated blood levels of glucose, increased production and accumulation of advanced glycation endproducts, and a greater systemic inflammatory burden. This mechanism has been associated with increased severity of periodontitis.[139]

Recognizing that cigarette smoking is the most important environmental risk factor for periodontal disease, the relationship between body weight (assessed by BMI) and periodontitis has been assessed in a group of nonsmoking older adults.[140] In a fully adjusted model, there was no significant association between BMI and periodontitis. Compared with individuals with a BMI of less than 25, the relative risk of having a greater extent of periodontitis was 0.7 (95% CI = 0.6 to 0.9) for those individuals with a BMI of 25 through 29 and 1.1 (95% CI = 0.8 to 1.4) for those with a BMI of 30 or higher. This study should be interpreted cautiously because of the other risk factors that would occur in this population, including advanced age,[140] as well as a very lenient definition of periodontitis.

Conflicting findings were also reported in younger individuals, based on data from a longitudinal study.[141] Measures of obesity, including BMI, waist circumference, and a history of being identified as obese or overweight in earlier examinations, were related to measures of peri-

odontal disease, including bleeding following periodontal probing, the presence of calculus, and the number of teeth with a probing depth of 5 mm or greater. While there was an association between gingival bleeding and obesity, this relationship did not remain in a fully adjusted model. Further, no association was observed between deeper probing depths and obesity. A relationship of obesity to dental calculus was observed. Unfortunately, while the larger parent study was longitudinal, the periodontal variables were only collected at one time point.

As noted, one of the drawbacks of this body of literature is the cross-sectional nature of many studies. Longitudinal data are available from a study from the US Veterans Administration. An analysis sought to determine if body weight could predict the progression of periodontitis.[142] Changes in weight, waist circumference, and arm fat were related to changes in periodontal disease over a period of nearly 30 years. Progression of periodontal disease was defined as an increase in probing depth greater than 3 mm or tooth loss associated with periodontitis. Men were categorized at baseline as being normal weight (BMI 18.5 to 24.9 kg/m²), overweight (BMI 25.0 to 29.9 kg/m²), or obese (BMI ≥ 30.0 kg /m²), and weight gain over time in these groups was divided into tertiles.

In general, greater weight gain over time was associated with greater progression of periodontitis.[142] For men with normal weight at baseline, both the greatest weight gain and greatest increase in waist circumference were associated with greater progression of periodontitis than was found in those with the least weight gain or the smallest increase in waist circumference (Fig 8-4). An increase in arm fat was associated with greater progression of periodontal disease in men in the normal weight group. Similar trends were seen for obese men, but differences did not reach significance for this subgroup because there were a small number of obese men in this study. This is an important contribution to the literature on oral changes related to excessive weight and confirms the association between weight gain and progression of periodontitis.

Similar findings were reported in a study of the relationship of BMI at baseline to the devel-

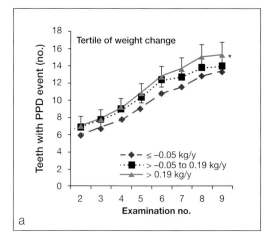

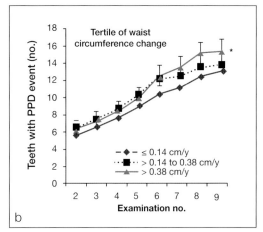

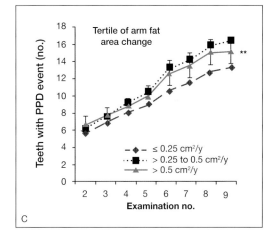

Fig 8-4 Mean cumulative number of teeth with probing pocket depth (PPD) events in men who were normal weight at baseline, by *(a)* change in weight, *(b)* change in waist circumference, and *(c)* change in arm fat area. Overall mean in *(c)* significantly different from that in *(a)* (*P < .05, **P < .01). (Reprinted from Gorman et al[142] with permission.)

opment of periodontal disease during the following 5 years.[143] In a fully adjusted model, the relative risk of developing periodontitis for men who were overweight (BMI 25.0 to 29.9) was 1.30 (P < .001), and for men who were obese (BMI ≥ 30.0) the risk was 1.44 (P = .072). The risks for women in these two groups were 1.70 (P < .01) and 3.24 (P < .05), respectively.

More recently, a systematic review and meta-analysis has examined the relationship of metabolic syndrome to periodontitis.[144] Metabolic syndrome is a complex of clinical and physiologic alterations that include excessive weight and obesity, insulin resistance, dyslipidemia, and elevated blood pressure. Metabolic syndrome places individuals at risk for devel-

opment of diabetes mellitus and cardiovascular disease. Periodontitis has been linked to a number of the criteria that are part of metabolic syndrome. A total of 20 studies were examined for this review. Most were cross-sectional in design, and together they yielded an OR of 1.71 (95% CI = 1.42 to 2.03) that a patient with metabolic syndrome would have periodontitis. The OR increased to 2.09 (95% CI = 1.28 to 3.44) when a more precise diagnosis of metabolic syndrome was required. Approximately 40% of patients with metabolic syndrome also presented with periodontitis.

This review[144] identified an association between metabolic syndrome and periodontitis. However, the direction of this association (metabolic syndrome affecting periodontitis or periodontitis affecting metabolic syndrome) could not be assessed because of a lack of longitudinal data. Further, metabolic syndrome includes a number of criteria that are risk factors for periodontitis, emphasizing the complex nature of these associations.

There is also preliminary evidence to suggest that treatment of periodontal disease in patients with metabolic syndrome reduces CRP level and the white blood cell count and raises the level of high-density lipoproteins.[145] Therefore, it was concluded that patients with metabolic syndrome should have a dental evaluation and that treatment is warranted if periodontitis is present. In addition, patients presenting to the dental office with periodontitis and signs and symptoms of metabolic syndrome should be referred to a medical provider for appropriate treatment.

Levels of inflammatory mediators in biologic fluids from patients with obesity and periodontitis can provide insight into the systemic and local inflammatory responses. Progranulin is a proinflammatory mediator that has been associated with an influx of polymorphonuclear leukocytes and macrophages and neovascularization in wound healing sites.[146] CRP levels are closely linked to levels of progranulin, and elevations in BMI are associated with elevations in progranulin. Four groups of patients were evaluated: Individuals who were not obese and were without periodontitis (group 1), those who were obese but were without periodontitis (group 2), those who were not obese but had periodontitis (group 3), and those who were obese and had periodontitis (group 4). The concentration of both mediators were determined both in serum and GCF. The concentrations of CRP in serum and GCF were highest in group 4, followed by groups 2, 3, and then 1, indicating that levels of both mediators were more closely associated with obesity than with periodontitis.

A panel of inflammatory markers and adipocytokines were evaluated in serum and GCF from individuals in four groups (with or without obesity and with or without periodontitis).[147] Levels of resistin, adiponectin, leptin, TNF-α, and IL-6 were determined. Both obesity and periodontal disease appeared to influence the concentration of the inflammatory mediators in serum and GCF. The levels of adiponectin, which is considered to be anti-inflammatory, were lower in the serum of patients with periodontitis and were not influenced by obesity. TNF-α levels were influenced by both obesity and periodontitis. Higher levels of TNF-α were found in obese patients than in normal-weight patients when periodontitis was not present. Periodontitis also increased the levels of TNF-α. These data emphasize that the effect of periodontitis and obesity on local and systemic levels of inflammatory mediators is complex.[147]

Treatment effects can also be used to assess the importance of these relationships. The effect of conservative periodontal therapy on circulating levels of inflammatory mediators has been studied in obese and normal-weight individuals with periodontitis.[148] All individuals received a complete periodontal examination, evaluation of the lipid profile, and assessment of the levels of CRP, blood glucose, insulin, IL-6, TNF-α, and leptin. Insulin resistance was also determined. All parameters were recorded prior to treatment and 3 months after root planing and scaling (which also included extraction of hopeless teeth) and a protocol for complete-mouth disinfection that relied on subgingival irrigation and rinsing with chlorhexidine.

Both groups demonstrated a pronounced improvement in clinical parameters following treatment.[148] The obese group demonstrated a significant reduction in the concentration of IL-6, TNF-α, and leptin following treatment, while the normal-weight individuals demonstrated a reduction in the concentration of IL-6. Further, insulin resistance decreased in the obese individuals. This was a small study, but results suggested that periodontal disease and periodontal inflammation can both adversely affect the concentration of inflammatory mediators in blood and induce insulin resistance in patients with obesity and periodontitis.

Dental caries

Studies of the relationship between dental caries and BMI in children are not conclusive. A systematic review of the literature in 2012 examined 48 articles that were published between 2004 and 2011.[149] The studies fell into three categories with respect to the association between BMI and dental caries: The authors reported that 23 studies found no association, 17 found a positive relationship, and 9 found that caries decreased with increasing BMI.

Another systematic review and meta-analysis analyzed results from 14 studies.[150] A significant relationship was observed between obesity and caries overall but not when the permanent and primary dentitions were analyzed separately. Obesity and caries were positively correlated in children from industrialized countries but not in newly industrialized countries. Socioeconomic status and age were significant risk factors. These authors observed that the method of measuring weight affected the results. Use of standardized measures, such as BMI-for-age percentile, revealed a significant correlation more often.

The expectation that caries and weight status should be correlated is based on the assumption and, in many cases, the observation that overweight individuals consume greater quantities of sugary foods, sodas, and other cariogenic foods. Dietary patterns such as the frequent eating of cariogenic foods have been shown to increase the risk for dental caries.[151,152] Children with severe early childhood caries have been shown to ingest food and beverages more frequently than caries-free children. Affected children also consume foods with greater cariogenic potential.[151] Several studies have noted that there is an association between consumption of sugar-sweetened beverages and obesity.[41,153,154] There is also evidence of a link between sugary drinks and dental caries.[155,156]

As the aforementioned systematic reviews demonstrate, there are many reports in the literature of associations between obesity and dental caries, particularly from outside the United States. A longitudinal study of more than 4,000 children (aged 4 to 8 years) in Australia examined the relationships among weight, caries, and diet.[157] Overweight and obesity and dental problems were associated with consumption of sweetened beverages and fatty foods.

In a cohort of 1,160 Mexican children aged 4 to 5 years, a significant association was found between caries in the primary dentition and be-

ing overweight or at risk for being overweight.[158] A study of 403 Swedish 15-year-olds who had been followed since the age of 1 year found that snacking habits reported in early childhood were associated with interproximal caries at age 15 years.[159] The overweight and obese adolescents in this group had more interproximal caries as well.

In a German study of 2,071 primary school pupils, a significant association between caries prevalence and BMI was found.[160] Low BMI was correlated with the absence of caries lesions ($P < .0001$), while high BMI was correlated with higher caries prevalence ($P = .0021$). The correlation between BMI and caries remained significant after data were adjusted for age.

Another Swedish study examined longitudinal data for 2,303 10-year-old children, including socioeconomic status; BMI at ages 4, 5, 7, and 10 years; and caries at ages 6, 10, and 12 years.[161] Caries prevalence decreased with higher socioeconomic status, but this variable was not associated with BMI. Obese children in this study had more caries than normal and overweight children. The authors concluded that there was a significant, but weak, association between being overweight and caries prevalence.

Another group of studies, many of them from the United States, did not find an association between body weight and caries. A systematic review by Kantovitz et al[162] reported that only one of seven cross-sectional studies with children showed an association between obesity and caries. In addition, analyses of oral health and body measurement data from the 1999 to 2002 NHANES indicated that, for the 6,000 children between the ages of 2 and 17 years, there was no statistically significant association between caries and BMI-for-age percentile.[163] This was true for both the permanent dentition and the primary dentition after researchers controlled for age, sex, race or ethnicity, and poverty status. Furthermore, overweight children with a history of caries had fewer decayed, missing, and filled teeth than did their normal-weight counterparts.

A later study based on the same NHANES database focused on the data for 2- to 6-year-olds with at least 10 primary teeth.[164] No significant association was found between being overweight and caries for the 1,507 children included in the analyses. An association was noted for the subgroup of Hispanic and non-Hispanic black groups, but after data were controlled for age and family income, the association was not significant.

A third study of national data examined results from NHANES III (1988 to 1994) for 10,180 children and from the 1999 to 2000 NHANES for 7,568 children.[165] In both surveys, among children 2 to 5 years of age, there were no significant differences in caries prevalence by weight categories. The same held true for children aged 6 to 18 years from the 1999 to 2000 NHANES. However, in NHANES III, overweight children aged 6 to 18 years were actually less likely to have caries than the normal-weight group. In a much smaller convenience sample of 178 children 8 to 11 years of age, the lack of an overall association between BMI and caries was confirmed.[166] However, an association was found between interproximal caries affecting permanent molar teeth and higher BMI.

Studies conducted outside of the United States have also failed to identify an association between weight and dental caries. A study of 1,003 children from Iran found that a surprising 67% of the 6- to 11-year-olds were overweight.[167] However, the researchers found no association between BMI-for-age percentile and number of decayed and filled teeth in the primary or permanent dentitions. Further, they found a statistically significant association between BMI-for-age percentile and being caries free.

A 4-year longitudinal study of 110 Mexican children found that, despite having more erupted teeth, children in the higher BMI categories had a lower number of decayed, missing, and filled teeth.[168] Starting at age 7 years and ending at age 11 years, the study revealed that the proportion of children in the overweight categories rose from 29.6% to 45.5%. Similar findings were reported in 2012 study of 8,284 Kuwaiti children aged 9 to 11 years.[169] In this cross-sectional observation of caries and weight, researchers reported a statistically significant decrease in the prevalence of caries in permanent teeth with increasing BMI-for-age categories.

Clearly, there are conflicting findings in the literature with respect to caries and weight status, suggesting that this relationship is complex and affected by a multitude of factors. Diet, eating patterns, socioeconomic status, race and ethnicity, and psychosocial factors are important variables that are discussed in the literature. Systematic reviews note the inconsistencies in the measures of weight status[150] as a possible cause of the variation in findings. Physiologic factors, such as a reduced flow rate of whole saliva in obese children, have been suggested as a possible explanation for increased risk of caries.[170]

While risk factors associated with obesity have been shown to be associated with caries, it is not clear which factors are common to both conditions. Dental caries and sleep duration were significantly related in a pilot study of 90 10-year-old Kuwaiti girls.[171] Those who reported shorter weekday sleep duration had more decayed and filled teeth surfaces and reported consuming more sugary foods. However, elevated sugar consumption alone was not associated with caries prevalence or obesity.

More research is needed to address the conflicting findings in the relationship between caries and weight status. Identifying truly common risk factors would be a way to implement preventive measures for these two chronic conditions. Furthermore, exploring the reasons for differences between groups may allow researchers to develop innovative ways to decrease the negative impacts of both obesity and caries.

Tooth eruption

Evidence suggests that high body fat content affects hormonal metabolism and growth, such that obese children have accelerated linear growth and skeletal maturation before puberty.[172,173] Obesity is also associated with early puberty and paradoxically, a slowing of linear growth during puberty, particularly in girls.[173–175] Some studies suggest that obese children have early craniofacial growth, which leads to modifications in the timing and planning of orthodontic treatment.[176] Maxillomandibular prognathism and greater facial measurements have been found more often in obese adolescents than in those with normal weight.[177]

Given the association between obesity and acceleration in skeletal growth, it is possible that hormonal changes produced by obesity could modify the timing of tooth eruption. Many cross-sectional studies have shown that overweight or obese children have accelerated dental development, which can have implications for caries risk and orthodontic treatment.

Hilgers et al[178] determined dental ages for 104 children using the method described by Demirjian et al.[179] They subtracted each subject's chronologic age from the calculated dental age so that a positive value reflected accelerated dental development and a negative value reflected delayed development. The mean difference between estimated dental age and chronologic age for all subjects was 0.98 years. When analyzed by BMI-for-age percentile, the mean difference in dental age was 1.51 ± 1.22 years for the 22% of subjects who were overweight and 1.53 ± 1.28 years for the 17% who were obese. The researchers concluded that dental development was significantly accelerated in children with a higher BMI percentile even after data were adjusted for age and sex.[178]

Zangouei-Booshehri et al[180] followed the same study design in 100 children aged 8 to 12 years. Using the international BMI standards and collapsing the categories into normal and above-normal groups, they found that the mean eruptive age was 9.52 years for the children with normal BMI and 10.00 years for the 15% in the above-normal BMI group. They concluded that increased BMI is associated with increased dental eruptive age.

BMI percentile, skeletal maturation, and dental age of 540 orthodontic patients, 8 to 17 years of age, were assessed with a retrospective chart review.[181] Linear regression and logistic regression models assessed the effect of weight status on dental age and cervical vertebral stage. The results demonstrated that cervical vertebral stage and dental age were slightly, but significantly, greater in subjects with higher BMI percentiles. The coefficient for the BMI percentile was 0.005 year per 1 unit of increase in dental age ($P < .001$), and the OR for the effect of the BMI percentile on the cervical vertebral method was 1.02 ($P < .001$).

Using Demirjian's method[179] to compare chronologic and dental age, Weddell and Hartsfield[182] evaluated 257 panoramic radiographs of 5- to 17.5-year-old white children. Overweight and obese children were significantly more dentally advanced than normal-weight and underweight subjects.[182]

In the longitudinal study of 110 Mexican schoolchildren cited in the previous discussion of caries, the researchers found that while overweight children had fewer carious teeth, they had more erupted permanent teeth.[168] At 11 years of age, the children in the overweight group had an average of 5 more permanent teeth than did normal-weight children, having 21.6 erupted permanent teeth compared with 15.9 permanent teeth in children of normal weight.[168]

Looking at percentage of body fat as another measure of obesity, Costacurta et al[183] calculated BMI-for-age percentile, conducted a DEXA examination for body fat analysis, and assessed skeletal and dental age in 107 healthy children. The difference between chronologic and skeletal-dental age was statistically significant for preobese and obese children but not for underweight and normal-weight children. The results demonstrated that, in addition to BMI-for-age percentile, there is an association between accelerated skeletal-dental age and percentage of body fat as measured by DEXA.

The aforementioned studies were carried out in convenience samples, opening the possibility of biased or nongeneralizable findings. However, a study based on data from three NHANES databases collected from 2001 to 2006 also found that obesity was significantly associated with tooth eruption in children.[184] In this national proportional probability sample, designed to reflect the US population, obese children aged 5 to 14 years had a higher average number of erupted teeth during the mixed dentition period. Analyses of 5,434 participants found that, on average, obese children had 1.44 more erupted

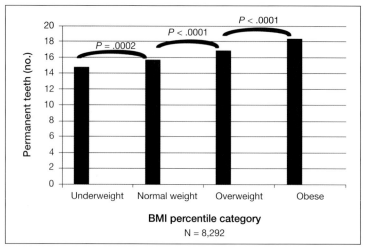

Fig 8-5 Number of permanent teeth by BMI percentiles for 8,292 Kuwaiti fourth and fifth grade children.[169]

permanent teeth than did nonobese children after data were adjusted for age, sex, and race and ethnicity.

The correlation between BMI-for-age percentile and the sequence of tooth eruption was examined in a cross-sectional highly homogenous sample of 8,292 children in Kuwait, where obesity, metabolic syndrome, and type 2 diabetes are highly prevalent.[169] Data from year 1 of a longitudinal study included BMI, waist circumference, and a count of decayed and filled teeth in the primary and permanent dentitions of fourth and fifth grade children, aged 9 to 11 years. Researchers found that 90% of children who were categorized as obese by waist circumference measurements were also obese according to BMI-for-age percentiles. According to the BMI-for-age percentiles, 29% of the children were obese and 18% were overweight.

When compared with the 53% of subjects who were normal weight or underweight, the obese and overweight children had significantly more permanent teeth when data were adjusted for age and sex: The overweight group had an average of 1.2 more teeth, and the obese group had 2.7 more teeth than did the normal-weight group (Fig 8-5). Moreover, this study demonstrated that there was a statistically significant difference in mean number of teeth between each discreet BMI category; the obese group had an average of 1.5 more teeth than the overweight group. Girls had significantly more permanent teeth than boys, regardless of BMI category. Furthermore, obese children were taller than nonobese children ($P < .0001$).[169]

Multiple study observations strongly support the evidence that obese and overweight children have an earlier tooth eruption sequence and have greater height than do nonobese children of the same age and sex, indicative of a pattern of earlier maturation. Mechanisms to explain accelerated skeletal maturation and early puberty in obese children are complex. In the literature, it has been suggested that leptin, a hormone produced by adipose tissue, can stimulate skeletal growth and accelerate pubertal development.[185,186]

Alternatively, leptin might act directly on the skeletal growth centers. Leptin receptors have been found in the cartilaginous growth centers that are involved in skeletal maturation. Therefore, an obese individual would have a mechanism of central resistance to leptin and an increased sensitivity to leptin at a peripheral level, causing increased differentiation and proliferation of chondrocytes, resulting in precocious skeletal maturation.[187] Leptin was strongly associated with fat mass as well as loss of eating control in a study of 7- to 18-year-olds.[188] The concentration of leptin in saliva was significantly higher in obese children than in nonobese children.[169]

Clearly, early tooth eruption and skeletal maturation are important considerations in dentistry. The correlation between early eruption and increased risk of caries has not been consistently found, and, in fact, there is evidence of an inverse correlation between caries and obesity.[168,169] However, for orthodontic therapy, knowledge of the stage of skeletal development is essential, because treatment is often implemented during the primary or mixed dentition period.[189] If not anticipated, discrepancies between skeletal-dental and chronologic age may jeopardize the outcome of treatment.

Masticatory efficiency

The relationship between body weight and masticatory efficiency may be an important determinant of the obesity–oral disease relationship.[190] If masticatory function is compromised, individuals may avoid hard-to-chew foods that contain fiber and instead choose processed foods or foods that are rich in carbohydrates with only limited amounts of fiber, protein, and other important nutrients. The results will be a greater caloric intake than what is expended and, consequently, weight gain.

Masticatory efficiency has been assessed in patients with a range of dental conditions.[190] In one study, participants chewed a test cylinder of silicone rubber, and particle size was evaluated after 20 chewing cycles. The swallowing trigger was also determined, participants were questioned about their ability to chew, and an oral examination was conducted to determine the number of occluding teeth. The participants' weights were assessed as the BMI.

Increased BMI was associated with the presence of fewer than 10 occluding pairs of teeth. Similarly, both reduced masticatory function and swallowing trigger were associated with a higher BMI. However, eating habits and masticatory function are complex processes, and the

authors emphasized the importance of a multidisciplinary health care approach to management of overweight and obese patients. They stressed that dentists can play different roles in this effort, including counseling patients about excessive weight and healthy eating as well as restoring masticatory function to enhance a patient's ability to eat a healthy diet.

Sleep, Obesity, and Sleep Apnea

The quality and duration of sleep are widely regarded as important, although not always obvious, factors in weight gain in children and adults.[191] In a 2011 study of 44,452 adults, those with sleep duration of less than 6 hours per night were significantly more likely to have signs of metabolic syndrome than were those with longer sleep duration.[192] The Nurses' Health Study found that adult women who slept 5 hours or less per night were 15% more likely to become obese over the course of the study than women who slept 7 hours or more each night.[193]

Children may be particularly vulnerable to the effects of too little sleep. In a prospective cohort study of 915 US children, those who slept less than 12 hours a day as infants had twice the chance of being overweight at age 3 years than did their counterparts who slept more than 12 hours.[194] A British study followed more than 8,000 children from birth and found that those who slept fewer than 10.5 hours a night at age 3 years had a 45% higher risk of becoming obese by age 7 years.[195] Some of the factors associated with shorter infant sleep duration include maternal depression during pregnancy, early introduction of solid foods (before age 4 months), and infant television viewing.[196]

Sleep duration has been related to elevated blood pressure.[197–201] There is also sufficient evidence that sleep duration could be an important marker of cardiovascular disease.[200] In an experiment in which healthy young men were sleep restricted for just 2 days, Spiegel et al[202] found decreased levels of the hormone leptin (which controls appetite) and increased levels of plasma ghrelin (which increases appetite and favors the accumulation of lipids in visceral fatty tissue). This finding is supported by a sleep laboratory study in which individuals who were deprived of sleep and surrounded by tasty snacks tended to eat more during the extra hours they were awake at night than when they had adequate sleep.[203] In a more recent study of healthy individuals, Buxton et al[204] reported that short and disrupted sleep altered insulin levels and slowed metabolism to a rate that could add more than 12 lb of weight in a year.

Population-based studies have revealed a strong relationship between obstructive sleep apnea (OSA) and obesity; more than 70% of individuals with OSA are clinically obese based on their BMI status.[205] OSA is associated with both obesity and diabetes, and a summary review of multiple studies suggests that weight loss can reduce OSA and have a positive effect on metabolic and cardiovascular risks.[206] Among patients attending a diabetes obesity clinic, 58% had OSA that was associated with worsening glycemic control.[207]

Obesity is a factor in both the development and severity of OSA. Obesity appears to affect control of the upper airway by alterations in upper airway structure and function, reductions in resting load volume, and negative effects on respiratory drive and load compensation.[208] Insulin resistance is also associated with OSA severity and may be linked with sleep deprivation or sympathetic activation.[209] A reciprocal relationship between OSA and obesity has been described by Ong et al,[208] who found that OSA has an impact on body weight in a variety of ways. OSA causes changes in energy expenditure during sleep and wakefulness, increases preference for energy-dense food, alters hormonal regulation specific to appetite and satiety, and affects sleep duration and quality, which may impact daytime physical activity, lethargy, and sleepiness.

Children are also affected by OSA. Kohler et al[210] found that, among adolescents, there was a 3.5-fold increase in OSA risk with each standard deviation increase in BMI percentile. Studies have demonstrated a relationship among OSA, inflammation, and insulin resistance in both obese and nonobese children.[211,212] In another study, imaging techniques revealed a strong relationship between visceral adiposity and OSA, independent of BMI.[213] The authors concluded that the quantity and location of adipose tissue were factors that might explain why some obese children do or do not develop OSA.

Dentists can play an active role in identifying children and adults with possible OSA and referring them for assessment.[214] Early detection, referral, and coordinated care with patients' physicians can prevent additional consequences and improve quality of life.[215] With the increasing interest in the use of oral appliances, more dentists are becoming involved in the care of patients with sleep-related breathing disorders.[216] Data suggest that mandibular advancement appliances can have a beneficial effect on sleep apnea. In a small crossover study, two different appliances were shown to be effective in improving symptoms in patients affected by mild to moderate sleep apnea.[217,218] In addition, use of a mandibular advancement appliance was associated with improvement in measures of quality of life for both patients and their bed partners.[219]

A position paper from the Canadian Sleep Society emphasized the importance of a team approach to caring for patients with OSA.[220] The report emphasized that physicians should make the diagnosis, and the appliance should only be fabricated by a dentist experienced in this clinical area. Further, treatment outcomes should be assessed by physicians using accepted methods, including polysomnography.

Conclusion

Obesity is now considered one of the most important health problems in the United States. The Institute of Medicine of the National Academy of Sciences has issued a number of reports in the last decade on this subject. In 2012, the institute issued a report that examined strategies for obesity prevention and made recommendations for the future.[221] The recommendations included an emphasis on exercise and

Fig 8-6 Decreasing obesity risk factors can improve oral health. (Reprinted from Tavares et al[10] with permission.)

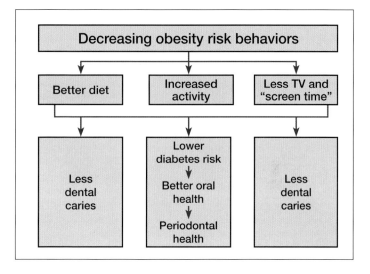

physical activity and how healthy living can be achieved, increased availability of healthy foods and beverages, an emphasis on obesity management as an important part of the work environment and a focus for health care personnel, and the important role that schools should play by focusing attention of younger individuals on health and healthy living.

Those recommendations clearly emphasize that obesity management is a national problem and that solutions must be societal. Considering their familiarity with dietary advice and messaging and the frequency with which they see patients, dental providers are in a position to make an important contribution in the effort to control obesity in the population.

The relationships between obesity and specific oral diseases and disorders (periodontal disease, dental caries, and early tooth eruption) are biologically plausible. The data supporting the relationship between obesity and periodontitis are the strongest. However, Chaffee and Weston[58] concluded that the cross-sectional nature of the majority of studies did not allow for determination of cause and effect, that is, the direction of the association.

Suvan et al[130] concluded that proinflammatory mechanisms associated with obesity (increased local inflammatory response, reduced insulin sensitivity, and elevated blood glucose levels leading to greater accumulation of advanced glycation endproducts) suggest that obesity can exacerbate periodontitis. However, they noted that many confounders, including smoking and diet, can influence both obesity and periodontitis. Further, a 5-year longitudinal study of weight gain and progression of periodontitis suggested that both weight gain and periodontal disease progression occurred concurrently.[142] The relationship of obesity and periodontal disease can be considered in the context of diabetes mellitus and periodontitis. That relationship is bidirectional, but the data supporting the notion that diabetes mellitus affects periodontitis are stronger than the data supporting the converse.

Oral health care professionals can make important contributions to the fight against obesity in different ways (Fig 8-6).[11] If periodontitis is present, treatment may help patients retain their dentition and thereby maintain a healthy diet. Furthermore, periodontal therapy can help to reduce the systemic inflammatory burden. In addition to treating oral disease and developing a preventive regimen to avoid future disease, dentists may provide appliance therapy to treat sleep apnea. Moreover, oral health care providers can advise patients regarding their diet and caloric intake.

It has been proposed that oral health care providers take an active role in obesity prevention and treatment. The frequency of dental visits for a significant segment of the population, as well as the fact that oral health care providers understand an appropriate diet that emphasizes reduced caloric intake, make this role a logical extension of dental practice. Nevertheless, treatment of obesity requires an interprofessional approach that includes physicians and other medical providers as well as dieticians.

In the future, dentists and dental hygienists should consider providing a broader health message to their patients, including the importance of a healthy lifestyle, exercise, diet control, smoking cessation (if necessary), and weight management. Adoption of this expanded range of responsibilities is in keeping with the training of oral health care providers, will place these providers in closer alignment with the health care system, and ultimately will result in improved oral health and health outcomes for patients.

Acknowledgment

The authors acknowledge the assistance of Lisa Lian, Harvard School of Dental Medicine, Class of 2016.

References

1. World Health Organization. Obesity and overweight. Fact sheet No. 311. March 2013. http://www.who.int/mediacentre/factsheets/fs311/en. Accessed 29 May 2013.
2. US Department of Health and Human Services, Centers for Disease Control and Prevention. The power of prevention: Chronic disease...The public health challenge of the 21st century. 2009. http://www.cdc.gov/chronicdisease/pdf/2009-Power-of-Prevention.pdf. Accessed 29 May 2013.
3. US Department of Health and Human Services. Centers for Disease Control and Prevention. Overweight and obesity, Causes and consequences. 2011. http://www.cdc.gov/obesity/adult/causes/index.html. Accessed 29 May 2013.
4. Finkelstein EA, Trogdon JG, Cohen JW, Dietz W. Annual medical spending attributable to obesity: Payer-and service-specific estimates. Health Aff (Millwood) 2009;28:w822–w831.
5. Hu FB. Measurements of adiposity and body composition. In: Hu FB (ed). Obesity Epidemiology. New York: Oxford University Press, 2008:53–83.
6. Mei Z, Grummer-Strawn LM, Pietrobelli A, Goulding A, Goran MI, Dietz WH. Validity of body mass index compared with other body-composition screening indexes for the assessment of body fatness in children and adolescents. Am J Clin Nutr 2002;75:978–985.
7. US Department of Health and Human Services, Centers for Disease Control and Prevention. Healthy weight—It's not a diet, it's a lifestyle! Child and teen—About BMI. 13 Sept 2011. http://www.cdc.gov/healthyweight/assessing/bmi/childrens_bmi/about_childrens_bmi.html. Accessed 29 May 2013.
8. Tchernof A, Despres JP. Pathophysiology of human visceral obesity: An update. Physiol Rev 2013;93:359–404.
9. Zimmet P, Magliano D, Matsuzawa Y, Alberti G, Shaw J. The metabolic syndrome: A global public health problem and a new definition. J Atheroscler Thromb 2005;12:295–300.
10. Tavares M, Dewundara A, Goodson JM. Obesity prevention and intervention in dental practice. Dent Clin North Am 2012;56:831–846.
11. Flegal KM, Carroll MD, Ogden CL, Curtin LR. Prevalence and trends in obesity among US adults, 1999–2008. JAMA 2010;303:235–241.
12. Al Rashdan I, Al Nesef Y. Prevalence of overweight, obesity, and metabolic syndrome among adult Kuwaitis: Results from community-based national survey. Angiology 2010;61:42–48.
13. de Onis M, Blossner M, Borghi E. Global prevalence and trends of overweight and obesity among preschool children. Am J Clin Nutr 2010;92:1257–1264.
14. Gerberding JL. Diabetes, disabling disease to double by 2050. 2007. http://www.cdc.gov/nccdphp/publications/aag/ddt.htm. Accessed 8 April 2013.
15. Ogden CL, Carroll MD, Kit BK, Flegal KM. Prevalence of obesity in the United States, 2009–2010. NCHS Data Brief 2012;(82):1–8.
16. Wang YC, McPherson K, Marsh T, Gortmaker SL, Brown M. Health and economic burden of the projected obesity trends in the USA and the UK. Lancet 2011;378:815–825.
17. Trust for America's Health and Robert Wood Johnson Foundation. F as in Fat: How Obesity Threatens America's Future. Sept 2012. http://www.healthyamericans.org/report/100. Accessed 29 May 2013.
18. US Department of Health and Human Services. HHS News. HHS Releases Assessment of Healthy People 2010 Objectives. Life Expectancy Rises, but Health Disparities Remain. Oct 2011. http://www.healthypeople.gov/2020/about/HP2010PressReleaseOct5.doc. Accessed 29 May 2013.

19. Ogden CL, Carroll MD, Curtin LR, Lamb MM, Flegal KM. Prevalence of high body mass index in US children and adolescents, 2007–2008. JAMA 2010; 303:242–249.

20. The NS, Suchindran C, North KE, Popkin BM, Gordon-Larsen P. Association of adolescent obesity with risk of severe obesity in adulthood. JAMA 2010;304:2042–2047.

21. Ritchie LD, Welk G, Styne D, Gerstein DE, Crawford PB. Family environment and pediatric overweight: What is a parent to do? J Am Diet Assoc 2005;105 (5 suppl 1):S70–S79.

22. Ogden CL, Carroll MD, Kit BK, Flegal KM. Prevalence of obesity and trends in body mass index among US children and adolescents, 1999–2010. JAMA 2012;307:483–490.

23. Skelton JA, Cook SR, Auinger P, Klein JD, Barlow SE. Prevalence and trends of severe obesity among US children and adolescents. Acad Pediatr 2009;9: 322–329.

24. Popkin BM, Duffey KJ. Does hunger and satiety drive eating anymore? Increasing eating occasions and decreasing time between eating occasions in the United States. Am J Clin Nutr 2010;91:1342–1347.

25. Ludwig DS, Currie J. The association between pregnancy weight gain and birthweight: A within-family comparison. Lancet 2010;376:984–990.

26. Oken E, Taveras EM, Kleinman KP, Rich-Edwards JW, Gillman MW. Gestational weight gain and child adiposity at age 3 years. Am J Obstet Gynecol 2007;196:322.e1–322.e8.

27. Hillier TA, Pedula KL, Schmidt MM, Mullen JA, Charles MA, Pettitt DJ. Childhood obesity and metabolic imprinting: The ongoing effects of maternal hyperglycemia. Diabetes Care 2007;30:2287–2292.

28. Oken E, Levitan EB, Gillman MW. Maternal smoking during pregnancy and child overweight: Systematic review and meta-analysis. Int J Obes (Lond) 2008; 32:201–210.

29. Willett WC, Leibel RL. Dietary fat is not a major determinant of body fat. Am J Med 2002;113(suppl 9B):47S–59S.

30. Melanson EL, Astrup A, Donahoo WT. The relationship between dietary fat and fatty acid intake and body weight, diabetes, and the metabolic syndrome. Ann Nutr Metab 2009;55:229–243.

31. Howard BV, Manson JE, Stefanick ML, et al. Low-fat dietary pattern and weight change over 7 years: The Women's Health Initiative Dietary Modification Trial. JAMA 2006;295:39–49.

32. Mozaffarian D, Hao T, Rimm EB, Willett WC, Hu FB. Changes in diet and lifestyle and long-term weight gain in women and men. N Engl J Med 2011;364: 2392–2404.

33. Barclay AW, Petocz P, McMillan-Price J, et al. Glycemic index, glycemic load, and chronic disease risk—A meta-analysis of observational studies. Am J Clin Nutr 2008;87:627–637.

34. Mente A, de Koning L, Shannon HS, Anand SS. A systematic review of the evidence supporting a causal link between dietary factors and coronary heart disease. Arch Intern Med 2009;169:659–669.

35. Thompson AK, Minihane AM, Williams CM. Trans fatty acids and weight gain. Int J Obes (Lond) 2011;35:315–324.

36. Koh-Banerjee P, Chu NF, Spiegelman D, et al. Prospective study of the association of changes in dietary intake, physical activity, alcohol consumption, and smoking with 9-y gain in waist circumference among 16 587 US men. Am J Clin Nutr 2003; 78:719–727.

37. Field AE, Willett WC, Lissner L, Colditz GA. Dietary fat and weight gain among women in the Nurses' Health Study. Obesity (Silver Spring) 2007;15:967–976.

38. Hu FB, Malik VS. Sugar-sweetened beverages and risk of obesity and type 2 diabetes: Epidemiologic evidence. Physiol Behav 2010;100:47–54.

39. Ogden CL, Kit BK, Carroll MD, Park S. Consumption of sugar drinks in the United States, 2005–2008. NCHS Data Brief 2011(71):1–8.

40. Vartanian LR, Schwartz MB, Brownell KD. Effects of soft drink consumption on nutrition and health: A systematic review and meta-analysis. Am J Public Health 2007;97:667–675.

41. Malik VS, Willett WC, Hu FB. Sugar-sweetened beverages and BMI in children and adolescents: Reanalyses of a meta-analysis. Am J Clin Nutr 2009;89:438–440.

42. Ebbeling CB, Feldman HA, Osganian SK, Chomitz VR, Ellenbogen SJ, Ludwig DS. Effects of decreasing sugar-sweetened beverage consumption on body weight in adolescents: A randomized, controlled pilot study. Pediatrics 2006;117:673–680.

43. Piernas C, Popkin BM. Food portion patterns and trends among U.S. children and the relationship to total eating occasion size, 1977–2006. J Nutr 2011; 141:1159–1164.

44. Poti JM, Popkin BM. Trends in energy intake among US children by eating location and food source, 1977–2006. J Am Diet Assoc 2011;111:1156–1164.

45. Juneau CE, Potvin L. Trends in leisure-, transport-, and work-related physical activity in Canada 1994–2005. Prev Med 2010;51:384–386.

46. Brownson RC, Boehmer TK, Luke DA. Declining rates of physical activity in the United States: what are the contributors? Annu Rev Public Health 2005; 26:421–443.

47. Petersen CB, Thygesen LC, Helge JW, Gronbaek M, Tolstrup JS. Time trends in physical activity in leisure time in the Danish population from 1987 to 2005. Scand J Public Health 2010;38:121–128.

48. Ng SW, Norton EC, Popkin BM. Why have physical activity levels declined among Chinese adults? Findings from the 1991–2006 China Health and Nutrition Surveys. Soc Sci Med 2009;68:1305–1314.

49. Lee IM, Djousse L, Sesso HD, Wang L, Buring JE. Physical activity and weight gain prevention. JAMA 2010;303:1173–1179.

50. Mekary RA, Feskanich D, Hu FB, Willett WC, Field AE. Physical activity in relation to long-term weight maintenance after intentional weight loss in premenopausal women. Obesity (Silver Spring) 2010; 18:167–174.

51. Lusk AC, Mekary RA, Feskanich D, Willett WC. Bicycle riding, walking, and weight gain in premenopausal women. Arch Intern Med 2010;170:1050–1056.

52. Hu FB. Physical activity, sedentary behaviors, and obesity. In: Hu FB (ed). Obesity Epidemiology. New York: Oxford University Press, 2008:301–319.

53. US Department of Health and Human Services. 2008 Physical Activity Guidelines for Americans. Oct 2008. http://www.health.gov/paguidelines/pdf /paguide.pdf. Accessed 5 Sept 2013.

54. Fantuzzi G. Adipose tissue, adipokines, and inflammation. J Allergy Clin Immunol 2005;115:911–919.

55. Trayhurn P. Adipocyte biology. Obes Rev 2007;8 (suppl 1):41–44.

56. Xu H, Barnes GT, Yang Q, et al. Chronic inflammation in fat plays a crucial role in the development of obesity-related insulin resistance. J Clin Invest 2003;112:1821–1830.

57. Liu KH, Chan YL, Chan WB, Chan JC, Chu CW. Mesenteric fat thickness is an independent determinant of metabolic syndrome and identifies subjects with increased carotid intima-media thickness. Diabetes Care 2006;29:379–384.

58. Chaffee BW, Weston SJ. Association between chronic periodontal disease and obesity: A systematic review and meta-analysis. J Periodontol 2010; 81:1708–1724.

59. Das UN. Is obesity an inflammatory condition? Nutrition 2001;17:953–966.

60. Weisberg SP, McCann D, Desai M, Rosenbaum M, Leibel RL, Ferrante AW Jr. Obesity is associated with macrophage accumulation in adipose tissue. J Clin Invest 2003;112:1796–1808.

61. Hotamisligil GS, Shargill NS, Spiegelman BM. Adipose expression of tumor necrosis factor-alpha: Direct role in obesity-linked insulin resistance. Science 1993;259(5091):87–91.

62. Weyer C, Yudkin JS, Stehouwer CD, Schalkwijk CG, Pratley RE, Tataranni PA. Humoral markers of inflammation and endothelial dysfunction in relation to adiposity and in vivo insulin action in Pima Indians. Atherosclerosis 2002;161:233–242.

63. Fried SK, Bunkin DA, Greenberg AS. Omental and subcutaneous adipose tissues of obese subjects release interleukin-6: Depot difference and regulation by glucocorticoid. J Clin Endocrinol Metab 1998;83:847–850.

64. Goerdt S, Politz O, Schledzewski K, et al. Alternative versus classical activation of macrophages. Pathobiology 1999;67:222–226.

65. Lumeng CN, Bodzin JL, Saltiel AR. Obesity induces a phenotypic switch in adipose tissue macrophage polarization. J Clin Invest 2007;117:175–184.

66. Lumeng CN, Deyoung SM, Bodzin JL, Saltiel AR. Increased inflammatory properties of adipose tissue macrophages recruited during diet-induced obesity. Diabetes 2007;56:16–23.

67. Fain JN, Tichansky DS, Madan AK. Most of the interleukin 1 receptor antagonist, cathepsin S, macrophage migration inhibitory factor, nerve growth factor, and interleukin 18 release by explants of human adipose tissue is by the non-fat cells, not by the adipocytes. Metabolism 2006;55:1113–1121.

68. Kershaw EE, Flier JS. Adipose tissue as an endocrine organ. J Clin Endocrinol Metab 2004;89:2548–2556.

69. Armellini F, Zamboni M, Bosello O. Hormones and body composition in humans: Clinical studies. Int J Obes Relat Metab Disord 2000;24(suppl 2):S18–S21.

70. Chan JL, Heist K, DePaoli AM, Veldhuis JD, Mantzoros CS. The role of falling leptin levels in the neuroendocrine and metabolic adaptation to short-term starvation in healthy men. J Clin Invest 2003; 111:1409–1421.

71. Lord GM, Matarese G, Howard JK, Baker RJ, Bloom SR, Lechler RI. Leptin modulates the T-cell immune response and reverses starvation-induced immunosuppression. Nature 1998;394:897–901.

72. Lord GM, Matarese G, Howard JK, Bloom SR, Lechler RI. Leptin inhibits the anti-CD3-driven proliferation of peripheral blood T cells but enhances the production of proinflammatory cytokines. J Leukoc Biol 2002;72:330–338.

73. Rodriguez L, Graniel J, Ortiz R. Effect of leptin on activation and cytokine synthesis in peripheral blood lymphocytes of malnourished infected children. Clin Exp Immunol 2007;148:478–485.

74. Loffreda S, Yang SQ, Lin HZ, et al. Leptin regulates proinflammatory immune responses. FASEB J 1998;12:57–65.

75. Caldefie-Chezet F, Poulin A, Vasson MP. Leptin regulates functional capacities of polymorphonuclear neutrophils. Free Radic Res 2003;37:809–814.

76. Fantuzzi G. Adiponectin and inflammation: Consensus and controversy. J Allergy Clin Immunol 2008; 121:326–330.

77. Barbosa Vde S, Rego J, Antonio da Silva N. Possible role of adipokines in systemic lupus erythematosus and rheumatoid arthritis. Rev Bras Reumatol 2012;52:278–287.

78. Chen X, Lu J, Bao J, Guo J, Shi J, Wang Y. Adiponectin: A biomarker for rheumatoid arthritis? Cytokine Growth Factor Rev 2013;24:83–89.

79. Ehling A, Schaffler A, Herfarth H, et al. The potential of adiponectin in driving arthritis. J Immunol 2006; 176:4468–4478.

80. Schaffler A, Ehling A, Neumann E, et al. Adipocytokines in synovial fluid [research letter]. JAMA 2003;290:1709–1710.

81. Bruun JM, Lihn AS, Verdich C, et al. Regulation of adiponectin by adipose tissue-derived cytokines: In vivo and in vitro investigations in humans. Am J Physiol Endocrinol Metab 2003;285:E527–E333.

82. Villarreal-Molina MT, Antuna-Puente B. Adiponectin: Anti-inflammatory and cardioprotective effects. Biochimie 2012;94:2143–2149.

83. Arita Y, Kihara S, Ouchi N, et al. Paradoxical decrease of an adipose-specific protein, adiponectin, in obesity. Biochem Biophys Res Commun 1999; 257:79–83.

84. Combs TP, Berg AH, Obici S, Scherer PE, Rossetti L. Endogenous glucose production is inhibited by the adipose-derived protein Acrp30. J Clin Invest 2001;108:1875–1881.

85. Ouchi N, Ohishi M, Kihara S, et al. Association of hypoadiponectinemia with impaired vasoreactivity. Hypertension 2003;42:231–234.

86. Yokota T, Oritani K, Takahashi I, et al. Adiponectin, a new member of the family of soluble defense collagens, negatively regulates the growth of myelomonocytic progenitors and the functions of macrophages. Blood 2000;96:1723–1732.

87. Masaki T, Chiba S, Tatsukawa H, et al. Adiponectin protects LPS-induced liver injury through modulation of TNF-α in KK-Ay obese mice. Hepatology 2004;40:177–184.

88. Ajuwon KM, Spurlock ME. Adiponectin inhibits LPS-induced NF-κB activation and IL-6 production and increases PPARγ2 expression in adipocytes. Am J Physiol Regul Integr Comp Physiol 2005; 288:R1220–R1225.

89. Fasshauer M, Kralisch S, Klier M, et al. Adiponectin gene expression and secretion is inhibited by interleukin-6 in 3T3-L1 adipocytes. Biochem Biophys Res Commun 2003;301:1045–1050.

90. Weyer C, Funahashi T, Tanaka S, et al. Hypoadiponectinemia in obesity and type 2 diabetes: Close association with insulin resistance and hyperinsulinemia. J Clin Endocrinol Metab 2001;86:1930–1935.

91. Berg AH, Combs TP, Du X, Brownlee M, Scherer PE. The adipocyte-secreted protein Acrp30 enhances hepatic insulin action. Nat Med 2001;7:947–953.

92. Hotamisligil GS. Inflammatory pathways and insulin action. Int J Obes Relat Metab Disord 2003;27(suppl 3):S53–S55.

93. Tsigos C, Papanicolaou DA, Kyrou I, Defensor R, Mitsiadis CS, Chrousos GP. Dose-dependent effects of recombinant human interleukin-6 on glucose regulation. J Clin Endocrinol Metab 1997;82: 4167–4170.

94. Yamauchi T, Kamon J, Ito Y, et al. Cloning of adiponectin receptors that mediate antidiabetic metabolic effects. Nature 2003;423:762–769.

95. Ouchi N, Walsh K. A novel role for adiponectin in the regulation of inflammation. Arterioscler Thromb Vasc Biol 2008;28:1219–1221.

96. Chen H, Montagnani M, Funahashi T, Shimomura I, Quon MJ. Adiponectin stimulates production of nitric oxide in vascular endothelial cells. J Biol Chem 2003;278:45021–45026.

97. Vaiopoulos AG, Marinou K, Christodoulides C, Koutsilieris M. The role of adiponectin in human vascular physiology. Int J Cardiol 2012;155:188–193.

98. Motoshima H, Wu X, Mahadev K, Goldstein BJ. Adiponectin suppresses proliferation and superoxide generation and enhances eNOS activity in endothelial cells treated with oxidized LDL. Biochem Biophys Res Commun 2004;315:264–271.

99. Sengenes C, Miranville A, Lolmede K, Curat CA, Bouloumie A. The role of endothelial cells in inflamed adipose tissue. J Intern Med 2007;262:415–421.

100. Salmi M, Jalkanen S. Cell-surface enzymes in control of leukocyte trafficking. Nat Rev Immunol 2005;5:760–771.

101. Kuldo JM, Ogawara KI, Werner N, et al. Molecular pathways of endothelial cell activation for (targeted) pharmacological intervention of chronic inflammatory diseases. Curr Vasc Pharmacol 2005;3:11–39.

102. Aoki S, Toda S, Sakemi T, Sugihara H. Coculture of endothelial cells and mature adipocytes actively promotes immature preadipocyte development in vitro. Cell Struct Funct 2003;28:55–60.

103. Hutley LJ, Herington AC, Shurety W, et al. Human adipose tissue endothelial cells promote preadipocyte proliferation. Am J Physiol Endocrinol Metab 2001;281:E1037–E1044.

104. Crandall DL, Busler DE, McHendry-Rinde B, Groeling TM, Kral JG. Autocrine regulation of human preadipocyte migration by plasminogen activator inhibitor-1. J Clin Endocrinol Metab 2000;85:2609–2614.

105. Fukumura D, Ushiyama A, Duda DG, et al. Paracrine regulation of angiogenesis and adipocyte differentiation during in vivo adipogenesis. Circ Res 2003;93(9):e88–e97.

106. Rupnick MA, Panigrahy D, Zhang CY, et al. Adipose tissue mass can be regulated through the vasculature. Proc Natl Acad Sci U S A 2002;99: 10730–10735.

107. Wood IS, de Heredia FP, Wang B, Trayhurn P. Cellular hypoxia and adipose tissue dysfunction in obesity. Proc Nutr Soc 2009;68:370–377.

108. Hosogai N, Fukuhara A, Oshima K, et al. Adipose tissue hypoxia in obesity and its impact on adipocytokine dysregulation. Diabetes 2007;56:901–911.

109. Ye J, Gao Z, Yin J, He Q. Hypoxia is a potential risk factor for chronic inflammation and adiponectin reduction in adipose tissue of ob/ob and dietary obese mice. Am J Physiol Endocrinol Metab 2007; 293:E1118–E1128.

110. Wang GL, Semenza GL. General involvement of hypoxia-inducible factor 1 in transcriptional response to hypoxia. Proc Natl Acad Sci U S A 1993;90:4304–4308.

111. Wang B, Wood IS, Trayhurn P. Hypoxia induces leptin gene expression and secretion in human pre-adipocytes: Differential effects of hypoxia on adipokine expression by preadipocytes. J Endocrinol 2008;198:127–134.

112. Oda T, Hirota K, Nishi K, et al. Activation of hypoxia-inducible factor 1 during macrophage differentiation. Am J Physiol Cell Physiol 2006;291:C104–C113.

113. Mendis S, Puska P, Norrving B (eds). Global Atlas on Cardiovascular Disease Prevention and Control. Geneva: World Health Organization, 2011.

114. Prospective Studies Collaboration (PSC), Clinical Trial Service Unit and Epidemiological Studies Unit (CTSU). Body-mass index and cause-specific mortality in 900,000 adults: Collaborative analyses of 57 prospective studies. Lancet 2009;373:1083–1096.

115. Pischon N, Heng N, Bernimoulin JP, Kleber BM, Willich SN, Pischon T. Obesity, inflammation, and periodontal disease. J Dent Res 2007;86:400–409.

116. Schiel R, Beltschikow W, Kramer G, Stein G. Overweight, obesity and elevated blood pressure in children and adolescents. Eur J Med Res 2006;11:97–101.

117. Freedman DS, Dietz WH, Srinivasan SR, Berenson GS. The relation of overweight to cardiovascular risk factors among children and adolescents: The Bogalusa Heart Study. Pediatrics 1999;103:1175–1182.

118. World Cancer Research Fund/American Institute for Cancer Research. Food, Nutrition, Physical Activity, and the Prevention of Cancer: A Global Perspective. Washington, DC: American Institute for Cancer Research, 2007.

119. Siegel R, Naishadham D, Jemal A. Cancer statistics, 2012. CA Cancer J Clin 2012;62:10–29.

120. Juonala M, Magnussen CG, Berenson GS, et al. Childhood adiposity, adult adiposity, and cardiovascular risk factors. N Engl J Med 2011;365:1876–1885.

121. Krakowiak P, Walker CK, Bremer AA, et al. Maternal metabolic conditions and risk for autism and other neurodevelopmental disorders. Pediatrics 2012;129:e1121–e1128.

122. De Niet JE, Naiman DI. Psychosocial aspects of childhood obesity. Minerva Pediatr 2011;63:491–505.

123. Puhl RM, Peterson JL, Luedicke J. Weight-based victimization: Bullying experiences of weight loss treatment-seeking youth. Pediatrics 2013;131:e1–e9.

124. Caliendo M, Lee WS. Fat chance! Obesity and the transition from unemployment to employment. Econ Hum Biol 2013;11:121–133.

125. Lightwood J, Bibbins-Domingo K, Coxson P, Wang YC, Williams L, Goldman L. Forecasting the future economic burden of current adolescent overweight: An estimate of the coronary heart disease policy model. Am J Public Health 2009;99:2230–2237.

126. Wang Y, Beydoun MA, Liang L, Caballero B, Kumanyika SK. Will all Americans become overweight or obese? Estimating the progression and cost of the US obesity epidemic. Obesity (Silver Spring) 2008;16:2323–2330.

127. Metabolic syndrome. A.D.A.M. Medical Encyclopedia. Updated 2 June 2012. http://www.ncbi.nlm.nih.gov/pubmedhealth/PMH0004546/. Accessed 10 July 2013.

128. Verzeletti GN, Gaio EJ, Linhares DS, Rosing CK. Effect of obesity on alveolar bone loss in experimental periodontitis in Wistar rats. J Appl Oral Sci 2012;20:218–121.

129. Cavagni J, Wagner TP, Gaio EJ, Rego RO, Torres IL, Rosing CK. Obesity may increase the occurrence of spontaneous periodontal disease in Wistar rats. Arch Oral Biol 2013;58:1034–1039.

130. Suvan J, D'Aiuto F, Moles DR, Petrie A, Donos N. Association between overweight/obesity and periodontitis in adults. A systematic review. Obes Rev 2011;12:e381–e404.

131. Buhlin K, Gustafsson A, Pockley AG, Frostegård J, Klinge B. Risk factors for cardiovascular disease in patients with periodontitis. Eur Heart J 2003;24:2099–2107.

132. Genco RJ, Grossi SG, Ho A, Nishimura F, Murayama Y. A proposed model linking inflammation to obesity, diabetes, and periodontal infections. J Periodontol 2005;76(11 suppl):2075–2084.

133. Nishida N, Tanaka M, Hayashi N, et al. Determination of smoking and obesity as periodontitis risks using the classification and regression tree method. J Periodontol 2005;76:923–928.

134. Saito T, Shimazaki Y, Kiyohara Y, et al. Relationship between obesity, glucose tolerance, and periodontal disease in Japanese women: The Hisayama study. J Periodontal Res 2005;40:346–353.

135. Kushiyama M, Shimazaki Y, Yamashita Y. Relationship between metabolic syndrome and periodontal disease in Japanese adults. J Periodontol 2009;80:1610–1615.

136. Han DH, Lim SY, Sun BC, Paek DM, Kim HD. Visceral fat area-defined obesity and periodontitis among Koreans. J Clin Periodontol 2010;37:172–179.

137. Bistrian B. Systemic response to inflammation. Nutr Rev 2007;65(suppl 3):S170–S172.

138. Lundin M, Yucel-Lindberg T, Dahllof G, Marcus C, Modeer T. Correlation between TNFα in gingival crevicular fluid and body mass index in obese subjects. Acta Odontol Scand 2004;62:273–277.

139. Schmidt AM, Weidman E, Lalla E, et al. Advanced glycation endproducts (AGEs) induce oxidant stress in the gingiva: A potential mechanism underlying accelerated periodontal disease associated with diabetes. J Periodontal Res 1996;31:508–515.

140. Oikarinen R, Syrjala AM, Komulainen K, et al. Body mass index and periodontal infection in a sample of non-smoking older individuals [epub ahead of print 22 March 2013]. Oral Dis doi: 10.1111/odi. 12108.

141. de Castilhos ED, Horta BL, Gigante DP, Demarco FF, Peres KG, Peres MA. Association between obesity and periodontal disease in young adults: A population-based birth cohort. J Clin Periodontol 2012;39:717–724.

142. Gorman A, Kaye EK, Nunn M, Garcia RI. Changes in body weight and adiposity predict periodontitis in men. J Dent Res 2012;91:921–926.

143. Morita I, Okamoto Y, Yoshii S, et al. Five-year incidence of periodontal disease is related to body mass index. J Dent Res 2011;90:199–202.

144. Nibali L, Tatarakis N, Needleman I, et al. Clinical review: Association between metabolic syndrome and periodontitis: A systematic review and meta-analysis. J Clin Endocrinol Metab 2013;98:913–920.

145. Acharya A, Bhavsar N, Jadav B, Parikh H. Cardio-protective effect of periodontal therapy in metabolic syndrome: A pilot study in Indian subjects. Metab Syndr Relat Disord 2010;8:335–341.

146. Pradeep AR, Priyanka N, Prasad MV, Kalra N, Kumari M. Association of progranulin and high sensitivity CRP concentrations in gingival crevicular fluid and serum in chronic periodontitis subjects with and without obesity. Dis Markers 2012;33:207–213.

147. Zimmermann GS, Bastos MF, Dias Goncalves TE, Chambrone L, Duarte PM. Local and circulating levels of adipocytokines in obese and normal weight individuals with chronic periodontitis. J Periodontol 2013;84:624–633.

148. Altay U, Gurgan CA, Agbaht K. Changes in inflammatory and metabolic parameters after periodontal treatment in patients with and without obesity. J Periodontol 2013;84:13–23.

149. Hooley M, Skouteris H, Boganin C, Satur J, Kilpatrick N. Body mass index and dental caries in children and adolescents: A systematic review of literature published 2004 to 2011. Syst Rev 2012;1:57.

150. Hayden C, Bowler JO, Chambers S, et al. Obesity and dental caries in children: A systematic review and meta-analysis. Community Dent Oral Epidemiol 2013;41:289–308.

151. Palmer CA, Kent R Jr, Loo CY, et al. Diet and caries-associated bacteria in severe early childhood caries. J Dent Res 2010;89:1224–1229.

152. Arcella D, Ottolenghi L, Polimeni A, Leclercq C. The relationship between frequency of carbohydrates intake and dental caries: A cross-sectional study in Italian teenagers. Public Health Nutr 2002;5:553–560.

153. Ludwig DS, Peterson KE, Gortmaker SL. Relation between consumption of sugar-sweetened drinks and childhood obesity: A prospective, observational analysis. Lancet 2001;357:505–508.

154. Schulze MB, Manson JE, Ludwig DS, et al. Sugar-sweetened beverages, weight gain, and incidence of type 2 diabetes in young and middle-aged women. JAMA 2004;292:927–934.

155. Marshall TA, Levy SM, Broffitt B, et al. Dental caries and beverage consumption in young children. Pediatrics 2003;112:e184–e191.

156. Ismail AI, Burt BA, Eklund SA. The cariogenicity of soft drinks in the United States. J Am Dent Assoc 1984;109:241–245.

157. Hooley M, Skouteris H, Millar L. The relationship between childhood weight, dental caries and eating practices in children aged 4-8 years in Australia, 2004-2008. Pediatr Obes 2012;7:461–470.

158. Vazquez-Nava F, Vazquez-Rodriguez EM, Saldivar-Gonzalez AH, Lin-Ochoa D, Martinez-Perales GM, Joffre-Velazquez VM. Association between obesity and dental caries in a group of preschool children in Mexico. J Public Health Dent 2010;70:124–130.

159. Alm A, Fahraeus C, Wendt LK, Koch G, Andersson-Gare B, Birkhed D. Body adiposity status in teenagers and snacking habits in early childhood in relation to approximal caries at 15 years of age. Int J Paediatr Dent 2008;18:189–196.

160. Willershausen B, Moschos D, Azrak B, Blettner M. Correlation between oral health and body mass index (BMI) in 2071 primary school pupils. Eur J Med Res 2007;12:295–299.

161. Gerdin EW, Angbratt M, Aronsson K, Eriksson E, Johansson I. Dental caries and body mass index by socio-economic status in Swedish children. Community Dent Oral Epidemiol 2008;36:459–465.

162. Kantovitz KR, Pascon FM, Rontani RM, Gaviao MB. Obesity and dental caries—A systematic review. Oral Health Prev Dent 2006;4:137–144.

163. Macek MD, Mitola DJ. Exploring the association between overweight and dental caries among US children. Pediatr Dent 2006;28:375–380.

164. Hong L, Ahmed A, McCunniff M, Overman P, Mathew M. Obesity and dental caries in children aged 2–6 years in the United States: National Health and Nutrition Examination Survey 1999–2002. J Public Health Dent 2008;68:227–233.

165. Kopycka-Kedzierawski DT, Auinger P, Billings RJ, Weitzman M. Caries status and overweight in 2- to 18-year-old US children: Findings from national surveys. Community Dent Oral Epidemiol 2008; 36:157–167.

166. Hilgers KK, Kinane DE, Scheetz JP. Association between childhood obesity and smooth-surface caries in posterior teeth: A preliminary study. Pediatr Dent 2006;28:23–28.

167. Sadeghi M, Alizadeh F. Association between dental caries and body mass index-for-age among 6–11-year-old children in Isfahan in 2007. J Dent Res Dent Clin Dent Prospects 2007;1:119–124.

168. Sanchez-Perez L, Irigoyen ME, Zepeda M. Dental caries, tooth eruption timing and obesity: A longitudinal study in a group of Mexican schoolchildren. Acta Odontol Scand 2010;68:57–64.

169. Tavares M, Goodson JM, Cugini M, et al. Tooth eruption and BMI percentile in Kuwaiti fifth grade children [abstract 2887]. J Dent Res 2013;92(special issue A).

170. Modeer T, Blomberg CC, Wondimu B, Julihn A, Marcus C. Association between obesity, flow rate of whole saliva, and dental caries in adolescents. Obesity (Silver Spring) 2010;18:2367–2373.

171. Tavares M, Goodson JM, Cugini M, et al. Kuwait Healthy Lifestyle Study: Sleep as a health factor [abstract 514]. J Dent Res 2012;91(special issue A).

172. He Q, Karlberg J. BMI in childhood and its association with height gain, timing of puberty, and final height. Pediatr Res 2001;49:244–251.

173. De Simone M, Farello G, Palumbo M, et al. Growth charts, growth velocity and bone development in childhood obesity. Int J Obes Relat Metab Disord 1995;19:851–857.

174. De Leonibus C, Marcovecchio ML, Chiavaroli V, de Giorgis T, Chiarelli F, Mohn A. Timing of puberty and physical growth in obese children: A longitudinal study in boys and girls [epub ahead of print 27 May 2013]. Pediatr Obes doi: 10.1111/j.2047-6310. 2013.00176.x.

175. Aksglaede L, Juul A, Olsen LW, Sorensen TI. Age at puberty and the emerging obesity epidemic. PLoS One 2009;4:e8450.

176. Ohrn K, Al-Kahlili B, Huggare J, Forsberg CM, Marcus C, Dahllof G. Craniofacial morphology in obese adolescents. Acta Odontol Scand 2002;60:193–197.

177. Sadeghianrizi A, Forsberg CM, Marcus C, Dahllof G. Craniofacial development in obese adolescents. Eur J Orthod 2005;27:550–555.

178. Hilgers KK, Akridge M, Scheetz JP, Kinane DE. Childhood obesity and dental development. Pediatr Dent 2006;28:18–22.

179. Demirjian A, Goldstein H, Tanner JM. A new system of dental age assessment. Hum Biol 1973;45:211–227.

180. Zangouei-Booshehri M, Ezoddini-Ardakani F, Agha Aghili H, Sharifi A. Assessment of the relationship between body mass index (BMI) and dental age. Health 2011;3:253–257.

181. Mack KB, Phillips C, Jain N, Koroluk LD. Relationship between body mass index percentile and skeletal maturation and dental development in orthodontic patients. Am J Orthod Dentofacial Orthop 2013;143:228–234.

182. Weddell LS, Hartsfield JK Jr. Dental maturity of Caucasian children in the Indianapolis area. Pediatr Dent 2011;33:221–227.

183. Costacurta M, Sicuro L, Di Renzo L, Condo R, De Lorenzo A, Docimo R. Childhood obesity and skeletal-dental maturity. Eur J Paediatr Dent 2012; 13:128–132.

184. Must A, Phillips SM, Tybor DJ, Lividini K, Hayes C. The association between childhood obesity and tooth eruption. Obesity (Silver Spring) 2012;20: 2070–2074.

185. Halaas JL, Gajiwala KS, Maffei M, et al. Weight-reducing effects of the plasma protein encoded by the obese gene. Science 1995;269:543–546.

186. Shalitin S, Phillip M. Role of obesity and leptin in the pubertal process and pubertal growth—A review. Int J Obes Relat Metab Disord 2003;27:869–874.

187. Maor G, Rochwerger M, Segev Y, Phillip M. Leptin acts as a growth factor on the chondrocytes of skeletal growth centers. J Bone Miner Res 2002; 17:1034–1043.

188. Miller R, Tanofsky-Kraff M, Shomaker LB, et al. Serum leptin and loss of control eating in children and adolescents [epub ahead of print 9 July 2013]. Int J Obes (Lond) doi: 10.1038/ijo.2013.126.

189. Giuca MR, Pasini M, Tecco S, Marchetti E, Giannotti L, Marzo G. Skeletal maturation in obese patients. Am J Orthod Dentofacial Orthop 2012; 142:774–779.

190. Sanchez-Ayala A, Campanha NH, Garcia RC. Relationship between body fat and masticatory function. J Prosthodont 2013;22:120–125.

191. Patel SR, Hu FB. Short sleep duration and weight gain: A systematic review. Obesity (Silver Spring) 2008;16:643–653.

192. Kobayashi D, Takahashi O, Deshpande GA, Shimbo T, Fukui T. Association between weight gain, obesity, and sleep duration: A large-scale 3-year cohort study. Sleep Breath 2012;16:829–833.

193. Pan A, Schernhammer ES, Sun Q, Hu FB. Rotating night shift work and risk of type 2 diabetes: Two prospective cohort studies in women. PLoS Med 2011;8:e1001141.

194. Taveras EM, Rifas-Shiman SL, Oken E, Gunderson EP, Gillman MW. Short sleep duration in infancy and risk of childhood overweight. Arch Pediatr Adolesc Med 2008;162:305–311.

195. Reilly JJ, Armstrong J, Dorosty AR, et al. Early life risk factors for obesity in childhood: Cohort study. BMJ 2005;330:1357.

196. Gillman MW, Rifas-Shiman SL, Kleinman K, Oken E, Rich-Edwards JW, Taveras EM. Developmental origins of childhood overweight: Potential public health impact. Obesity (Silver Spring) 2008;16: 1651–1656.

197. Buxton OM, Marcelli E. Short and long sleep are positively associated with obesity, diabetes, hypertension, and cardiovascular disease among adults in the United States. Soc Sci Med 2010;71:1027–1036.

198. Dean E, Bloom A, Cirillo M, et al. Association between habitual sleep duration and blood pressure and clinical implications: A systematic review. Blood Press 2012;21:45–57.

199. Kim J, Jo I. Age-dependent association between sleep duration and hypertension in the adult Korean population. Am J Hypertens 2010;23:1286–1291.

200. Sabanayagam C, Shankar A. Sleep duration and cardiovascular disease: Results from the National Health Interview Survey. Sleep 2010;33:1037–1042.

201. Wang H, Zee P, Reid K, et al. Gender-specific association of sleep duration with blood pressure in rural Chinese adults. Sleep Med 2011;12:693–699.

202. Spiegel K, Leproult R, L'Hermite-Baleriaux M, Copinschi G, Penev PD, Van Cauter E. Leptin levels are dependent on sleep duration: Relationships with sympathovagal balance, carbohydrate regulation, cortisol, and thyrotropin. J Clin Endocrinol Metab 2004;89:5762–5771.

203. Nedeltcheva AV, Kilkus JM, Imperial J, Kasza K, Schoeller DA, Penev PD. Sleep curtailment is accompanied by increased intake of calories from snacks. Am J Clin Nutr 2009;89:126–133.

204. Buxton OM, Cain SW, O'Connor SP, et al. Adverse metabolic consequences in humans of prolonged sleep restriction combined with circadian disruption. Sci Transl Med 2012;4:129ra43.

205. Malhotra A, White DP. Obstructive sleep apnoea. Lancet 2002;360:237–245.

206. Yu JC, Berger P 3rd. Sleep apnea and obesity. S D Med 2011;(special no.):28–34.

207. Pillai A, Warren G, Gunathilake W, Idris I. Effects of sleep apnea severity on glycemic control in patients with type 2 diabetes prior to continuous positive airway pressure treatment. Diabetes Technol Ther 2011;13:945–949.

208. Ong CW, O'Driscoll DM, Truby H, Naughton MT, Hamilton GS. The reciprocal interaction between obesity and obstructive sleep apnoea. Sleep Med Rev 2013;17:123–131.

209. Caples SM, Gami AS, Somers VK. Obstructive sleep apnea. Ann Intern Med 2005;142:187–197.

210. Kohler MJ, Thormaehlen S, Kennedy JD, et al. Differences in the association between obesity and obstructive sleep apnea among children and adolescents. J Clin Sleep Med 2009;5:506–511.

211. Verhulst SL, Schrauwen N, Haentjens D, et al. Sleep-disordered breathing and the metabolic syndrome in overweight and obese children and adolescents. J Pediatr 2007;150:608–612.

212. Verhulst SL, Schrauwen N, Haentjens D, et al. Sleep-disordered breathing in overweight and obese children and adolescents: Prevalence, characteristics and the role of fat distribution. Arch Dis Child 2007;92:205–208.

213. Canapari CA, Hoppin AG, Kinane TB, Thomas BJ, Torriani M, Katz ES. Relationship between sleep apnea, fat distribution, and insulin resistance in obese children. J Clin Sleep Med 2011;7:268–273.

214. Padmanabhan V, Kavitha PR, Hegde AM. Sleep disordered breathing in children — A review and the role of a pediatric dentist. J Clin Pediatr Dent 2010;35:15–21.

215. Simmons MS, Clark GT. The potentially harmful medical consequences of untreated sleep-disordered breathing: The evidence supporting brain damage. J Am Dent Assoc 2009;140:536–542.

216. Mohsenin N, Mostofi MT, Mohsenin V. The role of oral appliances in treating obstructive sleep apnea. J Am Dent Assoc 2003;134:442–449.

217. Zhou J, Liu YH. A randomised titrated crossover study comparing two oral appliances in the treatment for mild to moderate obstructive sleep apnoea/hypopnoea syndrome. J Oral Rehabil 2012;39:914–922.

218. Borrie F, Keightley A, Blacker S, Serrant P. Mandibular advancement appliances for treating sleep apnoea/hypopnoea syndrome. Evid Based Dent 2013;14:27–28.

219. Tegelberg A, Nohlert E, Bergman LE, Andren A. Bed partners' and patients' experiences after treatment of obstructive sleep apnoea with an oral appliance. Swed Dent J 2012;36:35–44.

220. Gauthier L, Almeida F, Arcache JP, et al. Position paper by Canadian dental sleep medicine professionals on the role of different health care professionals in managing obstructive sleep apnea and snoring with oral appliances. Can Respir J 2012;19:307–309.

221. Glickman D, Parker L, Sim LJ, Del Valle Cook H, Miller EA (eds). Accelerating Progress in Obesity Prevention: Solving the Weight of the Nation. Washington, DC: The National Academies Press, 2012.

Clinical Considerations:
What You Can Take Back to Your Practice

What is the effect of oral health on pulmonary diseases?

Poor oral hygiene fosters development of dental plaque, which, if aspirated, could lead to lung infection. Dental plaque could also be colonized by exogenous pathogens that can cause nosocomial lung infections, especially in hospital and nursing home patients.

Are oral infections independent risk factors for the development of pulmonary diseases?

Poor oral hygiene has been associated as a risk factor for nosocomial lung infections.

What is the biologic plausibility of the association between oral health and pulmonary diseases?

Bacteria isolated from lung aspirates in patients with suspected pneumonia have been shown to be genetically identical to those colonizing the oral cavity in the same patient.

Does the delivery of oral health care contribute to reduced incidence of pulmonary diseases?

A number of systematic reviews of randomized trials suggest that improved oral hygiene can contribute to prevention of pneumonia in hospital and nursing home patients.

Is it safe to provide dental care to patients with pulmonary diseases?

To date, there is no published evidence suggesting that oral care is harmful in patients with high risk for pneumonia.

What is the appropriate message to give to the public about the association between oral health and pulmonary diseases?

Maintaining good oral hygiene may prevent lung infections, especially in patients with high risk for pneumonia.

Pneumonia and Oral Pathogens

Frank A. Scannapieco, DMD, PhD

There has been increasing recognition that oral health status, particularly poor oral hygiene, can influence the course of several lung conditions. This should come as no surprise, because the surfaces of the oral cavity are contiguous with those of the trachea and lower airway. Bacteria that colonize the oral cavity are aspirated into the lower airway to cause infection. These bacteria could be endogenous, opportunistic commensal organisms or exogenous pathogens that are not normal members of the oral flora and that transiently colonize the oral cavity. Less well appreciated is the potential role played by biologic mediators such as cytokines and hydrolytic enzymes that are released from the periodontium as the result of periodontal inflammation that may also be aspirated into the airway to incite inflammation and increase susceptibility to infection.

This chapter focuses on the relationship between the oral microflora or oral inflammation and pneumonia. This subject has been reviewed in many book chapters and articles that the reader may find helpful.[1-6]

Definitions and Disease Classifications

Pneumonia is an infection of the lungs caused by bacteria, mycoplasma, viruses, fungi, or parasites. Bacterial pneumonia is a common and significant cause of mortality and morbidity in human populations. Pneumonia and influenza are together an important cause of morbidity and mortality throughout the world. Pneumonia also contributes to morbidity and decline in quality of life as well as to increased medical costs.

Pneumonia comprises several subtypes: community-acquired pneumonia (CAP), aspiration pneumonia, hospital-acquired (nosocomial) pneumonia (HAP), ventilator-associated pneumonia (VAP), and nursing home–associated pneumonia (NHAP). In all cases, connections have been made between these infections and oral health status.

Community-acquired pneumonia

CAP is an important cause of morbidity and mortality in individuals who have not recently been admitted to a hospital or other health care facility (eg, nursing home). Bacterial pneumonia is often preceded by viral infection or *Mycoplasma pneumoniae* infections, which diminishes the cough reflex, interrupts mucociliary clearance, and enhances the pathogenic bacterial adherence to respiratory mucosa to link the chain of events that may eventually lead to CAP.[7]

Viruses, for example respiratory syncytial virus or rhinovirus, are common etiologic agents of CAP. Bacterial causes of CAP include group B streptococci, gram-negative enteric bacteria, or *Streptococcus pneumoniae* early in life, while *S pneumoniae* and *Haemophilus influenzae* are often the cause of CAP in adults.

About 4 million cases of CAP occur in the United States each year.[8] Most of these patients are treated in the primary care setting. For example, a recent large, population-based cohort study of 46,237 seniors aged 65 years or older were observed over a 3-year period.[9] The overall rate of CAP ranged from 18.2 cases per 1,000 person-years among persons aged 65 to 69 years to 52.3 cases per 1,000 person-years among those aged 85 years or older. In this population, 59.3% of all pneumonia episodes were treated on an outpatient basis. Overall, CAP results in more than 600,000 hospitalizations, 64 million days of restricted activity, and 45,000 deaths annually.

Risk factors for CAP include older age, male sex, chronic obstructive pulmonary disease, asthma, diabetes mellitus, congestive heart failure, and smoking.[9] In a study of 1,336 patients with CAP and 1,326 control subjects for risk factors recruited from a population of 859,033 inhabitants of a region in eastern Spain,[10] multivariate analysis found cigarette smoking, usual contact with children, sudden changes of temperature at work, inhalation therapy (particularly that containing steroids), oxygen therapy, asthma, and chronic bronchitis all to be independent risk factors for CAP. Interestingly, a visit to a dentist in the last month was an independent protective factor for CAP, presumably because it encourages improvements in oral hygiene, which could limit colonization by respiratory pathogens.

Common clinical symptoms of CAP include cough, fever, chills, fatigue, dyspnea, rigors, and pleuritic chest pain.[8] Depending on the pathogen, a patient's cough may be persistent and dry or it may produce sputum. Other presentations may include headache and myalgia. Certain bacteria, such as *Legionella*, may induce gastrointestinal symptoms.

The chest radiograph is a critical tool for the diagnosis of pneumonia. A typical chest radiograph with positive results shows consolidation within the lung lobe or a more diffuse infiltration.[8] However, chest radiography performed early in the course of the disease often proves negative for signs of pneumonia.

CAP is almost always treated with antibiotics. Typical antibiotic regimens include the use of oral azithromycin, clarithromycin, erythromycin, or doxycycline in otherwise healthy patients and oral moxifloxacin, gemifloxacin, or levofloxacin in patients with other comorbidities.

A worrisome recent development is the emergence of community-acquired methicillin-resistant *Staphylococcus aureus* (MRSA) infections, including CAP.[11] While still a rare infection, the median age of recent patients, four of whom died, was 21 years, and usually a short interval occurred between the development of respiratory symptoms and the detection of disease.[11]

While the focus for CAP is typically on short-term outcomes, it is becoming more apparent that there are sometimes long-term negative consequences of CAP, particularly in the elderly.[12] For example, a large study of a Medicare database used a matched case-control design to compare the 1-year mortality rate of 158,960 older CAP patients with that of 794,333 control subjects hospitalized for reasons other than CAP.[13] The 1-year mortality rate for CAP patients (40.9%) exceeded that of control subjects (29.1%); the differences could not be explained by the types of underlying disease. These findings suggest that the consequences of CAP in the elderly are important to long-term survival, and thus the infection should be prevented.[12]

A recent case-control study compared the periodontal status of 100 individuals hospitalized for the treatment of an acute respiratory disease (pneumonia, acute bronchitis, or a lung abscess) or an exacerbation of chronic obstructive pulmonary disease with a group of 100 control subjects without respiratory disease.[14] Among the patients with respiratory disease, 72% had chronic obstructive pulmonary disease, 17% had pneumonia, and 11% had a lung abscess. All periodontal parameters (Gingival Index, Plaque Index, Oral Hygiene Index, probing depth, and clinical attachment level) were significantly worse for the patients with respiratory disease than for the control subjects.

Aspiration pneumonia

Aspiration pneumonia is an infectious process caused by the inhalation of oropharyngeal secretions colonized by pathogenic bacteria.[15] This is differentiated from aspiration pneumonitis, which is typically caused by chemical injury following inhalation of sterile gastric contents. Aspiration pneumonia is often caused by anaerobic organisms derived from the oral cavity (gingival crevice) and often develops in patients with an elevated risk of aspiration of oral contents into the lung, such as those with dysphagia or depressed consciousness. Aspiration pneumonia is very common in the nursing home setting and may also occur in the community.

Most adults inhale small amounts of oropharyngeal secretions during sleep. However, the small number and typically avirulent nature of the commensal microflora, as well as defense mechanisms such coughing, ciliary action, and normal immune mechanisms, work together to prevent onset of infection. However, circumstances that increase the volume of aspirate, especially the number of organisms in the aspirate, will increase the risk of pneumonia. The risk of aspiration pneumonia is lower in patients without teeth as well as in patients who receive aggressive oral care (discussed later in the chapter). However, little information is available regarding the effect of periodontal therapy in the prevention of aspiration pneumonia in vulnerable populations.

It is well documented that potential respiratory pathogens such as *S aureus, Pseudomonas aeruginosa, Klebsiella pneumoniae,* and *Enterobacter cloacae* colonize the dental plaque of dependent elderly.[16,17] In some settings, more than half of the individuals assessed showed the presence of these bacteria in the dental plaque.

Nosocomial pneumonia

Hospital-acquired pneumonia originally was defined as pneumonia occurring with onset more than 48 hours after admission to the hospital. This classification scheme was straightforward and easy to apply. However, over the past decade there has been a shift in delivery of medical care from the hospital to the outpatient setting for delivery of services such as antibiotic therapy, cancer chemotherapy, wound management, outpatient dialysis centers, and short-term rehabilitation. As a result, the classification scheme for pneumonia has changed. This shift in care from the hospital to the outpatient home setting or nursing home leads to cases of pneumonia that occur outside the hospital setting but are clearly within other health care delivery settings. Thus, such pneumonia has been referred to as *health care–associated pneumonia.*[18]

Pneumonia is a common infection in the hospital, often causing considerable morbidity and mortality as well as extending the length of stay and increasing the cost of hospital care. HAP can be further divided into two subtypes: VAP and non–ventilator-associated pneumonia. Pneumonia is the most common infection in the intensive care unit (ICU) setting, accounting for 10% of infections in ICUs.[19]

VAP is the second most common hospital-acquired infection.[20,21] VAP is a leading cause of death in critically ill patients in the ICU, with estimated prevalence rates of 10% to 65% and mortality rates of 25% to 60% depending on the study, patient populations, and medical or surgical conditions involved.[19,22–27] VAP and other forms of HAP are independent risk factors for mortality in hospitalized patients irrespective of the severity and type of underlying illness.[28] An episode of HAP adds approximately 5 to 6 days to the length of hospital stay and thousands of dollars in cost to medical care.[22-27]

The risk of developing VAP in the medical and surgical ICUs varies from 5 to 21 per 1,000 ventilator days.[29] The onset of pneumonia easily can double the length of the patient's hospital stay, and the cost of VAP treatment has been estimated to average as high as US$40,000 per case.[30] The mortality rate of nosocomial pneumonia can be as high as 25%.

NHAP is the most important common infection affecting nursing home residents because of the high morbidity and mortality associated with this infection.[31] Pneumonia is also a common reason for transfer of residents from the nursing home to the hospital,[32] with nursing home residents representing 13% to 48% of all infections.[33]

The Oral Cavity As a Reservoir of Respiratory Infection

The oral cavity may be an important source of bacteria that cause infections of the lungs. Dental plaque, a tooth-borne biofilm that initiates periodontal disease and dental caries, may host bacterial species as part of the normal flora that are capable of causing respiratory infection or may become colonized by exogenous respiratory pathogens. Oral pathogens may then be shed from the oral biofilm and released into the oral secretions, where they can attach to the endotracheal tube in ventilated patients to form pathogenic biofilms.[34] Bacteria can be released from the biofilms either on the teeth or on the tube to be aspirated into the respiratory tract.

The bacteria that cause CAP are typically species that normally colonize the oropharynx, such as S pneumoniae, H influenzae, and M pneumoniae. In contrast, nosocomial pneumonia is often caused by bacteria that are not common members of the oropharyngeal flora, such as P aeruginosa, S aureus, and enteric gram-negative bacteria. These organisms colonize the oral cavity in certain settings, for

example in institutionalized individuals and in people living in areas served by unsanitary water supplies.[1] Respiratory pathogens, such as S aureus, P aeruginosa, and Escherichia coli, are found to be present in substantial numbers on the teeth in both institutionalized elders[35] and intensive care patients.[36]

Just 1 mm³ of dental plaque contains about 100 million bacteria and may serve as a persistent reservoir for potential pathogens, both oral and respiratory bacteria. It is likely that oral and respiratory bacteria in the dental plaque are shed into the saliva and are then aspirated into the lower respiratory tract and the lungs to cause infection.[1,37] Indeed, the commensal, or normal, microflora of the oral cavity, especially the anaerobic bacteria that are associated with periodontal disease and reside in the subgingival space, often cause aspiration pneumonia in patients who have high risk for aspiration, such as those with dysphagia or neurologic impairment affecting the swallowing apparatus.

Cytokines and enzymes induced from the periodontally inflamed tissues by the oral biofilm may also be aspirated into the lungs, where they may stimulate local inflammatory processes before colonization by pathogens and the actual lung infection.[1,37] Other possible mechanisms to explain pulmonary infection are inhalation of airborne pathogens and translocation of bacteria from local infections via bacteremia.

In a healthy subject, the respiratory tract is able to defend itself against aspirated bacteria. Patients with diminished salivary flow, decreased cough reflex, swallowing disorders, poor ability to perform good oral hygiene, or other physical disabilities have a high risk for pulmonary infections. Mechanically ventilated patients in ICUs, who have no ability to clear oral secretions by swallowing or by coughing, are at particularly high risk for VAP, especially if the ventilation lasts for more than 48 hours.[38]

Oral bacterial load increases during intubation, and higher dental plaque scores predict risk of pneumonia.[39] Anaerobic bacteria are frequently found to colonize the lower respiratory tract in mechanically ventilated patients.[38] Colonization of bacteria in the digestive tract has been suggested to be a source for nosocomial pneumonia, but recently oral and dental bacterial colonization has been proposed to be the major source of bacteria implicated in the etiology of VAP.[40] It is likely that bacteria that first colonize the dental plaque can be shed and attach to the tubing that passes through the oral cavity into the lung.

In the institutionalized elderly, aspiration of saliva seems to be the main route by which bacteria enter the lungs to cause aspiration pneumonia. Dysphagia seems to be an important risk factor, even a predictor, for aspiration pneumonia.[41] For example, the major oral and dental risk factors for aspiration pneumonia in veteran residents of nursing homes were the number of carious teeth, periodontitis, oral *S aureus* colonization, and requirement of help with feeding.[42] In another study of 613 elderly nursing home patients, inadequate oral care and swallowing difficulties were also associated with pneumonia.[43]

Recent systematic reviews of the literature support the link between poor oral health and pneumonia.[44–46] Dentate status may put individuals at risk for pneumonia and respiratory tract infections: Patients with natural teeth develop aspiration pneumonia more often than do edentulous subjects.[47,48] The presence of cariogenic bacteria and periodontal pathogens in saliva or dental plaque have also been shown to be risk factors for aspiration pneumonia in nursing home patients.[41,42] It is well known that the teeth and gingival margin favor bacterial colonization, and periodontal pockets may serve as reservoirs for potential respiratory pathogens. Previous studies have shown that enteric bacteria colonize periodontal pockets.[49,50] Periodontitis, along with abundant dental plaque, may together facilitate colonization of dental plaque by respiratory pathogens and therefore promote pneumonia.

Several recently published studies have clearly demonstrated the genetic identity of bacterial strains from dental plaques with isolates from the lower airway from mechanically ventilated patients with suspected pneumonia. For example, strains of potential respiratory pathogens recovered from lung fluid were compared by pulsed field gel electrophoresis with isolates of the same species from the dental plaque of critically ill residents of long-term care

facilities transferred to an ICU.[51] Of 13 isolates recovered from protected bronchoalveolar lavage fluid, 9 respiratory pathogens appeared genetically identical to isolates of the same species recovered from the corresponding dental plaque.

A subsequent study also assessed the genetic relationship between strains of respiratory pathogens first isolated from the oral cavity and later isolated from bronchoalveolar lavage fluid obtained from patients who had been admitted to a trauma critical care unit, were undergoing mechanical ventilation, and were suspected to have VAP.[52] Pulsed field gel electrophoresis and multilocus sequence typing were used to determine the genetic relatedness of strains obtained from oral, tracheal, and bronchoalveolar lavage samples. Isolates of *S aureus*, *P aeruginosa*, *Acinetobacter* species, and enteric species recovered from plaque from most patients were indistinguishable from isolates recovered from bronchoalveolar lavage fluid.

These studies suggest that respiratory pathogens isolated from the lung are often genetically indistinguishable from strains of the same species isolated from the oral cavity in patients who receive mechanical ventilation and who are admitted to the hospital from both nursing homes and the community. Thus, dental plaque is an important reservoir for VAP infection.

Oral Interventions to Prevent VAP

Antiseptics

The most common approach to improve oral hygiene in ventilated patients is the use of antiseptics such as oral topical chlorhexidine (CHX). A large number of studies have tested the effectiveness of CHX to reduce VAP rates; most of these studies have been included in several recent meta-analyses and systematic reviews.[44–46,53,54] Several studies have suggested that oral topical application of CHX prevents pneumonia in mechanically ventilated patients (Table 9-1) and may even decrease the need

Table 9-1	Effect of oral antiseptic use on the prevalence of VAP and a subanalysis of chlorhexidine versus povidone-iodine use*					
	Antiseptic		**Control**			**Risk ratio**
Study or subgroup	**Events**	**Total**	**Events**	**Total**	**Weight**	**M-H [random, 95% CI]**
Povidone-iodine						
Chua et al[55]	6	22	8	20	6.8%	0.68 [0.29, 1.62]
Seguin et al[56]	3	36	25	62	4.7%	0.21 [0.07, 0.64]
Subtotal (95% CI)		58		82	11.5%	0.39 [0.11, 1.36]
Total events	9		33			
Heterogeneity: Tau² = 0.54; Chi² = 3.05; df = 1 (P = .08); I² = 67%. Test for overall effect: Z = 1.47 (P = .14).						
Chlorhexidine						
DeRiso et al[57]	3	173	9	180	3.8%	0.35 [0.10, 1.26]
Fourrier et al[58]	5	30	18	30	7.0%	0.28 [0.12, 0.65]
Houston et al[59]	4	270	9	291	4.4%	0.48 [0.15, 1.54]
MacNaughton et al[60]	32	91	28	88	14.1%	1.11 [0.73, 1.67]
Grap et al[61]	4	7	3	5	5.9%	0.95 [0.36, 2.49]
Fourrier et al[62]	13	114	12	114	8.3%	1.08 [0.52, 2.27]
Koeman et al[63]	13	127	23	130	9.9%	0.58 [0.31, 1.09]
Bopp et al[64]	0	2	1	3	0.9%	0.44 [0.03, 7.52]
Tantipong et al[65]	5	102	12	105	5.5%	0.43 [0.16, 1.17]
Bellissimo-Rodrigues et al[66]	16	64	17	69	10.6%	1.01 [0.56, 1.83]
Scannapieco et al[67]	14	116	12	59	8.8%	0.59 [0.29, 1.20]
Panchabhai et al[68]	14	88	15	83	9.4%	0.88 [0.45, 1.71]
Subtotal (95% CI)		1,184		1,157	88.5%	0.72 [0.55, 0.94]
Total events	123		159			
Heterogeneity: Tau² = 0.06; Chi² = 15.54; df = 11 (P = .16); I² = 29%. Test for overall effect: Z = 2.40 (P = .02).						
Total (95% CI)		**1,242**		**1,239**	**100.0%**	**0.67 [0.50, 0.88]**
Total events	**132**		**192**			
Heterogeneity: Tau² = 0.10; Chi² = 20.96; df = 13 (P = .07); I² = 38%. Test for overall effect: Z = 2.89 (P = .004). Test for subgroup differences: Not applicable.						*(continued on next page)*

*From Labeau et al.[54] Reprinted with permission.
M-H, Mantel-Haenszel test; CI, confidence interval.

for systemic intravenous antibiotics or shorten the duration of mechanical ventilation in the ICU.[57,58,63,69] In addition, oral application of CHX in the early postintubation period lowers the numbers of cultivable oral bacteria and may delay the development of VAP.[61]

Not all studies, however, have validated the effectiveness of oral CHX in preventing pneumonia. For example, the rate of oropharyngeal colonization by pathogenic bacteria was significantly reduced by gingival decontamination with CHX gel, but this was not sufficient to reduce the incidence of respiratory infections in venti-

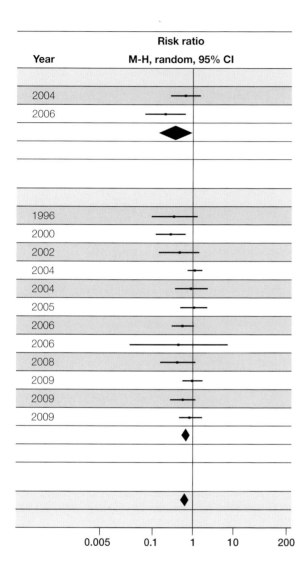

Year	Risk ratio M-H, random, 95% CI
2004	
2006	
1996	
2000	
2002	
2004	
2004	
2005	
2006	
2006	
2008	
2009	
2009	
2009	

0.005   0.1   1   10   200

lated patients.[62] Another study reported that the use of CHX rinse achieved a significant reduction in pneumonia in ICU patients after only 24 hours of intubation.[59] A recent randomized trial compared twice-daily oral topical application of 0.2% CHX with application of 0.01% potassium permanganate (control) solution in 512 cardiac surgery patients.[68] No differences were found between the groups with respect to the incidence of nosocomial pneumonia, median day of development of pneumonia, median ICU stay, or mortality among patients.

In addition to CHX, other antiplaque agents have been investigated. The use of antimicrobial gels, including polymyxin B sulfate, neomycin sulfate, and vancomycin hydrochloride[70] or a combination of gentamicin, colistin, and vancomycin,[71] also reduces the incidence of VAP.

Toothbrushing

The first study showing that mechanical oral care in combination with application of povidone-iodine significantly decreases the incidence of pneumonia in ventilated ICU patients was published in 2006.[72] This suggested that toothbrushing, combined with application of a topical antimicrobial agent, could be a promising method for oral cleansing of mechanically ventilated patients.

However, randomized trials have tested the specific effectiveness of toothbrushing for prevention of VAP.[73,74] Both studies tested the effect of the use of an electric toothbrush in addition to CHX rinse. While the addition of toothbrushing reduced the amount of visible dental plaque on the teeth,[74] it did not reduce the incidence of VAP.[73]

Oral Interventions to Prevent NHAP

Institutionalized but nonventilated patients, mainly the elderly living in nursing homes, appear to also benefit from improved oral care by showing lower levels of oral bacteria and fewer pneumonia episodes and febrile days. Daily toothbrushing and topical oral swabbing with povidone-iodine significantly decreased the frequency of pneumonia in residents in long-term care facilities.[75-77] However, in an earlier study by the same research group, oral care with both toothbrushing and antimicrobial gargling had an effect only on the number of febrile days but not on the incidence of pneumonia.[78]

Professional cleaning by a dental hygienist once a week significantly reduced the prevalence of fever and fatal pneumonia in 141 elderly patients in nursing homes.[79] Similar once-a-week professional oral cleaning significantly reduced the incidence of influenza infections in an elderly population.[80] Dental plaque is known to form clearly visible masses in the teeth in a few days, but these studies suggest that improved oral care, even without chemical agents and even if not performed daily, not only reduces the oral bacterial, viral, and fungal loads but also may have an effect on reducing the risk of pneumonia.

A systematic review of randomized controlled trials assessed the role of oral care in the prevention of NHAP.[81] This analysis suggested that oral hygiene interventions reduced rates of pneumonia and respiratory tract infection in elderly nursing home residents, with absolute risk reductions ranging from 6.6% to 11.7% and reductions in numbers needed to treat ranging from 8.6 to 15.3 individuals. Mechanical oral hygiene has a preventive effect on mortality from pneumonia and nonfatal pneumonia in hospitalized elderly people and elderly nursing home residents. These authors estimated that approximately 1 in 10 cases of death from pneumonia among elderly nursing home residents could be prevented by improving oral hygiene.

Oral cleansing reduces pneumonia in both edentulous and dentate subjects, suggesting that oral colonization of bacteria contributes to nosocomial pneumonia to a greater extent than periodontitis. However, intervention studies to assess the effect of treatment of periodontitis on the incidence of pneumonia have not been performed because of the complexities associated with investigating ICU or bed-bound nursing home patients. In edentulous people, dentures, similar to teeth, may easily serve as a reservoir for oral and respiratory bacteria if not cleaned properly and daily.

Clinical Guidelines for Oral Hygiene in Vulnerable Patients

An important development over the past 10 years has been the establishment of "ventilator bundles," or sets of evidence-based thera-

Box 9-1	Recommendations for oral care of critically ill patients[87]

- Provision of effective oral care is an important strategy in reducing nosocomial pneumonia.
- The use of a designated oral care protocol can increase compliance and assessment of mouth care.
- Systematic clinical assessment of the oral cavity using standardized methods is important in the planning and evaluation of oral care in the critically ill (to include the condition of the teeth, gingiva, tongue, mucous membranes, and lips).
- The use of a soft-bristled brush can remove debris and subsequent plaque.
- Mouth swabs (foam and cotton) should be used where toothbrushing is contraindicated (eg, bleeding gingiva associated with thrombocytopenia).
- At the present, there is no evidence to support the use of one oral rinse over another (with the exception of 0.12% CHX gluconate in cardiac surgical patients).
- Tap water should not be used for oral hygiene in the critically ill because it is often contaminated with potential respiratory pathogens.
- Subglottic suctioning in mechanically ventilated patients is recommended to limit aspiration of contaminated secretions.
- Although the optimal frequency for oral hygiene has never been evaluated, toothbrushing at least twice a day is suggested.
- Although the optimal duration of oral care has never been evaluated, oral cleansing for 3 to 4 minutes with a toothbrush that allows access to all areas of the mouth is suggested.
- Although no evidence is available to support the use of individual, clean storage devices for oral hygiene tools, the use of designated containers is recommended.

pies instituted within health care settings to reduce the rate of VAP.[82] These bundles include a number of actions, including semirecumbent patient positioning; stress ulcer prophylaxis to decrease gastrointestinal bleeding; prophylaxis to decrease deep venous thrombosis; adjustment of sedation until the patient can follow commands; and daily assessment of readiness to extubate, to reduce the duration of mechanical ventilation. Implementation of these bundles has been shown to greatly reduce VAP rates.[82] In some cases, oral hygiene care, including topical application of CHX, has been included as part of the bundles.[83]

Many studies have demonstrated that improved oral hygiene can reduce the risk of pneumonia in vulnerable patients. Therefore, the present status of oral hygiene practice in hospitals and nursing homes is of great importance. The type and frequency of oral care provided in ICUs in the United States, as well as the attitudes, beliefs, and knowledge of health care personnel have been evaluated.[84] While 512 (92%) of 556 respondents perceived oral care to be a high priority, the primary oral care procedures involved the use of foam swabs, moisturizers, and mouthwash. Interventions thought to reduce oral colonization by respiratory pathogens, such as toothbrushing and the use of antiseptic rinses such as CHX gluconate, appear to be used infrequently in critical care settings.[85] This is complicated by the fact that dental plaque formation is more robust on posterior teeth, and posterior plaque is more difficult to assess and remove by conventional methods, especially in patients who are intubated.[86]

A recent article described clinical practice guidelines for oral hygiene in critically ill patients based on a systematic literature review followed by prospective consideration of the evidence at a consensus development conference.[87] Several recommendations were offered to guide clinicians in the care of vulnerable patients (Box 9-1).

Other measures for consideration for intubated patients may include removal of all dental appliances on admission to the critical care unit, periodic repositioning of the tube, or deflation of the cuff. If possible, removal of hard deposits (eg, calculus) from the teeth should be considered prior to admission (for example, in the case of elective surgery). Placing the patient's head to the side or the patient's body in the semi-Fowler (semireclined) body position will also minimize inadvertent aspiration.

Conclusion

It is now established that bacteria that colonize dental plaque can influence the initiation and/or progression of respiratory infections such as pneumonia. Further research is required to determine the simplest and most cost-effective oral intervention strategies to prevent respiratory disease in vulnerable populations.

References

1. Scannapieco FA. Role of oral bacteria in respiratory infection. J Periodontol 1999;70:793–802.
2. Shay K, Scannapieco FA, Terpenning MS, Smith BJ, Taylor GW. Nosocomial pneumonia and oral health. Spec Care Dentist 2005;25:179–187.
3. Scannapieco FA. Pneumonia in nonambulatory patients. The role of oral bacteria and oral hygiene. J Am Dent Assoc 2006;137(suppl):21S–25S.
4. Paju S, Scannapieco FA. Oral biofilms, periodontitis, and pulmonary infections. Oral Dis 2007;13:508–512.
5. Raghavendran K, Mylotte JM, Scannapieco FA. Nursing home-associated pneumonia, hospital-acquired pneumonia and ventilator-associated pneumonia: The contribution of dental biofilms and periodontal inflammation. Periodontol 2000 2007; 44:164–177.
6. Scannapieco FA, Mylotte JM. Oral health and diseases of the respiratory tract. In: Genco RJ, Williams RC (eds). Periodontal Disease and Overall Health: A Clinician's Guide. Yardley, PA: Professional Audience Communications, 2010:147–161.
7. Stein RT, Marostica PJ. Community-acquired pneumonia. Paediatr Respir Rev 2006;7(suppl 1):S136–S137.
8. Lutfiyya MN, Henley E, Chang LF, Reyburn SW. Diagnosis and treatment of community-acquired pneumonia. Am Fam Physician 2006;73:442–450.
9. Jackson ML, Neuzil KM, Thompson WW, et al. The burden of community-acquired pneumonia in seniors: Results of a population-based study. Clin Infect Dis 2004;39:1642–1650.
10. Almirall J, Bolíbar I, Serra-Prat M, et al. New evidence of risk factors for community-acquired pneumonia: A population-based study. Eur Respir J 2008;31:1274–1284.
11. Durrington HJ, Summers C. Recent changes in the management of community acquired pneumonia in adults. BMJ 2008;336:1429–1433.
12. Niederman MS. Recent advances in community-acquired pneumonia: Inpatient and outpatient. Chest 2007;131:1205–1215.
13. Kaplan V, Clermont G, Griffin MF, et al. Pneumonia: Still the old man's friend? Arch Intern Med 2003; 163:317–323.
14. Sharma N, Shamsuddin H. Association between respiratory disease in hospitalized patients and periodontal disease: A cross-sectional study. J Periodontol 2011;82:1155–1160.
15. Marik PE. Aspiration pneumonitis and aspiration pneumonia. N Engl J Med 2001;344:665–671.
16. Russell SL, Boylan RJ, Kaslick RS, Scannapieco FA, Katz RV. Respiratory pathogen colonization of the dental plaque of institutionalized elders. Spec Care Dentist 1999;19:128–134.
17. Sumi Y, Miura H, Michiwaki Y, Nagaosa S, Nagaya M. Colonization of dental plaque by respiratory pathogens in dependent elderly. Arch Gerontol Geriatr 2007;44:119–124.
18. Tablan OC, Anderson LJ, Besser R, et al. Guidelines for preventing health-care–associated pneumonia, 2003: Recommendations of CDC and the Healthcare Infection Control Practices Advisory Committee. MMWR Recomm Rep 2004;53(RR-3):1–36.
19. Vincent JL, Bihari DJ, Suter PM, et al. The prevalence of nosocomial infection in intensive care units in Europe. Results of the European Prevalence of Infection in Intensive Care (EPIC) Study. EPIC International Advisory Committee. JAMA 1995;274:639–644.
20. Richards MJ, Edwards JR, Culver DH, Gaynes RP. Nosocomial infections in medical intensive care units in the United States. National Nosocomial Infections Surveillance System. Crit Care Med 1999;27:887–892.
21. Arozullah AM, Khuri SF, Henderson WG, Daley J. Participants in the National Veterans Affairs Surgical Quality Improvement Program. Development and validation of a multifactorial risk index for predicting postoperative pneumonia after major noncardiac surgery. Ann Intern Med 2001;135:847–857.
22. Horan TC, White JW, Jarvis WR. Nosocomial infection surveillance, 1984. MMWR CDC Surveill Summ 1986;35:17SS–29SS.

23. Craven DE, Barber TW, Steger KA, Montecalvo MA. Nosocomial pneumonia in the 1990s: Update of epidemiology and risk factors. Semin Respir Infect 1990;5:157–172.

24. Craven DE, Steger KA, Barber TW. Preventing nosocomial pneumonia: State of the art and perspectives for the 1990s. Am J Med 1991;91(3B):44S–53S.

25. Craven DE, Steger KA. Epidemiology of nosocomial pneumonia. New perspectives on an old disease. Chest 1995;108(suppl 2):1S–16S.

26. Kollef MH. The identification of ICU-specific outcome predictors: A comparison of medical, surgical, and cardiothoracic ICUs from a single institution. Heart Lung 1995;24:60–66.

27. Kollef MH. Prevention of hospital-associated pneumonia and ventilator-associated pneumonia. Crit Care Med 2004;32:1396–1405.

28. Fagon JY, Chastre J, Hance AJ, Montravers P, Novara A, Gibert C. Nosocomial pneumonia in ventilated patients: A cohort study evaluating attributable mortality and hospital stay. Am J Med 1993;94:281–288.

29. Lynch J, Lama V. Diagnosis and therapy of nosocomial ventilator associated pneumonia. AFC 2000;4:19–26.

30. Rello J, Ollendorf DA, Oster G, et al. Epidemiology and outcomes of ventilator-associated pneumonia in a large US database. Chest 2002;122:2115–2121.

31. Mylotte JM. Nursing home-acquired pneumonia. Clin Infect Dis 2002;35:1205–1211.

32. Muder RR. Pneumonia in residents of long-term care facilities: Epidemiology, etiology, management, and prevention. Am J Med 1998;105:319–330.

33. Crossley KB, Thurn JR. Nursing home-acquired pneumonia. Semin Respir Infect 1989;4:64–72.

34. Gil-Perotin S, Ramirez P, Marti V, et al. Implications of endotracheal tube biofilm in ventilator-associated pneumonia response: A state of concept. Crit Care 2012;16:R93.

35. Russell SL, Boylan RJ, Kaslick RS, Scannapieco FA, Katz RV. Respiratory pathogen colonization of the dental plaque of institutionalized elders. Spec Care Dentist 1999;19:128–134.

36. Scannapieco FA, Stewart EM, Mylotte JM. Colonization of dental plaque by respiratory pathogens in medical intensive care patients. Crit Care Med 1992;20:740–745.

37. Scannapieco FA, Wang B, Shiau HJ. Oral bacteria and respiratory infection: Effects on respiratory pathogen adhesion and epithelial cell proinflammatory cytokine production. Ann Periodontol 2001;6:78–86.

38. Estes RJ, Meduri GU. The pathogenesis of ventilator-associated pneumonia. 1. Mechanisms of bacterial translocation and airway inoculation. Intensive Care Med 1995;21:365–383.

39. Munro CL, Grap MJ, Elswick RK Jr, McKinney J, Sessler CN, Hummel RS 3rd. Oral health status and development of ventilator-associated pneumonia: A descriptive study. Am J Crit Care 2006;15:453–460.

40. Garcia R. A review of the possible role of oral and dental colonization on the occurrence of health care–associated pneumonia: Underappreciated risk and a call for interventions. Am J Infect Control 2005;33:527–541.

41. Langmore SE, Terpenning MS, Schork A, et al. Predictors of aspiration pneumonia: How important is dysphagia? Dysphagia 1998;13:69–81.

42. Terpenning MS, Taylor GW, Lopatin DE, Kerr CK, Dominguez BL, Loesche WJ. Aspiration pneumonia: Dental and oral risk factors in an older veteran population. J Am Geriatr Soc 2001;49:557–563.

43. Quagliarello V, Ginter S, Han L, Van Ness P, Allore H, Tinetti M. Modifiable risk factors for nursing home-acquired pneumonia. Clin Infect Dis 2005;40:1–6.

44. Scannapieco FA, Bush RB, Paju S. Associations between periodontal disease and risk for nosocomial bacterial pneumonia and chronic obstructive pulmonary disease. A systematic review. Ann Periodontol 2003;8:54–69.

45. Azarpazhooh A, Leake JL. Systematic review of the association between respiratory diseases and oral health. J Periodontol 2006;77:1465–1482.

46. Chan EY, Ruest A, Meade MO, Cook DJ. Oral decontamination for prevention of pneumonia in mechanically ventilated adults: Systematic review and meta-analysis. BMJ 2007;334(7599):889.

47. Terpenning M, Bretz W, Lopatin D, Langmore S, Dominguez B, Loesche W. Bacterial colonization of saliva and plaque in the elderly. Clin Infect Dis 1993;16(suppl 4):314–316.

48. Mojon P, Budtz-Jørgensen E, Michel JP, Limeback H. Oral health and history of respiratory tract infection in frail institutionalised elders. Gerodontol 1997;14:9–16.

49. Rams TE, Babalola OO, Slots J. Subgingival occurence of enteric rods, yeasts and staphylococci after systemic doxycycline therapy. Oral Microbiol Immunol 1990;5:166–168.

50. Slots J, Rams TE, Listgarten MA. Yeasts, enteric rods and psuedomonads in the subgingival flora of severe adult periodontitis. Oral Microbiol Immunol 1988;3:47–52.

51. El-Solh AA, Pietrantoni C, Bhat A, et al. Colonization of dental plaques: A reservoir of respiratory pathogens for hospital-acquired pneumonia in institutionalized elders. Chest 2004;126:1575–1582.

52. Heo SM, Haase EM, Lesse AJ, Gill SR, Scannapieco FA. Genetic relationships between respiratory pathogens isolated from dental plaque and bronchoalveolar lavage fluid from patients in the intensive care unit undergoing mechanical ventilation. Clin Infect Dis 2008;47:1562–1570.

53. Roberts N, Moule P. Chlorhexidine and tooth-brushing as prevention strategies in reducing ventilator-associated pneumonia rates. Nurs Crit Care 2011;16:295–302.

54. Labeau SO, Van de Vyver K, Brusselaers N, Vogelaers D, Blot SI. Prevention of ventilator-associated pneumonia with oral antiseptics: A systematic review and meta-analysis. Lancet Infect Dis 2011;11: 845–854.

55. Chua JV, Dominguez EA, Sison CMC, Berba RP. The efficacy of povidone-iodine oral rinse in preventing ventilator-associated pneumonia: A randomized, double-blind, placebo-controlled (VAPOR) trial: Preliminary report. Philipp J Microbiol Infect Dis 2004;33:153–161.

56. Seguin P, Tanguy M, Laviolle B, Tirel O, Malledant Y. Effect of oropharyngeal decontamination by povidone-iodine on ventilator-associated pneumonia in patients with head trauma. Crit Care Med 2006;34: 1514–1519.

57. DeRiso AJ 2nd, Ladowski JS, Dillon TA, Justice JW, Peterson AC. Chlorhexidine gluconate 0.12% oral rinse reduces the incidence of total nosocomial respiratory infection and nonprophylactic systemic antibiotic use in patients undergoing heart surgery. Chest 1996;109:1556–1561.

58. Fourrier F, Cau-Pottier E, Boutigny H, Roussel-Delvallez M, Jourdain M, Chopin C. Effects of dental plaque antiseptic decontamination on bacterial colonization and nosocomial infections in critically ill patients. Intensive Care Med 2000;26:1239–1247.

59. Houston S, Hougland P, Anderson JJ, LaRocco M, Kennedy V, Gentry LO. Effectiveness of 0.12% chlorhexidine gluconate oral rinse in reducing prevalence of nosocomial pneumonia in patients undergoing heart surgery. Am J Crit Care 2002;11:567–570.

60. MacNaughton PD, Bailey J, Donlin N, Branfield P, Williams A, Rowswell H. A randomised controlled trial assessing the efficacy of oral chlorhexidine in ventilated patients. Intensive Care Med 2004;30 (suppl):S12.

61. Grap MJ, Munro CL, Elswick RK Jr, Sessler CN, Ward KR. Duration of action of a single, early oral application of chlorhexidine on oral microbial flora in mechanically ventilated patients: A pilot study. Heart Lung 2004;33:83–91.

62. Fourrier F, Dubois D, Pronnier P, et al. Effect of gingival and dental plaque antiseptic decontamination on nosocomial infections acquired in the intensive care unit: A double-blind placebo-controlled multicenter study. Crit Care Med 2005;33:1728–1735.

63. Koeman M, van der Ven AJ, Hak E, et al. Oral decontamination with chlorhexidine reduces the incidence of ventilator-associated pneumonia. Am J Respir Crit Care Med 2006;173:1348–1355.

64. Bopp M, Darby M, Loftin KC, Broscious S. Effects of daily oral care with 0.12% chlorhexidine gluconate and a standard oral care protocol on the development of nosocomial pneumonia in intubated patients: A pilot study. J Dent Hyg 2006;80:1–13.

65. Tantipong H, Morkchareonpong C, Jaiyindee S, Thamlikitkul V. Randomized controlled trial and meta-analysis of oral decontamination with 2% chlorhexidine solution for the prevention of ventilator-associated pneumonia. Infect Control Hosp Epidemiol 2008;29:131–136.

66. Bellissimo-Rodrigues F, Bellissimo-Rodrigues WT, Viana JM, et al. Effectiveness of oral rinse with chlorhexidine in preventing nosocomial respiratory tract infections among intensive care unit patients. Infect Control Hosp Epidemiol 2009;30:952–958.

67. Scannapieco F, Yu J, Raghavendran K, et al. A randomized trial of chlorhexidine gluconate on oral bacterial pathogens in mechanically ventilated patients. Crit Care 2009;13(4):R117.

68. Panchabhai TS, Dangayach NS, Krishnan A, Kothari VM, Karnad DR. Oropharyngeal cleansing with 0.2% chlorhexidine for prevention of nosocomial pneumonia in critically ill patients: An open-label randomized trial with 0.01% potassium permanganate as control. Chest 2009;135:1150–1156.

69. Genuit T, Bochicchio G, Napolitano LM, McCarter RJ, Roghman MC. Prophylactic chlorhexidine oral rinse decreases ventilator-associated pneumonia in surgical ICU patients. Surg Infect (Larchmt) 2001; 2:5–18.

70. Pugin J, Auckenthaler R, Lew DP, Suter PM. Oropharyngeal decontamination decreases incidence of ventilator-associated pneumonia. A randomized, placebo-controlled, double-blind clinical trial. JAMA 1991;265:2704–2710.

71. Bergmans DC, Bonten MJ, Gaillard CA, et al. Prevention of ventilator-associated pneumonia by oral decontamination: A prospective, randomized, double-blind, placebo-controlled study. Am J Respir Crit Care Med 2001;164:382–388.

72. Mori H, Hirasawa H, Oda S, Shiga H, Matsuda K, Nakamura M. Oral care reduces incidence of ventilator-associated pneumonia in ICU populations. Intensive Care Med 2006;32:230–236.

73. Pobo A, Lisboa T, Rodriguez A, et al. A randomized trial of dental brushing for preventing ventilator-associated pneumonia. Chest 2009;136:433–439.

74. Needleman IG, Hirsch NP, Leemans M, et al. Randomized controlled trial of toothbrushing to reduce ventilator-associated pneumonia pathogens and dental plaque in a critical care unit. J Clin Periodontol 2011;38:246–252.

75. Yoshida M, Yoneyama T, Akagawa Y. Oral care reduces pneumonia of elderly patients in nursing homes, irrespective of dentate or edentate status [in Japanese]. Nihon Ronen Igakkai Zasshi 2001; 38:481–483.

76. Yoneyama T, Yoshida M, Matsui T, Sasaki H. Oral care and pneumonia [letter]. Oral Care Working Group. Lancet 1999;354:515.

77. Yoneyama T, Yoshida M, Ohrui T, et al. Oral care reduces pneumonia in older patients in nursing homes. J Am Geriatr Soc 2002;50:430–433.

78. Yoneyama T, Hashimoto K, Fukuda H, et al. Oral hygiene reduces respiratory infections in elderly bed-bound nursing home patients. Arch Gerontol Geriatr 1996;22:11–19.

79. Adachi M, Ishihara K, Abe S, Okuda K, Ishikawa T. Effect of professional oral health care on the elderly living in nursing homes. Oral Surg Oral Med Oral Pathol Oral Radiol Endod 2002;94:191–195.

80. Abe S, Ishihara K, Adachi M, Sasaki H, Tanaka K, Okuda K. Professional oral care reduces influenza infection in elderly. Arch Gerontol Geriatr 2006;43: 157–164.

81. Sjögren P, Nilsson E, Forsell M, Johansson O, Hoogstraate J. A systematic review of the preventive effect of oral hygiene on pneumonia and respiratory tract infection in elderly people in hospitals and nursing homes: Effect estimates and methodological quality of randomized controlled trials. J Am Geriatr Soc 2008;56:2124–2130.

82. Berenholtz SM, Pham JC, Thompson DA, et al. Collaborative cohort study of an intervention to reduce ventilator-associated pneumonia in the intensive care unit. Infect Control Hosp Epidemiol 2011;32:305–314.

83. Caserta RA, Marra AR, Durão MS, et al. A program for sustained improvement in preventing ventilator associated pneumonia in an intensive care setting. BMC Infect Dis 2012;12:234.

84. Binkley C, Furr LA, Carrico R, McCurren C. Survey of oral care practices in US intensive care units. Am J Infect Control 2004;32:161–169.

85. Grap MJ, Munro CL, Ashtiani B, Bryant S. Oral care interventions in critical care: Frequency and documentation. Am J Crit Care 2003;12:113–118.

86. Jones DJ, Munro CL, Grap MJ. Natural history of dental plaque accumulation in mechanically ventilated adults: A descriptive correlational study. Intensive Crit Care Nurs 2011;27:299–304.

87. Berry AM, Davidson PM, Nicholson L, Pasqualotto C, Rolls K. Consensus based clinical guideline for oral hygiene in the critically ill. Intensive Crit Care Nurs 2011;27:180–185.

Clinical Considerations:
What You Can Take Back to Your Practice

What is the effect of pregnancy on periodontal health?

The significant increase in sex steroids during pregnancy affects the periodontal tissues via multiple mechanisms, and their net effect is manifested as an increase in the prevalence, extent, and severity of gingival inflammation *(pregnancy gingivitis)*. These changes are infrequently associated with loss of connective tissue attachment and usually revert after parturition.

Are oral infections independent risk factors for the development of adverse pregnancy outcomes?

Epidemiologic studies demonstrate an association between poor maternal periodontal health and adverse pregnancy outcomes (preterm birth, low birth weight, and preeclampsia). The magnitude of this effect is moderate but independent of other confounders.

What is the biologic plausibility of the association between oral health and adverse pregnancy outcomes?

Oral bacteria and bacterial products can gain access to the fetoplacental unit via hematogenous spread, where they may elicit inflammatory responses that contribute to adverse pregnancy outcomes.

Does the delivery of oral health care contribute to an improvement of pregnancy outcomes?

Well-conducted studies providing periodontal therapy during the second trimester of pregnancy have shown no accompanying improvements in adverse pregnancy outcomes.

Is dental care during pregnancy safe for both mother and child?

Dental care during pregnancy has been shown to be safe for both mother and child.

What is the appropriate message to give to the public about the association between oral health and pregnancy?

Oral health is an integral part of overall health and should be maintained at all times, pregnancy included.

10 Periodontal Infections and Adverse Pregnancy Outcomes

Yiorgos A. Bobetsis, DDS, PhD
Wenche S. Borgnakke, DDS, MPH, PhD
Panos N. Papapanou, DDS, PhD

For the past two decades, the association between periodontal diseases and adverse pregnancy outcomes has been the focus of investigation in a variety of studies, ranging from experimental animal models to epidemiologic association studies and intervention trials in humans. Yet several uncertainties still remain, and oral health care professionals and the public alike are exposed to frequently contradictory information that must be clarified. This chapter addresses the following specific questions:

- What is the effect of pregnancy on the periodontal tissues?
- What is the biologic plausibility of the association between periodontal diseases and adverse pregnancy outcomes?
- Are periodontal diseases independent risk factors for the development of adverse pregnancy outcomes?
- Does the delivery of periodontal therapy in pregnant women contribute to an improvement in pregnancy outcomes?
- Is periodontal therapy during pregnancy safe for both mother and child?
- What is the appropriate message to give to the public about this association?

The impact of adverse pregnancy outcomes on society cannot be overestimated. A recent Global Burden of Disease Study[1] identified neonatal disorders and specifically *preterm birth* (PTB), defined as the live birth of an infant before completion of the 37th gestational week, as significant contributors to global mortality. More than 15 million babies (1 in every 10 live births) are born too soon every year around the world,[2] and more than 1 million children die each year as a result of complications of PTB.[3] Surviving PTB infants often face multiple lifelong challenges, including respiratory distress, impaired motor skills, cognitive and intellectual impairment, and visual and learning difficulties.[4,5]

PTB largely occurs for three different reasons: medically indicated PTB, spontaneous PTB, and preterm premature rupture of membranes. The rate of PTB varies greatly: Among 39 countries with a Very High Human Development Index ranking, the PTB rate ranges from a low of 5.3% (Latvia) to a high of 14.7% (Cyprus).[5] The United States (US) ranks 37th on this list (Fig 10-1) but 54th highest among 184 countries.[6] Despite a decline since its peak of 12.9% in 2006, with an estimated rate of 11.7% for 2011 (ie, more than 1 in 8 live births), infants in the United States are still born preterm at double the rate of the Western industrialized countries in Northern Europe (around 5%) and at a higher rate than in Canada (7.8%).[7] The US PTB rate is highest for non-Hispanic black infants (16.8%

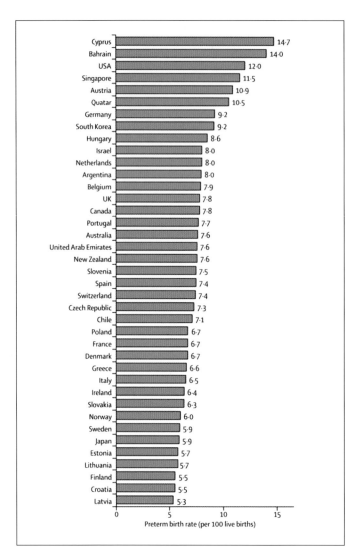

Fig 10-1 PTB rates in 2010 for 39 countries with a Very High Human Development Index ranking. (Reprinted from Chang et al[5] with permission.)

Preterm birth rate (per 100 live births)

Cyprus	14·7
Bahrain	14·0
USA	12·0
Singapore	11·5
Austria	10·9
Quatar	10·5
Germany	9·2
South Korea	9·2
Hungary	8·6
Israel	8·0
Netherlands	8·0
Argentina	8·0
Belgium	7·9
UK	7·8
Canada	7·8
Portugal	7·7
Australia	7·6
United Arab Emirates	7·6
New Zealand	7·6
Slovenia	7·5
Spain	7·4
Switzerland	7·4
Czech Republic	7·3
Chile	7·1
Poland	6·7
France	6·7
Denmark	6·7
Greece	6·6
Italy	6·5
Ireland	6·4
Slovakia	6·3
Norway	6·0
Sweden	5·9
Japan	5·9
Estonia	5·7
Lithuania	5·7
Finland	5·5
Croatia	5·5
Latvia	5·3

of live births), followed by Native American (13.5%), Hispanic (11.7%), non-Hispanic white (10.5%), and Asian/Pacific Islander (10.4%) infants.[7] In 2010, the US had the 6th highest number of PTB of the world's 184 countries, only surpassed by India, China, Nigeria, Pakistan, and Indonesia.[6]

PTB babies are further subdivided into the categories extremely preterm (born before 28 weeks), severely premature (between 28 and 31 weeks), moderately premature (between 32 and 33 weeks), and near term (between 34 and 36 weeks). Additional neonatal disorders or pregnancy complications include *low birth weight*, defined as weight at birth of less than 2,500 g (5 lb 8 oz), approximately one-third less than the average weight of a term infant (3.5 kg/7 lb); *intrauterine growth restriction* or *small for gestational age*, defined as weight at less than the 10th percentile at any given gestational age; preeclampsia, ie, high maternal blood pressure (higher than 140/90 mmHg) and sig-

---

Box 10-1   **Risk factors or markers of PTB and low birth weight[8]**

- Young maternal age
- African American or Afro-Caribbean maternal genotype
- Intrauterine infections
- Interpregnancy interval of less than 6 months
- Drugs and heavy alcohol use
- Tobacco use
- Multiple gestation
- In vitro fertilization
- Psychologic and social stress
- Depression
- Obesity-related preeclampsia
- Diabetes
- Hypertension
- Low prepregnancy body mass index
- Low socioeconomic status
- Low educational status
- Fetal genotype
- History of previous PTB

---

nificant proteinuria (300 mg/24 h) after the 20th gestational week; eclampsia, ie, occurrence of life-threatening maternal seizures; and gestational diabetes, ie, glucose intolerance with onset or first recognition during pregnancy, most commonly during the second trimester.

There is a close association between gestational age and weight at birth, both of which are important predictors for future morbidity and mortality. For example, in 2008, 24.0% of infants with very low birth weight (less than 1,500 g/3 lb 5 oz) died within their first year of life, compared with 1.4% of infants born with moderately low birth weight (1,500 to 2,500 g) and 0.2% of infants with a birth weight of more than 2,500 g.[7]

Several risk factors have been associated with adverse pregnancy outcomes, some of which involve infectious or inflammatory pathways (Box 10-1). The diverse nature of the exposures and phenotypic characteristics associated with PTB have led to the proposal to classify it as a syndrome, the development of which depends on the interaction of environmental exposures and genotypic characteristics.[9]

Effects of Pregnancy on the Periodontal Tissues

While dental plaque is the primary etiology for the development of periodontitis, the presence of the bacterial biofilm is necessary but not always sufficient for the initiation and progression of the disease. A number of systemic factors may increase the susceptibility of the host to the microbial challenge and may hence impact the extent and severity of periodontitis. Several hormones, including the sex steroids, have an influence on the cellular components of the periodontal tissues and may thus interfere with the mechanisms involved in the pathobiology of periodontitis. Fluctuations in the levels of these hormones in physiologic or nonphysiologic conditions may result in significant alterations in the periodontium, especially in the presence of preexisting, plaque-induced gingival inflammation.

Natural sex steroids, also known as *gonadal steroids*, are steroid hormones produced by the gonads (ovaries or testes), by adrenal glands, or by conversion from other sex steroids in other tissues such as the liver or adipose depots. The main classes of sex steroids are androgens, estrogens, and progestogens, of which the most important human derivatives include testosterone, estradiol, and progesterone, respectively. In general, androgens are considered "male sex hormones," since they have masculinizing effects, while estrogens and progestogens are considered "female sex hormones"; however, all three types are present in both sexes, albeit at different levels.

Because periodontal tissues possess receptors for sex steroids, researchers have extensively studied the effects of these hormones on the periodontium, which include:

- An impact on the degree of keratinization of the gingival epithelium and, thus, its barrier function as a first line of defense against bacterial pathogens.[10]
- Involvement in vascular functions such as angiogenesis and vascular permeability. Specifically, higher estrogen levels stimulate angiogenesis, while elevated circulating progesterone enhances capillary permeability and dilation, resulting in increased gingival exudate that may facilitate the recruitment of inflammatory cells in the gingival area and the crevicular fluid. The enhanced vascular permeability also may be partly due to stimulating effects of progesterone on prostaglandin synthesis.[11]
- Involvement in periodontal connective tissue turnover,[12] because estrogen has been shown to enhance the proliferation of fibroblasts and the production and maturation of collagen, while progesterone has the opposite effects.[13]
- An effect of estrogen on salivary peroxidases, which are active against a variety of microorganisms. Estrogen changes the redox potential of the salivary peroxidases.[14]
- Estrogen-mediated suppression of leukocyte production in the bone marrow and inhibition of polymorphonuclear leukocyte chemotaxis and phagocytosis.[15]
- Progesterone-induced reduction of the anti-inflammatory effects of glucocorticoids either directly via receptor binding on osteoblasts or indirectly by antagonizing glucocorticoid receptors.[16]

Therefore, periods of hormonal flux during puberty, menstruation, pregnancy, menopause, hormone replacement therapy, or use of contraceptives have been associated with periodontal manifestations.

There is a significant rise in the amount of sex steroids produced during the course of pregnancy; secreted near-term levels of estradiol, estriol, and progesterone reach 20.0, 80.0, and 300.0 mg/d, respectively, compared with normal secretion levels of 0.6, 3.0, and 19.0 mg/d, respectively, in nonpregnant women.[17] This temporary hormonal elevation correlates with an increase in the prevalence, extent, and severity of gingival inflammation, commonly referred to as *pregnancy gingivitis*, which occurs in approximately 50% of pregnant women[18,19] and usually affects interdental papillae of anterior areas. The severity of gingival inflammation is accentuated from the second gestational month and as pregnancy progresses under consistent plaque colonization.[20] After the eighth gestational month, and especially after delivery, gingival inflammation subsides and reverts to the levels of the first trimester. This spontaneous improvement in the absence of periodontal therapy correlates closely with the concomitant dramatic reduction in the secretion of sex steroids.[21] However, despite this exacerbated inflammatory response and accompanying increases in sulcular depth, gingival crevicular fluid flow, and bleeding on probing,[12] loss of clinical attachment is infrequent.[20]

In a small percentage of pregnant women (at frequencies ranging between 0.5% and 10.0% in the literature), the combined stimulatory effects of sex steroids on angiogenesis and extracellular matrix can lead to an exaggerated inflammatory response to dental plaque and the formation of a localized mass of highly vascularized granulation tissue, referred to as *pregnancy granuloma* or *epulis* (Fig 10-2). This lesion commonly arises from the proximal gingival tissues of the maxillary anterior, does not exceed 2 cm in diameter, has a pedunculated base, and resembles the clinical and histologic appearance of a pyogenic granuloma, or rather a telangiectatic granuloma, since it is usually not purulent. It is characterized by rapid growth and a bright red, hyperemic, and edematous

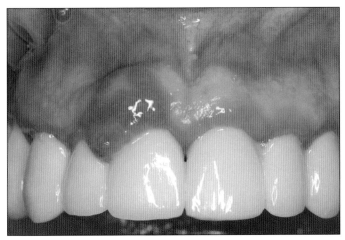

Fig 10-2 Clinical presentation of pregnancy granuloma or epulis.

appearance because of increased vascularization and may show ulceration of its thin epithelial lining. The lesion is typically not painful but may bleed spontaneously or when traumatized.

Occasionally, surgical removal of the granuloma may be necessary, especially when it interferes with mastication or normal speech, but full excision should be accompanied by thorough debridement and meticulous oral hygiene to minimize the risk of recurrence. However, in most cases, its removal is best deferred until after parturition, when there is often considerable regression in its size.[22]

In parallel to the clinical manifestations, pregnancy results in altered periodontal microbial colonization profiles, including an increase in the proportion of anaerobic over aerobic bacteria during the second trimester. In comparison with nonpregnant women, pregnant women harbor higher levels of *Prevotella intermedia*, *Prevotella nigrescens*, and *Porphyromonas gingivalis*,[23] and colonization by the aforementioned species was shown to be enhanced throughout gestation.[24-26] Although the exact mechanisms underlying these shifts are unclear, hormone-enhanced inflammation and gingival bleeding appear to increase the bioavailability of nutrients, augment bacterial growth, and facilitate the proliferation of hemolytic bacteria, such as *P gingivalis*.[27]

Local immunologic modifications may also underlie the occurrence of pregnancy gingivitis. Sex steroids were shown to decrease the production of interleukin 6 (IL-6) by fibroblasts and to reduce the levels of plasminogen activator inhibitor 2 in the gingival crevicular fluid.[28-30] High levels of estrogen and progesterone inhibit polymorphonuclear leukocyte chemotaxis and phagocytosis and suppress antibody and T-cell responses because of the reduction of B lymphocytes and CD3 and CD4 cells,[31] suggesting that pregnant women may experience a state of compromised immunity that may also facilitate bacterial growth.

Biologic Plausibility

The hypothesis that a number of local or systemic pathologic conditions such as tonsillitis, pneumonia, endocarditis, and septicemia originated from oral foci of infection was first formulated by Miller in 1891,[32] but lack of scientific evidence condemned the theory of focal infection to dormancy. Almost 100 years later, the landmark experimental studies in the pregnant hamster by Collins et al[33] paved the way for an intense research effort focusing on the role of periodontal infection and inflammation in adverse pregnancy outcomes.

To better appreciate the pathogenic mechanisms that may underlie the association between periodontal infection and inflammation and adverse pregnancy outcomes, some basic knowledge of the physiology of normal and complicated pregnancies is essential. After conception, the fetus is nourished by the mother through the vessel-rich placenta and via the umbilical cord that connects the fetus with the placenta. Provided with the necessary nutrients, the fetus grows in the amniotic fluid, which is contained by the amniotic sac. The walls of this cavity consist of the amnion and the chorion, both of which are attached to the uterus through the decidua (the uterine lining or endometrium) and the myometrium (the middle layer of the uterine wall). As the fetus grows, satisfying the increasing needs for nutrients and coping successfully with the decreasing space are critical for the survival of both the mother and fetus.

As pregnancy progresses, amniotic fluid levels of prostaglandin E_2 (PGE$_2$) and inflammatory cytokines such as tumor necrosis factor α (TNF-α) and IL-1β rise steadily until a critical threshold level is reached, at which point they induce rupture of the amniotic sac membranes, uterine contraction, cervical dilation, and delivery.[34] Thus, normal parturition is controlled by inflammatory signaling. This process represents a triggering mechanism that can be modified by external stimuli, including infection and inflammatory stressors.

In the medical literature, high levels of inflammatory mediators (such as IL-1β, IL-6, TNF-α, and PGE$_2$)[35–38] in the amniotic fluid and the serum have been associated with various pregnancy complications. Moreover, C-reactive protein (CRP), which is an acute-phase reactant synthesized by the liver in response to proinflammatory cytokines and hence a marker of systemic inflammation, has also been associated with an increased risk for PTB, low birth weight, and preeclampsia.[39,40] In addition, genitourinary tract infections have been implicated in intrauterine infections. Microorganisms mainly gain access to various sites of the fetoplacental compartment by ascending from the vagina and the cervix or by hematogenous dissemination through the placenta. This microbial invasion is frequently associated with intra-amniotic inflammation and fetal inflammatory responses, which are both linked to adverse pregnancy outcomes.[41] Finally, several non–genital tract infections, such as pyelonephritis, asymptomatic bacteriuria, pneumonia, and appendicitis, have also been associated with, and probably predispose to, PTB.[42]

Periodontal diseases are also infectious, and although they occur at a distance from the fetoplacental unit, inflammatory mediators produced at the gingiva, periodontal pathogens, and bacterial products may enter the blood circulation and disseminate throughout the body. This low-grade bacteremia may trigger the induction of systemic inflammatory responses and/or the establishment of ectopic infections.[43–45]

A mechanistic model potentially explaining the biologic association between periodontal infection and inflammation and adverse pregnancy outcomes[44,45] is illustrated in Fig 10-3. The model consists of two alternative pathways, one direct and one indirect. In a direct pathway, periodontal bacteria and/or their products disseminate to the fetoplacental unit, where they establish an ectopic infection and/or trigger a local inflammatory response that results in the elevation of inflammatory cytokines and mediators that contribute to pregnancy complications.

In an indirect pathway, inflammatory cytokines and mediators produced in the periodontal tissues in response to periodontal pathogens enter the blood circulation and reach (1) the fetoplacental unit and contribute to an enhanced concentration of these mediators in this compartment and (2) the liver, where they stimulate a systemic inflammatory response through the production of acute-phase reactants. In turn, these mediators enter the blood circulation and reach the fetoplacental unit, where they exacerbate intrauterine inflammation.

Interestingly, current evidence indicates that the majority of intrauterine infections originate in the lower genital tract, with the infectious

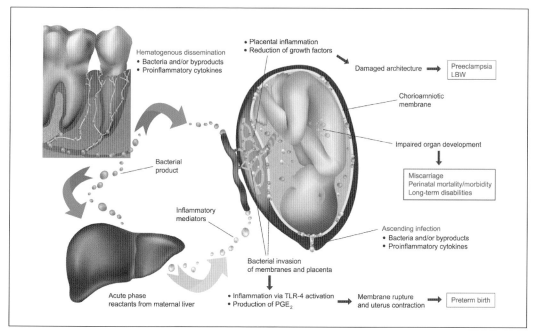

Fig 10-3 Biologic pathways associating periodontal infection and inflammation with adverse pregnancy outcomes. TLR-4, toll-like receptor 4; LBW, low birth weight. (Reprinted from Madianos et al[44,45] with permission.)

agents ascending into the otherwise sterile womb.[46] Hence, it is also possible that periodontal pathogens may reach the amniotic space as a result of ascending infection following oral-genital transfer. However, this third pathway is probably the least likely, because, from an ecologic point of view, it is difficult for oral bacteria to establish colonization in the vagina as a result of oral-genital contact due to colonization resistance.

Both the direct and indirect pathways have been extensively studied in humans and animal models. The two more common animal models used include the bacteremia infection model, in which periodontal pathogens are injected in the circulation to mimic bacteremia from periodontal pathogens in humans, and the chamber model, in which periodontal pathogens are injected in a subcutaneously implanted chamber to mimic a distant site of infection and inflammation such as periodontal infection. Although these experimental models are meant to simulate a periodontal infection in a simplified and reproducible manner, they have several key

limitations: The amount of bacteria injected in the circulation may not correspond to a transient bacteremia induced by periodontal infection, and the injection of a single bacterial species in the circulation or the chamber resembles a monoinfection rather than a mixed, biofilm-mediated infection such as periodontitis. The discussion that follows summarizes key research findings that support the biologic plausibility of each of the two pathways.

Direct pathway

Probably the strongest evidence in favor of a hematogenous dissemination of periodontal pathogens to the amniotic cavity derives from two case reports of women with adverse pregnancy outcomes: In the first, the same clonal type of uncultivable oral *Bergeyella* was identified in the subgingival plaque as well as the amniotic fluid of a woman with PTB, while no *Bergeyella* was detected in the mother's vaginal tract.[47] In the second case, an oral strain of

Fusobacterium nucleatum was identified as the cause of a term stillbirth and was isolated from the lung and stomach of the infant. Interestingly, the same clonal type of *F nucleatum* was present in the subgingival plaque of the mother but not in her vaginal or rectal microflora.[48]

Immunologic studies in humans are also supportive of the direct pathway: In these studies, serum from the umbilical cord was collected, and levels of immunoglobulin (Ig) M and IgG were evaluated against specific periodontal pathogens. The idea behind these experiments is that fetal exposure to periodontal pathogens and/or their byproducts would result in specific antibody responses against these bacteria. Presence of IgM antibodies in the umbilical cord blood would suggest direct exposure of the fetus in utero, because the fetus is not immunocompetent, and the size of the IgM molecule prevents its passage through the placental barrier and thus precludes the possibility that the antibodies would be of maternal origin. In contrast, IgG antibodies against the periodontal pathogens would have maternal origin, indicating a chronic exposure of the mother to these bacteria and/or their byproducts.

Studies evaluating IgM antibodies against specific periodontal bacteria have revealed a higher prevalence of umbilical cord IgM seropositivity for one or more organisms of the "red complex" (*P gingivalis*, *Tannerella forsythia*, and *Treponema denticola*) or the "orange complex" (*Campylobacter rectus*, *F nucleatum*, *Peptostreptococcus micros*, *P intermedia*, and *P nigrescens*) in women who experienced preterm or vaginal bleeding.[49,50] The concomitant presence of these bacteria in the dental plaque of pregnant women with pregnancy complications implies a hematogenous dissemination of these pathogens to the amniotic cavity and fetal exposure.

However, findings from maternal serum IgG antibody levels are not always consistent: For example, data from the large Obstetrics and Periodontal Therapy trial indicated that mothers who delivered preterm had significantly lower serum IgG levels against *P gingivalis* or other red complex bacteria than did mothers who delivered at term.[51] In another study, the highest rate of PTB occurred in mothers with low or no IgG responses to red complex species and high IgG responses to orange complex species.[49] Other studies have found elevated serum IgG antibodies against *F nucleatum* in women who suffered a fetal loss, while higher IgG levels against *P gingivalis* were associated with more low–birth weight infants.[52] These seemingly contradictory findings from seroepidemiologic studies may indicate that low levels of maternal serum IgG antibodies to periodontal bacteria signify an inadequate protection against the disseminating oral pathogens, thus allowing them to translocate to the fetoplacental unit and contribute to pregnancy complications. Alternatively, elevated maternal serum IgG could indicate either an increase in systemic exposure by oral pathogens or a hyperinflammatory phenotype, which may predispose these women to an increased fetal inflammatory response and injury.

Additional evidence indicating that periodontal pathogens may translocate to the fetoplacental unit derives from studies that detected bacterial DNA in this compartment. Indeed, DNA from several periodontal pathogens, such as *P gingivalis, Aggregatibacter actinomycetemcomitans*, *F nucleatum,* and *Bergeyella* species has been identified in the amniotic fluid, placenta, and even neonatal gastric aspirates obtained from complicated pregnancies.[47,53] Similar results have also been obtained in experiments with animal models. Specifically, using the chamber model in mice, researchers found DNA from *P gingivalis* and *C rectus* in the maternal liver and uterus of infected pregnant animals and in the placenta of fetuses showing intrauterine growth restriction.[54,55] However, intravenous infection of mice with *F nucleatum* was restricted inside the uterus without spreading systemically.[56]

Nevertheless, to fully appreciate the significance of these findings, it must be remembered that periodontal pathogens have been detected in human amniotic fluid and fetoplacental tissues in normal pregnancies as well.[57] Hence, it is still unclear which factors determine whether fetal exposure to periodontal bacteria will contribute to pregnancy complications. It is likely that varying levels of host susceptibility to periodontal pathogens may render some pregnant women more vulnerable to adverse pregnancy outcomes than others.

Another possibility is that variation in virulence properties within a single species may enable some, but not all, strains to colonize the amniotic cavity and induce pregnancy complications. This notion is further supported by mechanistic studies. Indeed, in mice, *F nucleatum* was shown to reach the placental blood vessels after hematogenous dissemination and to invade the endothelial cell lining the vessels, cross the endothelium, proliferate in the surrounding tissues, and finally spread to the amniotic fluid.[56] Intravenous injection of *P gingivalis* into pregnant rats resulted in strain-dependent colonization in the placenta.[58] In vitro studies showed that specific *C rectus* strains were able to invade human trophoblast cells.[59] Thus, it appears that the ability of bacteria to invade the fetoplacental unit may be an important property in the context of induction of adverse pregnancy outcomes.

Infection of the placenta with periodontal pathogens may result in the induction of local inflammatory responses, such as elevated levels of IL-2 and interferon γ and a decrease in IL-10.[54] These responses are probably mediated by the release of major components of the bacterial cell wall, such as lipopolysaccharide or outer membrane vesicles, and are dependent on both the potency of these virulence factors and the inflammatory profile of the host. In pregnancy, the innate proinflammatory immune response is strictly regulated within the uterus to prevent immunologic rejection of the fetal allograft. However, the local increase in proinflammatory mediators may disrupt this delicate balance and elicit an inflammatory burden that may contribute to preterm rupture of the membranes and uterine contraction, which in turn may lead to miscarriage or PTB.[60] Histologically, this inflammatory response is accompanied by an increase in the inflammatory infiltrate, predominantly by neutrophils, and in decidual necrosis.[61]

Moreover, *C rectus* infection in mice induces major alterations in the structure of the placenta as indicated by the decrease in the size of the labyrinth.[61] This may be partly due to the attenuation in the expression of genes related to placental and fetal growth, such as placental growth factor (*Pgf*) and insulinlike growth factor 2 (*Igf2*).[62] Because the labyrinth is the area of the placenta where the exchange of nutrients and waste between the mother and the fetus takes place, its diminished volume may result in insufficient nutrition for the fetus, resulting in restricted fetal growth and low birth weight. Furthermore, structural damage in the placenta may disrupt the normal blood flow between the fetus and the mother, affecting maternal blood pressure, and may thus lead to preeclampsia.

Finally, *C rectus* infection in mice results in an increased rate of neonatal mortality. In the surviving pups, *C rectus* can be detected in the brain and may induce a local inflammatory response, which is accompanied by increased apoptosis and defects in nerve myelination.[61] Comparable effects have also been reported in humans; neonates exposed to both *C rectus* and *P gingivalis* infection are twice as likely to be admitted to the neonatal intensive care unit.[63] It has also been established that preterm infants demonstrate an increased risk for developing neurodevelopmental, behavioral, and learning problems. Thus, fetal exposure to periodontal pathogens may induce tissue damage to fetal organs, and, depending on the extent of this damage, the fetus may die, or the neonate may demonstrate an increased risk for perinatal mortality or morbidity. Importantly, detrimental exposures during fetal development may manifest themselves later in life.

Indirect pathway

Patients with periodontal infection and/or inflammation show an increased production of proinflammatory cytokines and mediators from periodontal tissues. Once released, these cytokines may diffuse in the gingival crevicular fluid or enter the blood circulation and reach the fetoplacental unit. Inflammatory cytokines (such as IL-1β, IL-6, and TNF-α) could then stimulate the production of prostaglandins in the chorion and hence exacerbate cervical ripening and uterine contraction, leading to an increased risk for PTB. However, there is limited evidence available to date to suggest an association between these cytokines in the gingival crevicular fluid, serum, or amniotic fluid and pregnancy complications in women with periodontitis.[64]

Another possibility is that proinflammatory cytokines released in the maternal circulation, along with disseminated bacteria or bacterial products from the periodontal tissues, may induce a low-grade systemic inflammation by stimulating hepatic production of acute-phase reactants, such as CRP and fibrinogen. Elevated plasma CRP could then augment the inflammatory responses at the fetoplacental interface through complement activation, tissue damage, and induction of proinflammatory cytokines. Although elevated levels of CRP have been associated with PTB, intrauterine growth retardation, preeclampsia, and gestational diabetes mellitus, there are only a few studies evaluating the association between pregnancy complications and CRP levels in pregnant women with periodontitis, and the findings are inconsistent.[65]

Thus, there is much more evidence to support the direct pathway than the indirect pathway.

Epidemiologic Studies of Maternal Periodontitis and Adverse Pregnancy Outcomes

Observational studies

Since the first case-control study of pregnant or postpartum women that showed that women giving birth to preterm, low–birth weight babies had significantly greater mean levels of clinical attachment loss than did mothers with full-term, normal–birth weight babies was published in the mid-1990s,[66] a large number of publications have reported on the association between maternal periodontal status and pregnancy outcomes. As expected, a number of studies corroborated and extended these early observations, while others failed to detect an association. At least 10 systematic reviews

have been carried out so far on this topic, the most recent published by Ide and Papapanou in 2013.[67,68] These authors screened approximately 700 articles using predefined criteria to evaluate the existing evidence associating maternal periodontitis, defined broadly and encompassing a variety of conditions ranging from gingivitis to aggressive periodontitis, and three primary pregnancy complications: PTB, low birth weight, and preeclampsia.

In their review, Ide and Papapanou[67,68] discussed in detail a number of features related to the methodology used and the overall quality of the studies, all of which could conceivably have an impact on the strength of the association between the putative exposure under investigation (ie, poor maternal periodontal status) and the outcome (adverse pregnancy outcomes). These study features included the type of periodontal examination performed (whether it was based on a complete-mouth or partial-mouth examination); the consistency in the timing of the examination with respect to gestational age (antepartum or postpartum); whether the study examiners were blinded with respect to the occurrence of the particular adverse pregnancy outcome, thus excluding the possibility of examination bias; and whether additional exposures with known or suspected roles in pregnancy outcome were also considered in the data analyses along with maternal periodontitis. In this context, accounting for the role of confounding factors (ie, additional exposures associated with both periodontitis and adverse gestational outcomes) was deemed to be critically important.

Another issue highlighted in the review[67,68] was the use of continuous versus categorical definitions of periodontitis: While some studies defined maternal periodontal status using continuous variables (eg, mean probing depth and clinical attachment loss, or percentage of sites with bleeding on probing), other studies used categorical (dichotomous) definitions to classify the women as having periodontitis or being periodontally healthy. Given the absence of universally accepted definitions of periodontitis in general and in women of childbearing age in particular, the threshold values used across studies to define a case of periodontitis varied substantially.

Finally, because of the generally low prevalence of adverse pregnancy outcomes in the population, the majority of the studies used a case-control design rather than the preferred longitudinal prospective cohort design. The latter is much better suited for the assessment of interactions among different exposures but requires recruitment of considerably larger numbers of participants and is therefore more demanding logistically.

The review[67,68] reiterated that there is a high degree of variability among the study populations involved in the available studies as well as in the methodologies used for recruitment and periodontitis assessment. More than 50 continuous parameters and 14 different definitions of cases (not specific to pregnancy) were applied in studies exploring relationships between periodontal disease and preterm delivery and/or low–birth weight infants.[69] Therefore, it is difficult to compare the findings of these reports with regard to the prevalence of periodontal disease among pregnant women. To illustrate the importance of choice of case definitions, Manau et al[69] calculated the prevalence of periodontal disease to be between 3.2% and 70.8% when 14 different case definitions were applied to the same data from 1,296 pregnant women.

Importantly, Ide and Papapanou[67,68] found that potentially detrimental exposures that may be shared between periodontitis and adverse pregnancy outcomes did not appear to have been adequately accounted for in all studies. Another observation that emerged was that studies that used categorical definitions of periodontitis were more likely to detect statistically significant associations between maternal periodontitis and adverse pregnancy outcomes than studies that used continuous measures of periodontitis. Likewise, studies using a case-control design were more likely to detect associations than the more robust prospective cohort studies. Nevertheless, and despite the aforementioned shortcomings in the existing evidence, the systematic review concluded that there is a positive association between poor maternal periodontal status and all three adverse pregnancy outcomes examined (PTB,

low birth weight, and preeclampsia).[67,68] With respect to the magnitude of the adverse effect, the review identified it as modest but as independent of other exposures. In other words, the identified association between periodontitis and adverse pregnancy outcomes cannot solely be ascribed to common risk factors that are also more prevalent in women with periodontitis, such as poor socioeconomic status, young maternal age, certain race or ethnicity characteristics, and tobacco smoking. Thus, the epidemiologic evidence from the association studies available so far is largely consistent with the biologically plausible role of periodontitis as a systemic stressor that was described in the first part of this chapter.

Intervention studies

Given the positive association between periodontitis and adverse pregnancy outcomes, an obvious question arises that is of major interest for both patients and clinicians: Can treatment of maternal periodontitis result in an improvement of gestational outcomes? The public health implications of such a possibility are obviously profound, because approximately half of the variance in the prevalence of PTB and low birth weight is unexplained by the currently established risk factors. Therefore, even if a relatively small proportion of the cases could be ascribed to maternal periodontitis, but this risk turned out to be modifiable by means of periodontal therapy, the benefits would be substantial.

This question is arguably one of the most thoroughly investigated in the field of dental medicine: At least 13 randomized controlled trials (RCTs) reported thus far have collectively enrolled in excess of 7,000 pregnant women with periodontitis or gingivitis. Approximately half of these women were randomized to receive scaling and root planing, occasionally accompanied by adjunctive antimicrobial pharmacotherapies, prior to the completion of the second trimester, while the other half received similar periodontal treatment after delivery. Table 10-1 summarizes the key features and study outcomes of RCTs with a sample size of at least 100 women.

Table 10-1	RCTs with a total sample size of at least 100 that examine the effect of periodontal treatment during gestation on PTB				

Study	Publication year	N randomized	Treatment (Tx) arm intervention	Study quality*	Improved pregnancy outcome in Tx arm
López et al[70]; Chile	2002	400	SRP and 0.12% chlorhexidine mouthwash[†]	Low	Yes
Jeffcoat et al[71]; USA	2003	366	SRP and adjunctive systemic metronidazole in approximately half of the treatment arm	High	No
López et al[72]; Chile	2005	870[‡]	SRP and 0.12% chlorhexidine mouthwash	Low	Yes
Michalowicz et al[73]; USA	2006	823	SRP	High	No
Offenbacher et al[74]; USA	2006	109	SRP	Low	Yes
Tarannum and Faizuddin[75]; India	2007	200	SRP and 0.2% chlorhexidine mouthwash	Low	Yes
Newnham et al[76]; Australia	2009	1,082	SRP and 0.12% chlorhexidine mouthwash	High	No
Offenbacher et al[77]; USA	2009	1,806	SRP	High	No
Macones et al[78]; USA	2010	759	SRP	High	No
Oliveira et al[79]; Brazil	2011	246	SRP	Low	No
Weidlich et al[80]; Brazil	2013	303	SRP	High	No

*As assessed by Michalowicz et al.[81]
[†]18% of the women in the test group also received adjunctive systemic antibiotics (amoxicillin and metronidazole).
[‡]Includes exclusively women with gingivitis.
SRP, scaling and root planing.

The data from these studies have been included in meta-analyses in recent systematic reviews[82,83] that concluded that nonsurgical treatment of periodontitis during the second trimester does not result in a decreased rate of preterm delivery or have a positive impact on birth weight. Although individual trials that reported improved gestational outcomes in pregnant women allocated to the active intervention arm do exist, the findings of the higher-quality studies and the outcomes of the aggregate analyses are unequivocal and do not support this notion. A thoughtful discussion of the potential reasons underlying these diverse findings was recently published by Michalowicz et al.[81] Given that the larger, high-quality RCTs were consistent in documenting that nonsurgical periodontal therapy provided during the second trimester has no positive effect on gestational outcomes, these authors questioned whether there is a need for additional studies of similar design.

A frequent criticism of the available RCTs is that the periodontal treatment rendered failed to result in adequate improvement of maternal periodontal status to the extent needed to impact pregnancy outcomes. Although this is indeed a possibility, given that periodontal inflammation was not eliminated in most studies, the subgroups of individuals in whom a pronounced resolution of periodontal inflammation was achieved did not appear to experience the best pregnancy outcomes. On the other hand, the induction of bacteremia[84] and the increase in systemic inflammation[85] shown to occur in conjunction with instrumentation of the periodontal tissues may have posed a significant challenge to the fetoplacental unit and negated the positive effects of the subsequent improvement in gingival inflammation.

It has therefore been argued that the ideal timing of delivery of the periodontal intervention is prior to conception. Obviously, the logistics involved in the conduct of such a trial are complicated, and the concept cannot be tested easily. However, it is noteworthy that a recent nonrandomized trial[86] that tested the effect of an antiseptic oral mouthrinse as the sole periodontal therapy indicated that interventions that are not likely to induce bacteremia and a rise in systemic inflammation may improve pregnancy outcomes.

Dental and Periodontal Therapy During Pregnancy

Dentists have a general reluctance to treat pregnant women, for reasons ranging from the relative paucity of objective data to support safety claims regarding specific dental procedures or use of adjunctive therapeutic agents to a genuine concern that they may cause harm to the pregnant woman or the fetus. In some countries, these attitudes are likely further promoted by a fear of litigation. Conversely, it is also known through surveys in a variety of populations that a relative minority of pregnant women (between 25% and 50%) receive any dental care, including prophylaxis, even when insured. All types of dental services decrease during pregnancy and increase after pregnancy, compared with prepregnancy usage.[87] Utilization of dental services is still lower by pregnant women of low socioeconomic status[88] or women of certain cultural backgrounds in whom the fear of harm to the fetus as a result of dental care is deeply rooted.[89]

The first study that addressed issues of safety of dental treatment in pregnant women as part of an RCT was the Obstetrics and Periodontal Therapy study,[90] which randomly assigned 823 women with periodontitis to receive scaling and root planing, either at 13 to 21 weeks' gestation or up to 3 months after delivery. All women were evaluated for essential dental treatment needs, defined as the presence of moderate to severe caries and fractured or abscessed teeth, and 351 women received essential dental care prior to the completion of the second trimester. The study demonstrated that the rates of serious adverse events, defined as spontaneous abortions or stillbirths, fetal or congenital anomalies, and PTBs, were not statistically different between groups of women that received essential dental care alone, essential dental care combined with nonsurgical periodontal therapy, or no dental treatment during pregnancy. Thus, this study provided high-quality evidence demonstrating that dental and periodontal treatment that also involved use of local anesthetics is safe during the second trimester. These findings have been further corroborated by the additional large RCTs mentioned earlier (see Table 10-1), none of which reported a statistically higher incidence of adverse pregnancy outcomes among women who received periodontal therapy during gestation than among those who received periodontal treatment after delivery.

Based on a thorough review of all existing scientific evidence, a national consensus statement developed by the national Oral Health Care During Pregnancy Expert Workgroup[91] concluded that "Oral health care, including use of radiographs, pain medication, and local anesthesia, is safe throughout pregnancy." The statement calls for interprofessional collaboration between health care providers throughout the pregnancy and on delivery to ensure the best possible health of the mother and child. All health care providers, including physicians and their assistants, nurses, midwives, nurse practitioners, dentists, and dental hygienists, are encouraged to educate themselves regarding oral health and dental care in pregnancy, to provide pertinent oral health education, and to collaborate to ensure that both pregnant women and new mothers attain and maintain oral health that is as good as possible.

The national consensus statement also contains step-by-step guidance targeting prenatal care health professionals, oral health care professionals, pregnant women, and new mothers. Moreover, it provides a user-friendly table-form overview of pharmaceutical agents with their indications, contraindications, and special considerations. It also includes a reference to informative brochures in English and Spanish.[92,93]

The statement also introduces the *dental home concept*, developed by the American Association of Public Health Dentistry[94] and supported by the American Association of Pediatric Dentists. The dental home model delineates an ongoing relationship between the dentist and the patient, inclusive of all aspects of oral health care, delivered in a comprehensive, continuously accessible, coordinated, and family-centered way. Pregnant women should be encouraged to obtain periodontal and restorative treatment to attain and maintain good periodontal health throughout their pregnancy and beyond.

For the newborn child, parental awareness of oral health concepts should translate into oral health–promoting practices (toothcleaning and healthy dietary habits) already at the time of eruption of the first primary tooth. According to the American Academy of Pediatric Dentistry (AAPD), every infant should receive an oral health risk assessment from his or her primary health care provider or qualified health care professional by 6 months of age.[95] During this initial assessment, the practitioner should evaluate the infant's risk of developing oral diseases of soft and hard tissues, including caries risk assessment, provide education on infant oral health, and evaluate and optimize fluoride exposure. Furthermore, the AAPD recommends

that parents or caregivers establish a dental home for infants by 12 months of age.[96]

On a different note, because teenage mothers are those at the highest risk for preterm delivery, the AAPD has developed guidelines on oral health care for pregnant adolescents.[97] The advice is aimed at not only the future mother but also the dental professionals who must be familiar with state statutes that govern consent for care for a pregnant woman who is not an adult. If a pregnant adolescent's parents are unaware of the pregnancy and state laws require parental consent for dental treatment, the practitioner should encourage the adolescent to inform her parents so that the appropriate informed consent for dental treatment can occur. The AAPD recommends incorporating positive youth development that goes beyond traditional care and suggests that a strong interpersonal relationship be cultivated between the adolescent and her dental care providers. Through positive youth development, the dentist can promote healthy lifestyles, teach positive patterns of social interaction, and provide a safety net in times of need.

Conclusion

The association between poor maternal periodontal status and adverse pregnancy outcomes is biologically plausible, and multiple lines of evidence support a number of mechanistic links through which maternal periodontal infection and inflammation may contribute to an increased incidence of PTB, low birth weight, and preeclampsia. Meta-analyses of the available epidemiologic association studies also support the notion that maternal periodontal infections have a negative impact on pregnancy outcomes, independent of known confounders. However, the strength of this association is rather modest and may vary in different populations.

The effect of maternal periodontal treatment during pregnancy on the incidence of adverse pregnancy outcomes has been investigated in several high-quality RCTs, all of which have administered nonsurgical periodontal therapy prior to the completion of the second trimester. The preponderance of evidence from these trials indicates that periodontal therapy does not improve pregnancy outcomes. Thus, at first glance, the findings from the mechanistic and the epidemiologic association studies on the one hand and those from the intervention studies on the other appear to be conflicting. However, a strict and appropriate interpretation of the RCTs is that the particular intervention tested (ie, nonsurgical periodontal therapy administered after the first trimester and prior to the completion of the second) does *not* result in improved pregnancy outcomes.

This conclusion is clearly not synonymous with a conclusion suggesting that maternal periodontal infections are *unrelated* to adverse pregnancy outcomes. What the RCTs merely suggest is that any increased risk for adverse pregnancy outcomes documented in the mechanistic and the epidemiologic association studies cannot be reversed by the particular interventions performed.

Importantly, the possible effects of different interventions with respect to either timing or intensity have not been examined. Therefore, it is unknown whether alternative therapeutic approaches may or may not yield improved outcomes. However, the primary reason RCTs are conducted is to identify the best therapies, to update standards of care, and to inform stakeholders responsible for public health policy. RCTs are not designed to accept or refute a hypothesized causal relationship between an exposure and an outcome. Instead, they focus on whether any risk conferred by the exposure can be modified by means of the tested intervention. In the case of maternal periodontal infections and adverse pregnancy outcomes, it may be argued that the central question from a public health point of view—that is, whether treatment of pregnant women with periodontitis will result in improved pregnancy outcomes—has been addressed already by several high-quality trials, and the answer is no.

It is probably not very meaningful to focus on the fact that periodontal treatment in the existing RCTs improved, but clearly did not eliminate, periodontal inflammation in the treated women and thus to advocate that more intensive interventions would have resulted in improved outcomes. Indeed, the pragmatic therapeutic approach adopted by the available RCTs (ie, complete-mouth scaling and root planing followed by regular periodontal maintenance until delivery) is probably what the majority of pregnant women can tolerate and accommodate within the busy prenatal period. The improvement in periodontal status that is typically achieved by this type of intervention in pregnant women falls short of eliminating (or even substantially suppressing) gingival inflammation. Therefore, it is probably not productive to speculate about what more intensive interventions would have achieved or to focus on pregnancy outcomes occurring in the subset of women who were the most compliant with the research protocol or those whose periodontal health improved most. It is the mainstream response that occurs in the majority of women that is interesting from a public health point of view, not what occurs in small subgroups that may be atypical and may not represent the source population. Although valuable conclusions can still be drawn from a biologic point of view, based on the pregnancy outcomes achieved in the most compliant women or in those whose periodontal inflammation was most effectively suppressed, recommendations regarding prenatal care policy cannot be based on subgroup findings but must adhere to the intent-to-treat principle that is the cornerstone of RCTs.

The possibility that the optimal time point to provide periodontal interventions in women with periodontitis is prior to conception is certainly compatible with current understanding of the effects of maternal periodontal infection and inflammation on the fetoplacental unit. Indeed, periodontal therapy results in a substantial, short-term increase in systemic inflammation. Findings from an RCT of the effects of periodontal treatment on vascular endothelial function demonstrated that periodontal therapy results in immediate, significant impairment of endothelial function that is restored to pretreatment levels within approximately 1 month after intervention, while the beneficial effects of therapy are manifested 6 months after intervention.[98] This timeline may be too extended to translate into any tangible improvements in the context of pregnancy outcomes. Therefore, restoration of maternal periodontal health prior to conception makes biologic sense. However, a formal assessment of the potential effects of periodontal treatment administered prior to conception in a randomized controlled trial is logistically difficult, and such a study may not be available in the near future.

In the meantime, while it is not justified to recommend that pregnant women be treated periodontally for the sole purpose of improving pregnancy outcomes, maternal periodontal therapy is safe for both the mother and the unborn child. It improves oral health and is an indispensable part of a holistic approach geared toward the advancement of general health, risk factor control, and enhancement of health-promoting behaviors.

References

1. Lozano R, Naghavi M, Foreman K, et al. Global and regional mortality from 235 causes of death for 20 age groups in 1990 and 2010: A systematic analysis for the Global Burden of Disease Study 2010. Lancet 2012;380:2095–2128.
2. March of Dimes, PMNCH, Save the Children, WHO. Born too soon: The global action report on preterm birth. 2012. http://whqlibdoc.who.int/publications/2012/9789241503433_eng.pdf. Accessed 23 June 2013.
3. Liu L, Johnson HL, Cousens S, et al. Global, regional, and national causes of child mortality: An updated systematic analysis for 2010 with time trends since 2000. Lancet 2012;379:2151–2161.
4. Saigal S, Doyle LW. An overview of mortality and sequelae of preterm birth from infancy to adulthood. Lancet 2008;371:261–269.
5. Chang HH, Larson J, Blencowe H, et al. Preventing preterm births: Analysis of trends and potential reductions with interventions in 39 countries with very high human development index. Lancet 2013;381:223–234.
6. Blencowe H, Cousens S, Oestergaard MZ, et al. National, regional, and worldwide estimates of preterm birth rates in the year 2010 with time trends since 1990 for selected countries: A systematic analysis and implications. Lancet 2012;379:2162–2172.
7. Hamilton BE, Martin JA, Ventura SJ. Births: Preliminary data for 2011. Natl Vital Stat Rep 2012;61:1–20. http://www.cdc.gov/nchs/data/nvsr/nvsr61/nvsr61_05.pdf. Accessed 23 June 2013.
8. Villar J, Papageorghiou AT, Knight HE, et al. The preterm birth syndrome: A prototype phenotypic classification. Am J Obstet Gynecol 2012;206:119–123.
9. Goldenberg RL, Culhane JF, Iams JD, Romero R. Epidemiology and causes of preterm birth. Lancet 2008;371:75–84.
10. Abraham-Inpijn L, Polsacheva OV, Raber-Durlacher JE. The significance of endocrine factors and microorganisms in the development of gingivitis in pregnant women [in Russian]. Stomatologiia (Mosk) 1996;75:15–18.
11. Miyagi M, Morishita M, Iwamoto Y. Effects of sex hormones on production of prostaglandin E2 by human peripheral monocytes. J Periodontol 1993;64:1075–1078.
12. Soory M. Targets for steroid hormone mediated actions of periodontal pathogens, cytokines and therapeutic agents: Some implications on tissue turnover in the periodontium. Curr Drug Targets 2000;1:309–325.
13. Mealey BL, Moritz AJ. Hormonal influences: Effects of diabetes mellitus and endogenous female sex steroid hormones on the periodontium. Periodontol 2000 2003;32:59–81.
14. Kimura S, Elce JS, Jellinck PH. Immunological relationship between peroxidases in eosinophils, uterus and other tissues of the rat. Biochemic J 1983;213:165–169.
15. Ito I, Hayashi T, Yamada K, Kuzuya M, Naito M, Iguchi A. Physiological concentration of estradiol inhibits polymorphonuclear leukocyte chemotaxis via a receptor mediated system. Life Sci 1995;56:2247–2253.
16. Gallagher JC, Kable WT, Goldgar D. Effect of progestin therapy on cortical and trabecular bone: Comparison with estrogen. Am J Med 1991;90:171–178.
17. Soory M. Hormonal factors in periodontal disease. Dent Update 2000;27:380–383.
18. Machuca G, Khoshfeiz O, Lacalle JR, Machuca C, Bullón P. The influence of general health and sociocultural variables on the periodontal condition of pregnant women. J Periodontol 1999;70:779–785.
19. Gürsoy M, Gürsoy UK, Sorsa T, Pajukanta R, Könönen E. High salivary estrogen and risk of developing pregnancy gingivitis. J Periodontol 2013;84:1281–1289.
20. Tilakaratne A, Soory M, Ranasinghe AW, Corea SM, Ekanayake SL, de Silva M. Periodontal disease status during pregnancy and 3 months post-partum, in a rural population of Sri-Lankan women. J Clin Periodontol 2000;27:787–792.
21. Bieri RA, Adriaens L, Spörri S, Lang NP, Persson GR. Gingival fluid cytokine expression and subgingival bacterial counts during pregnancy and postpartum: A case series. Clin Oral Investig 2013;17:19–28.

22. Wang PH, Chao HT, Lee WL, Yuan CC, Ng HT. Severe bleeding from a pregnancy tumor. A case report. J Reprod Med 1997;42:359–362.

23. Carrillo-de-Albornoz A, Figuero E, Herrera D, Cuesta P, Bascones-Martínez A. Gingival changes during pregnancy. 3. Impact of clinical, microbiological, immunological and socio-demographic factors on gingival inflammation. J Clin Periodontol 2012;39:272–283.

24. Jensen J, Liljemark W, Bloomquist C. The effect of female sex hormones on subgingival plaque. J Periodontol 1981;52:599–602.

25. Gürsoy M, Haraldsson G, Hyvönen M, Sorsa T, Pajukanta R, Könönen E. Does the frequency of Prevotella intermedia increase during pregnancy? Oral Microbiol Immunol 2009;24:299–303.

26. Carrillo-de-Albornoz A, Figuero E, Herrera D, Bascones-Martínez A. Gingival changes during pregnancy. 2. Influence of hormonal variations on the subgingival biofilm. J Clin Periodontol 2010;37:230–240.

27. Di Placido G, Tumini V, D'Archivio D, Di Peppe G. Gingival hyperplasia in pregnancy. 2. Etiopathogenic factors and mechanisms [in Italian]. Minerva Stomatol 1998;47:223–229.

28. Miyagi M, Aoyama H, Morishita M, Iwamoto Y. Effects of sex hormones on chemotaxis of human peripheral polymorphonuclear leukocytes and monocytes. J Periodontol 1992;63:28–32.

29. Ferris GM. Alteration in female sex hormones: Their effect on oral tissues and dental treatment. Compendium 1993;14:1558–1564, 1566.

30. Kinnby B, Matsson L, Astedt B. Aggravation of gingival inflammatory symptoms during pregnancy associated with the concentration of plasminogen activator inhibitor type 2 (PAI-2) in gingival fluid. J Periodontal Res 1996;31:271–277.

31. Raber-Durlacher JE, van Steenbergen TJ, Van der Velden U, de Graaff J, Abraham-Inpijn L. Experimental gingivitis during pregnancy and post-partum: Clinical, endocrinological, and microbiological aspects. J Clin Periodontol 1994;21:549–558.

32. Miller WD. The human mouth as a focus of infection. Dent Cosmos 1891;33:689–709.

33. Collins JG, Smith MA, Arnold RR, Offenbacher S. Effects of Escherichia coli and Porphyromonas gingivalis lipopolysaccharide on pregnancy outcome in the golden hamster. Infect Immun 1994;62:4652–4655.

34. Haram K, Mortensen JH, Wollen AL. Preterm delivery: An overview. Acta Obstet Gynecol Scand 2003;82:687–704.

35. Inglis SR. Biochemical markers predictive of preterm delivery. Infect Dis Obstet Gynecol 1997;5:158–164.

36. Gücer F, Balkanli-Kaplan P, Yüksel M, Yüce MA, Türe M, Yardim T. Maternal serum tumor necrosis factor-alpha in patients with preterm labor. J Reprod Med 2001;46:232–236.

37. Greig PC, Murtha AP, Jimmerson CJ, Herbert WN, Roitman-Johnson B, Allen JR. Maternal serum interleukin-6 during pregnancy and during term and preterm labor. Obstet Gynecol 1997;90:465–469.

38. von Minckwitz G, Grischke EM, Schwab S, et al. Predictive value of serum interleukin-6 and -8 levels in preterm labor or rupture of the membranes. Acta Obstet Gynecol Scand 2000;79:667–672.

39. Pitiphat W, Gillman MW, Joshipura KJ, Williams PL, Douglass CW, Rich-Edwards JW. Plasma C-reactive protein in early pregnancy and preterm delivery. Am J Epidemiol 2005;162:1108–1113.

40. Tjoa ML, van Vugt JM, Go AT, Blankenstein MA, Oudejans CB, van Wijk IJ. Elevated C-reactive protein levels during first trimester of pregnancy are indicative of preeclampsia and intrauterine growth restriction. J Reprod Immunol 2003;59:29–37.

41. Romero R, Mazor M. Infection and preterm labor. Clin Obstet Gynecol 1988;31:553–584.

42. Goldenberg RL, Culhane JF, Johnson DC. Maternal infection and adverse fetal and neonatal outcomes. Clin Perinatol 2005;32:523–559.

43. Han YW, Wang X. Mobile microbiome: Oral bacteria in extra-oral infections and inflammation. J Dent Res 2013;92:485–491.

44. Madianos PN, Bobetsis YA, Offenbacher S. Adverse pregnancy outcomes (APOs) and periodontal disease: Pathogenic mechanisms. J Clin Periodontol 2013;40(suppl 14):S170–S180.

45. Madianos PN, Bobetsis YA, Offenbacher S. Adverse pregnancy outcomes (APOs) and periodontal disease: Pathogenic mechanisms. J Periodontol 2013;84(4 suppl):S170–S180.

46. Han YW. Oral health and adverse pregnancy outcomes—What's next? J Dent Res 2011;90:289–293.

47. Han YW, Ikegami A, Bissada NF, Herbst M, Redline RW, Ashmead GG. Transmission of an uncultivated Bergeyella strain from the oral cavity to amniotic fluid in a case of preterm birth. J Clin Microbiol 2006;44:1475–1483.

48. Han YW, Fardini Y, Chen C, et al. Term stillbirth caused by oral Fusobacterium nucleatum. Obstet Gynecol 2010;115:442–445.

49. Madianos PN, Lieff S, Murtha AP, et al. Maternal periodontitis and prematurity. 2. Maternal infection and fetal exposure. Ann Periodontol 2001;6:175–182.

50. Boggess KA, Moss K, Murtha A, Offenbacher S, Beck JD. Antepartum vaginal bleeding, fetal exposure to oral pathogens, and risk for preterm birth at <35 weeks of gestation. Am J Obstet Gynecol 2006;194:954–960.

51. Ebersole JL, Novak MJ, Michalowicz BS, et al. Systemic immune responses in pregnancy and periodontitis: Relationship to pregnancy outcomes in the Obstetrics and Periodontal Therapy (OPT) study. J Periodontol 2009;80:953–960.

52. Dasanayake AP, Chhun N, Tanner AC, et al. Periodontal pathogens and gestational diabetes mellitus. J Dent Res 2008;87:328–333.

53. Ercan E, Eratalay K, Deren O, et al. Evaluation of periodontal pathogens in amniotic fluid and the role of periodontal disease in pre-term birth and low birth weight. Acta Odontol Scand 2013;71:553–559.

54. Lin D, Smith MA, Elter J, et al. *Porphyromonas gingivalis* infection in pregnant mice is associated with placental dissemination, an increase in the placental Th1/Th2 cytokine ratio, and fetal growth restriction. Infect Immun 2003;71:5163–5168.

55. Yeo A, Smith MA, Lin D, et al. *Campylobacter rectus* mediates growth restriction in pregnant mice. J Periodontol 2005;76:551–557.

56. Han YW, Redline RW, Li M, Yin L, Hill GB, McCormick TS. *Fusobacterium nucleatum* induces premature and term stillbirths in pregnant mice: Implication of oral bacteria in preterm birth. Infect Immun 2004;72:2272–2279.

57. Katz J, Chegini N, Shiverick KT, Lamont RJ. Localization of *P. gingivalis* in preterm delivery placenta. J Dent Res 2009;88:575–578.

58. Bélanger M, Reyes L, von Deneen K, Reinhard MK, Progulske-Fox A, Brown MB. Colonization of maternal and fetal tissues by *Porphyromonas gingivalis* is strain-dependent in a rodent animal model. Am J Obstet Gynecol 2008;199:86.e1–86.e7.

59. Arce RM, Diaz PI, Barros SP, et al. Characterization of the invasive and inflammatory traits of oral *Campylobacter rectus* in a murine model of fetoplacental growth restriction and in trophoblast cultures. J Reprod Immunol 2010;84:145–153.

60. Africa CW. Oral colonization of gram-negative anaerobes as a risk factor for preterm delivery. Virulence 2011;2:498–508.

61. Offenbacher S, Riché EL, Barros SP, Bobetsis YA, Lin D, Beck JD. Effects of maternal *Campylobacter rectus* infection on murine placenta, fetal and neonatal survival, and brain development. J Periodontol 2005;76(11 suppl):2133–2143.

62. Bobetsis YA, Barros SP, Lin DM, Arce RM, Offenbacher S. Altered gene expression in murine placentas in an infection-induced intrauterine growth restriction model: A microarray analysis. J Reprod Immunol 2010;85:140–148.

63. Jared H, Boggess KA, Moss K, et al. Fetal exposure to oral pathogens and subsequent risk for neonatal intensive care admission. J Periodontol 2009;80:878–883.

64. Stadelmann P, Alessandri R, Eick S, Salvi GE, Surbek D, Sculean A. The potential association between gingival crevicular fluid inflammatory mediators and adverse pregnancy outcomes: A systematic review. Clin Oral Investig 2013;17:1453–1463.

65. Pitiphat W, Joshipura KJ, Rich-Edwards JW, Williams PL, Douglass CW, Gillman MW. Periodontitis and plasma C-reactive protein during pregnancy. J Periodontol 2006;77:821–825.

66. Offenbacher S, Katz V, Fertik G, et al. Periodontal infection as a possible risk factor for preterm low birth weight. J Periodontol 1996;67(10 suppl):1103–1113.

67. Ide M, Papapanou PN. Epidemiology of association between maternal periodontal disease and adverse pregnancy outcomes—Systematic review. J Clin Periodontol 2013;40(suppl 14):S181–S194.

68. Ide M, Papapanou PN. Epidemiology of association between maternal periodontal disease and adverse pregnancy outcomes—Systematic review. J Periodontol 2013;84(suppl 4):S181–S194.

69. Manau C, Echeverria A, Agueda A, Guerrero A, Echeverria JJ. Periodontal disease definition may determine the association between periodontitis and pregnancy outcomes. J Clin Periodontol 2008;35:385–397.

70. López NJ, Smith PC, Gutierrez J. Periodontal therapy may reduce the risk of preterm low birth weight in women with periodontal disease: A randomized controlled trial. J Periodontol 2002;73:911–924.

71. Jeffcoat MK, Hauth JC, Geurs NC, et al. Periodontal disease and preterm birth: Results of a pilot intervention study. J Periodontol 2003;74:1214–1218.

72. López NJ, Da Silva I, Ipinza J, Gutiérrez J. Periodontal therapy reduces the rate of preterm low birth weight in women with pregnancy-associated gingivitis. J Periodontol 2005;76(11 suppl):2144–2153.

73. Michalowicz BS, Hodges JS, DiAngelis AJ, et al. Treatment of periodontal disease and the risk of preterm birth. N Engl J Med 2006;355:1885–1894.

74. Offenbacher S, Lin D, Strauss R, et al. Effects of periodontal therapy during pregnancy on periodontal status, biologic parameters, and pregnancy outcomes: A pilot study. J Periodontol 2006;77:2011–2024.

75. Tarannum F, Faizuddin M. Effect of periodontal therapy on pregnancy outcome in women affected by periodontitis. J Periodontol 2007;78:2095–2103.

76. Newnham JP, Newnham IA, Ball CM, et al. Treatment of periodontal disease during pregnancy: A randomized controlled trial. Obstet Gynecol 2009;114:1239–1248.

77. Offenbacher S, Beck JD, Jared HL, et al. Effects of periodontal therapy on rate of preterm delivery: A randomized controlled trial. Obstet Gynecol 2009;114:551–559.

78. Macones GA, Parry S, Nelson DB, et al. Treatment of localized periodontal disease in pregnancy does not reduce the occurrence of preterm birth: Results from the Periodontal Infections and Prematurity Study (PIPS). Am J Obstet Gynecol 2010;202:147.e1–147.e8.

79. Oliveira AM, de Oliveira PA, Cota LO, Magalhães CS, Moreira AN, Costa FO. Periodontal therapy and risk for adverse pregnancy outcomes. Clin Oral Investig 2011;15:609–615.

80. Weidlich P, Moreira CH, Fiorini T, et al. Effect of non-surgical periodontal therapy and strict plaque control on preterm/low birth weight: A randomized controlled clinical trial. Clin Oral Investig 2013;17:37–44.

81. Michalowicz BS, Gustafsson A, Thumbigere-Math V, Buhlin K. The effects of periodontal treatment on pregnancy outcomes. J Clin Periodontol 2013;40 (suppl 14):S195–S208.

82. Polyzos NP, Polyzos IP, Zavos A, et al. Obstetric outcomes after treatment of periodontal disease during pregnancy: Systematic review and meta-analysis. BMJ 2010;341:c7017.

83. Boutin A, Demers S, Roberge S, Roy-Morency A, Chandad F, Bujold E. Treatment of periodontal disease and prevention of preterm birth: Systematic review and meta-analysis. Am J Perinatol 2013;30: 537–544.

84. Zhang W, Daly CG, Mitchell D, Curtis B. Incidence and magnitude of bacteraemia caused by flossing and by scaling and root planing. J Clin Periodontol 2013;40:41–52.

85. D'Aiuto F, Parkar M, Tonetti MS. Acute effects of periodontal therapy on bio-markers of vascular health. J Clin Periodontol 2007;34:124–129.

86. Jeffcoat M, Parry S, Gerlach RW, Doyle MJ. Use of alcohol-free antimicrobial mouth rinse is associated with decreased incidence of preterm birth in a high-risk population. Am J Obstet Gynecol 2011;205:382. e1–382.e6.

87. Jiang P, Bargman EP, Garrett NA, Devries A, Springman S, Riggs S. A comparison of dental service use among commercially insured women in Minnesota before, during and after pregnancy. J Am Dent Assoc 2008;139:1173–1180 [erratum 2008;139:1312].

88. Milgrom P, Lee RS, Huebner CE, Conrad DA. Medicaid reforms in Oregon and suboptimal utilization of dental care by women of childbearing age. J Am Dent Assoc 2010;141:688–695.

89. Ressler-Maerlender J, Krishna R, Robison V. Oral health during pregnancy: Current research. J Womens Health (Larchmt) 2005;14:880–882.

90. Michalowicz BS, DiAngelis AJ, Novak MJ, et al. Examining the safety of dental treatment in pregnant women. J Am Dent Assoc 2008;139:685–695.

91. Oral Health Care During Pregnancy Expert Workgroup. Oral health care during pregnancy: A national consensus statement. Washington, DC: National Maternal and Child Oral Health Resource Center, 2012. http://www.mchoralhealth.org/PDFs/OralHealth PregnancyConsensus.pdf. Accessed 23 June 2013.

92. Holt K, Clark M, Barzel R. Two healthy smiles: Tips to keep you and your baby healthy (rev.). Washington, DC: National Maternal and Child Oral Health Resource Center, 2009. http://www.mchoralhealth.org/PDFs/ pregnancybrochure.pdf. Accessed 23 June 2013.

93. Holt K, Clark M, Barzel R. Dos sonrisas saludables: Consejos para mantenerte a ti y a tu bebé sanos (rev.). Washington, DC: National Maternal and Child Oral Health Resource Center, 2009. http://www. mchoralhealth.org/PDFs/pregnancybrochure_sp .pdf. Accessed 23 June 2013.

94. American Association of Public Health Dentistry, Alves-Dunkerson J, Amini H, et al. Toward a comprehensive health home: Integrating the mouth to the body. http://www.aaphd.org/docs/AAPHD%20 Final%20Health%20Home%20Resolution%20 -%20Last%20Revision%20Oct%202011.pdf. Accessed 23 June 2013.

95. American Academy of Pediatric Dentistry, Clinical Affairs Committee - Infant Oral Health Subcommittee. Guideline on infant oral health care. Reference Manual 2012;34:132–136. http://www.aapd.org /media/Policies_Guidelines/G_InfantOralHealth Care.pdf. Accessed 23 June 2013.

96. American Academy of Pediatric Dentistry, Council on Clinical Affairs. Guideline on perinatal oral health care. Reference Manual 2011;34:126–131.http://www .aapd.org/media/Policies_Guidelines/G_Perinatal OralHealthCare.pdf. Accessed 23 June 2013.

97. American Academy of Pediatric Dentistry, Council on Clinical Affairs, Committee on the Adolescent. Guideline on oral health care for the pregnant adolescent. Reference Manual 2012;34:145–151. http://www .aapd.org/media/Policies_Guidelines/G_Pregnancy .pdf. Accessed 23 June 2013.

98. Tonetti MS, D'Aiuto F, Nibali L, et al. Treatment of periodontitis and endothelial function. N Engl J Med 2007;356:911–920.

Clinical Considerations:
What You Can Take Back to Your Practice

What is the effect of immunosuppression in oncology patients on oral health?

The myelosuppression and immunosuppression associated with high-dose cancer therapies can exert direct and indirect injury to oral tissues. Oral mucositis is a direct consequence of the cancer treatments, which cause a complex inflammatory cascade that affects oral epithelium as well as connective tissue. Indirect toxicities such as acute mucosal infection can occur in the setting of decreased host immune response.

Is an immunosuppressed status in oncology patients an independent risk factor for the development of oral infections?

As indicated above, acute oral mucosal infections can occur as a result of the compromised immune surveillance and function. Thus, the immunosuppression can be viewed as an independent risk factor in these patients. The infections can be caused by either colonizing microorganisms, acquired pathogens, or reactivation of latent viruses.

What is the biologic plausibility of the association between oral health and immunosuppressed oncology patients?

A fully intact immune response is an essential component of maintaining the homeostasis that is a prerequisite to oral health. The oncology patient who is experiencing chemotherapy-induced myelosuppression serves as a key prototype for how compromised host defenses can lead to emergence of clinically significant oral toxicities. There is thus a profound biologic plausibility regarding the association between oral health and the immunosuppressed oncology patient.

Does the delivery of oral health care contribute to improvement of an immunosuppressed status in oncology patients?

Delivery of medically necessary oral health care prior to and during the period of myelosuppression can mitigate selected constituents of the oral toxicity profile. Examples of this benefit to patients include prevention of acute exacerbations of preexisting chronic inflammatory periodontitis as well as reduced risk for opportunistic mucosal infection in the setting of oral mucositis caused by the cancer chemotherapy.

Is it safe to provide dental care to immunosuppressed oncology patients?

Clear and evidence-based consultation between the dental provider and the oncology team is essential to provide safe and effective, medically necessary oral care in these patients. Considerations include the potential risks and benefits associated with each specific dental intervention, the patient's hematologic trajectory including maximum nadir of white blood cells, and the degree to which normal immune function is projected to recover in the future.

What is the appropriate message to give to the public about the association between oral health and immunosuppressed oncology patients?

Acute oral complications arising in myelosuppressed oncology patients can cause considerable morbidity and, in selected cases, can be fatal. The high-quality basic, translational, and clinical research evidence base that has emerged in recent years provides an excellent foundation for providing state-of-the-science, medically necessary dental care to these patients in ways that are both safe as well as effective.

Oral Complications in Immunocompromised Patients: The Oncology Prototype

Douglas E. Peterson, DMD, PhD, FDS RCSEd

Oral complications in cancer patients can have considerable adverse impact on both the clinical condition of the cancer patient and the cost of cancer care.[1,2] This dynamic occurs for a number of reasons, including the intensity of cancer treatment regimens as well as the extent of preexisting oral disease, which can evolve into acute and/or chronic toxicity.

However, substantive advances in the field of oral oncology over the past two decades have resulted in reduced incidence and severity of selected oral toxicities. Key drivers for this progress include the increasingly effective modeling of molecular science into clinical practice as well as the leading role that scientists and clinicians from dental medicine have taken in interprofessional research, production of clinical guidelines, and education of health professionals. These advances have occurred even as combination cancer therapies for advanced stages of oral cancer have become increasingly prominent:

- *Neoadjuvant (debulk)*: sole use prior to surgery (eg, 5-fluorouracil, which can cause oral mucositis)
- *Adjuvant (curative)*: use after surgery and before radiation therapy (eg, 5-fluorouracil, which can cause oral mucositis)
- *Concurrent/concomitant (synergistic)*: combination with radiation therapy (eg, head and neck radiation therapy plus weekly cisplatin)

Although considerable evidence exists about treatment-based oral toxicity in relation to tumor type, new frontiers in research are beginning to delineate patient-based factors with more precision. This evolving evidence base continues to more precisely define the interrelationships between the more classic modeling of disease (and its treatment) and new knowledge directed to patient-based risk determinants[3,4] (Fig 11-1). This line of research represents a promising foundation for future implementation of personalized medicine in which customized oral prevention and management interventions are developed for each individual patient.

The management of acute myelogenous leukemia is utilized in this chapter as the principal prototype by which the science and its clinical translation can be applied to clinical decision making and patient care (Figs 11-2 and 11-3). The high-dose induction chemotherapy regimen that is used to treat patients with acute myelogenous leukemia is profoundly myelosuppressive and typically causes severe ulcerative oral mucositis of at least 2 weeks' duration. The interface of profound myelosuppression with disrup-

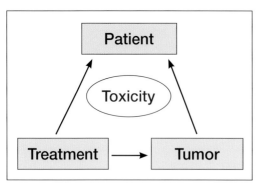

Fig 11-1 Toxicity of cancer treatment, including oral complications, occurs as a result of patient-based, tumor-based, and treatment-based components.

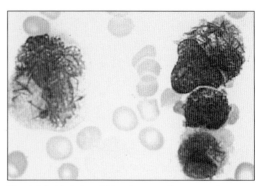

Fig 11-2 Peripheral blood smear from a patient with newly diagnosed acute myelogenous leukemia in blast crisis.

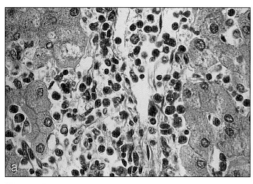
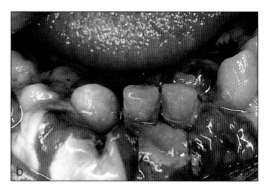

Fig 11-3 Acute leukemia can be considered "naturally metastatic" in that the neoplasm arises within the white blood cell progenitors produced in the bone marrow. Because of the inherent circulation of these cells, the disease is widespread by time of diagnosis. (a) Histopathology based on hepatic biopsy, demonstrating widespread infiltrate of the blast leukemic cells. (b) Gingival leukemic infiltrate in a patient newly diagnosed with acute myelogenous leukemia. Extensive gingival engorgement has been caused by the infiltrating leukemic cells. The resulting ischemia can contribute to development of tissue necrosis as well as opportunistic infection such as pseudomembranous candidiasis.

tion in integrity of the oral mucosal barrier can result in a risk of life-threatening bacteremia and/or sepsis.

Because of their high clinical importance and frequency, this chapter highlights the acute toxicities of mucosal injury and its associated pain, as well as oral infection, in the setting of multiple acute and chronic sequelae that can occur (Table 11-1). Because chronic toxicities caused by chemotherapy are not common, this aspect of oncology patient care will not be specifically addressed in detail.

Given the scientific and medical complexity of cancer and its treatment, the multidisciplinary oncology team has essential value in achieving optimal outcomes while minimizing side effects of that treatment. As a part of this team, the dental professional has vital responsibilities, including:

- Education of the patient and family members
- Education of the medical and nursing staff
- Diagnosis and treatment of oral complications
- Prevention of oral complications
- Oral health follow-up and maintenance

The interprofessional model as described for the oncology patient can also provide context for research and clinical management of pa-

Table 11-1	Oral toxicities in cancer patients*
Complication	**Weighted prevalence**
Bisphosphonate-induced osteonecrosis	All studies: 6.1% (mean)
	Studies with documented follow-up: 13.3%
	Studies with undocumented follow-up: 0.7%
	Epidemiologic studies: 1.2%
Dysgeusia	CT only: 56.3% (mean)
	RT only: 66.5% (mean)
	Combined CT and RT: 76% (mean)
Oral fungal infection	*Clinical oral fungal infection (all oral candidiasis)*
	Pretreatment: 7.5%
	During treatment: 39.1%
	Posttreatment: 32.6%
	Clinical oral candidiasis infection by cancer treatment
	During HNC RT: 37.4%
	During CT: 38%
Oral viral infection	*Patients treated with CT for hematologic malignancies*
	Patients with oral ulcerations/sampling oral ulcerations: 49.8%
	Patients sampling oral ulcerations: 33.8%
	Patients sampling independently of the presence of oral ulcerations: 0%
	Patients treated with RT
	Patients with RT only/sampling oral ulcerations: 0%
	Patients with RT and adjunctive CT/sampling oral ulcerations: 43.2%
Dental disease	*Dental caries in patients treated with cancer therapy*
	All studies: 28.1%
	CT only: 37.3%
	Post-RT: 24%
	Post-CT and post-RT: 21.4%
	Severe gingivitis in patients undergoing CT: 20.3%
	Dental infection/abscess in patients undergoing CT: 5.8%
Osteoradionecrosis	Conventional RT: 7.4%
	IMRT: 5.2%
	RT and CT: 6.8%
	Brachytherapy: 5.3%
Trismus	Conventional RT: 25.4%
	IMRT: 5%
	Combined RT and CT: 30.7%

(continued on next page)

Table 11-1 (cont) **Oral toxicities in cancer patients***

Complication	Weighted prevalence
Oral pain[†]	*VAS pain level (0–100) in HNC patients*
	Pretreatment: 12/100
	Immediately posttreatment: 33/100
	1 Mo posttreatment: 20/100
	EORTC QLQ-C30 pain level (0–100) in HNC patients
	Pretreatment: 27/100
	3 Mo posttreatment: 30/100
	6 Mo posttreatment: 23/100
	12 Mo posttreatment: 24/100
Salivary gland hypofunction and xerostomia (in HNC patients by type of RT)	*All studies*
	Pre-RT: 6%
	During RT: 93%
	1–3 Mo post-RT: 74%
	3–6 Mo post-RT: 79%
	6–12 Mo post-RT: 83%
	1–2 Y post-RT: 78%
	> 2 Y post-RT: 85%
	Conventional RT
	Pre-RT: 10%
	During RT: 81%
	1–3 Mo post-RT: 71%
	3–6 Mo post-RT: 83%
	6–12 Mo post-RT: 72%
	1–2 Y post-RT: 84%
	> 2 Y post-RT: 91%
	IMRT
	Pre-RT:12%
	During RT: 100%
	1–3 Mo post-RT: 89%
	3–6 Mo post-RT: 73%
	6–12 Mo post-RT: 90%
	1–2 Y post-RT: 66%
	> 2 Y post-RT: 68%

*Adapted from the National Cancer Institute website.[1]
†Pain is common in patients with HNCs and is reported by approximately half of patients before cancer therapy, by 81% during therapy, by 70% at the end of therapy, and by 36% at 6 months posttreatment.
CT, chemotherapy; EORTC QLQ-C30, European Organisation for Research and Treatment of Cancer Quality of Life Questionnaire C30; HNC, head and neck cancer; IMRT, intensity-modulated radiation therapy; RT, radiation therapy; VAS, visual analog scale.

Fig 11-4 Oral mucositis in a breast cancer patient receiving high-dose chemotherapy. Extensive pseudomembranous lesions can significantly impair normal oral function and represent a portal of entry for severe systemic infection. (Reprinted from Brennan et al[7] with permission.)

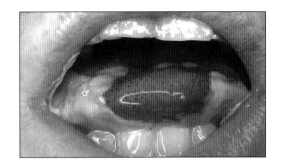

Box 11-1	Key developments in the field of oral mucositis over the past 20 years[2]

- Initiation of research studies into pathobiology and clinical trials
- The creation of international organizations of health professionals directed to the mission of supportive care in cancer
- The first two American Society of Clinical Oncology educational sessions addressing mucositis, held in 2003 and 2004
- Publication of the first evidence-based mucositis guidelines by the Multinational Association of Supportive Care in Cancer and International Society of Oral Oncology

(MASCC/ISOO), which have since been updated twice
- Incorporation of mucositis as a MeSH term by the National Library of Medicine
- The publication of clinical practice guidelines for mucositis by other organizations
- Comprehensive updating of the National Cancer Institute's Physician Data Query website[1] to include a section on oral complications of chemotherapy and head and neck radiation

---

tients whose immune function is attenuated as a result of systemic disease. Examples of these diseases include genetically based or acquired immunodeficiencies, as well as adverse outcomes of non-neoplastic disease treatment.

Acute Oral Toxicities in the Myelosuppressed Oncology Patient

Oral mucositis

Clinical impact

Oral mucositis can have a significant deleterious impact on the cancer patient receiving high-dose chemotherapy[2,4–6] (Fig 11-4). The lesion can be so painful that oral functions such as eating, speaking, and swallowing are se-

verely compromised. In cancer patients receiving multicycle chemotherapy regimens, the oral pain can necessitate subsequent dose delays or reductions to lessen the extent of oral injury and discomfort. In neutropenic cancer patients, ulcerative oral mucositis can be a portal of entry for systemic infection, resulting in bacteremia and/or sepsis. The collective sequelae of the lesion can require extensive use of health care resources,[8] including by some estimates approximately US$41,000 in the hematopoietic stem cell transplant (HSCT) population.[9] Oral mucositis can thus be clinically and economically consequential.

Despite the importance of the condition, however, until the early 1990s oral mucositis had been viewed by many clinicians and thus patients as an inevitable consequence of high-dose cancer therapy. Fortunately, substantial progress over the past 20 years at the research and clinical levels has set the stage for new opportunities for prevention and treatment (Box 11-1).[2]

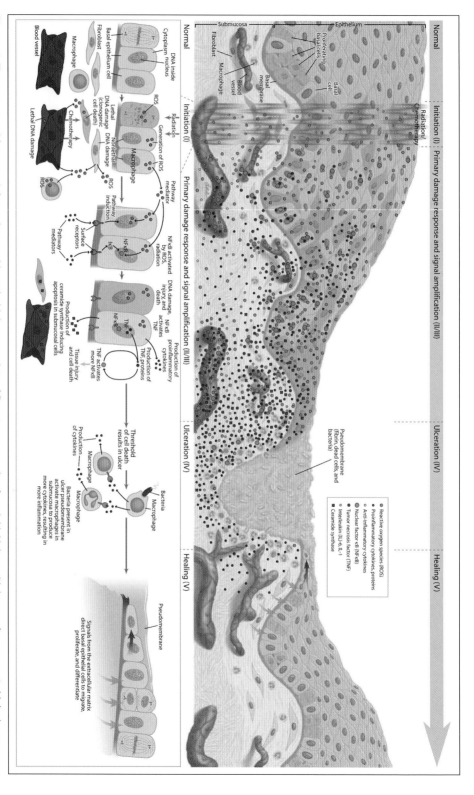

Fig 11-5 The conceptual framework for oral mucositis pathobiology consists of five stages, ranging from initial injury with hours of exposure to high-dose cancer therapy to eventual healing approximately 2 to 4 weeks after cessation of that treatment. Although the illustration depicts an orderly and sequential mechanistic process, the course of molecular and cellular events is more likely dysregulated and biologically chaotic. (Reprinted from Sonis[5] with permission.)

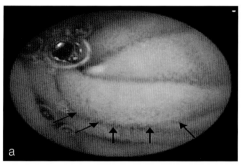
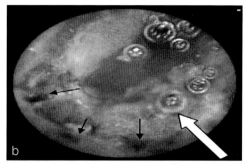

Fig 11-6 Systemic chemotherapy causes architectural and functional disturbances throughout the alimentary tract, including the intestine. *(a)* Normal jejunal mucosa in a healthy patient, as imaged by video-capsule endoscopy. *(black arrows)* Normal villi. *(b)* Extensive ulceration *(white arrow)* and hemorrhage *(black arrows)* of the intestine in a hematopoietic cell transplant patient approximately 7 days after the last dose of high-dose chemotherapy as a component of the conditioning regimen. This lesion of the gastrointestinal tract is not typically painful but can be associated with severe diarrhea, cramping, and compromised absorption of nutrients. (Reprinted from Triantafyllou et al[11] with permission.)

Pathobiology and future research directions

One of the key advances in the last two decades has been the delineation of a contemporary pathobiologic model that illustrates the complex interactions within and across oral epithelial and connective tissues[5,6,10] (Fig 11-5). An additional major advance in recent years has been the scientific and clinical linkage of oral mucositis with gastrointestinal mucositis[3,4,11,12] (Fig 11-6). This paradigm of alimentary tract mucositis has provided an essential foundation for new research frontiers that collectively could permit personalized medicine for each oncology patient based on a priori prediction of both risk for mucositis and likely response to therapeutics (Box 11-2).

Achievement of this goal is important because the incidence and severity of oral mucositis vary across cancer patient cohorts, from approximately 40% of patients receiving standard-dose chemotherapy to approximately 80% of patients receiving myeloablative conditioning regimens for HSCT.[2] There is thus a need to implement customized prevention and management for selected, but not all, cancer patients who are about to begin mucotoxic cancer treatment.

Patients with advanced stages of head and neck cancer typically receive multimodality treatment that includes approximately two cycles of induction chemotherapy followed by high-dose head and neck radiation with or without weekly concomitant chemotherapy (Fig 11-7). Decisions on types of oral cancer treatment typically incorporate multiple considerations, including the location and staging of the cancer, the age of the patient, and anticipated cure rates. Although the chemotherapy utilized in these treatment protocols is not highly myelosuppressive, it can cause oral mucositis that is clinically significant in some patients.

At present, the United States Food and Drug Administration has cleared only one nondevice intervention for oral mucositis.[13] This agent, palifermin, is a member of the keratinocyte growth factor family and is cleared for prevention of oral mucositis in HSCT patients receiving chemotherapy with or without total body

Box 11-2	Future research questions: Oral mucositis caused by cancer therapies*

Pathobiology
- What is the role of the oral microbiome relative to causation, progression, and/or healing of oral mucositis?
- What are the molecular bases for incidence and severity of pain in relation to degree of oral mucosal injury?
- Why do patients with comparable characteristics, including age, sex, cancer diagnosis, and treatment regimen, collectively exhibit variability of toxicity expression, including oral mucositis?
- How can delineation of molecular pathogenesis lead to novel models for prediction of incidence, severity, and response to therapeutics in individual patients, in contrast to a cohort-wide basis?
- What biologic characteristics contribute to native protection against development of mucositis at selected non–alimentary tract mucosal sites such as vaginal and conjunctival mucosa?
- What crosstalk occurs between at-risk mucosal and dermal sites for which common etiologies can be delineated?
- How can systems biology technology be optimally applied to study the regulatory function of gene clusters in comparison with single gene expression? In addition, how do these interrelated gene cluster functions translate to studies of symptom burden that are observed in many oncology patients undergoing high-dose cancer therapies?

Development of pharmacologics, biologics, and devices to manage oral mucositis
- What are the key molecular targets that, if successfully perturbed, are likely to permit achievement of a high degree of clinical efficacy with the least extent of side effects?
- What is the most efficient preclinical and clinical development strategy to bring new therapeutics to clinical practice in a cost-effective fashion?

Impact of evidence-based clinical practice guidelines
- What are the most effective ways to ascertain the impact of utilization of evidence-based oral mucositis clinical practice guidelines relative to enhanced clinical outcomes and reduced cost of cancer care?

*Reprinted from Peterson et al[2] with permission.

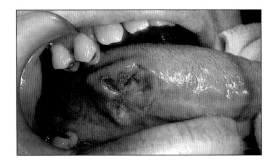

Fig 11-7 Advanced stage of squamous cell carcinoma on the right lateral side of the tongue. Advanced stages of oral squamous cell carcinoma typically warrant multimodality cancer treatment, including surgery and/or chemotherapy followed by high-dose head and neck radiation. The chemotherapeutic regimens utilized are not usually profoundly myelosuppressive, although they can cause clinically significant oral mucositis.

radiation in the autologous transplant setting. Despite phase IV studies, the agent has not demonstrated consistent efficacy in the non-autologous transplant setting.[14]

Additional preclinical and clinical development of drugs and biologics continues, directed to key molecular targets and network hubs (see Box 11-2). Notable among many current studies is work being conducted by investigators at

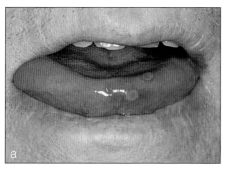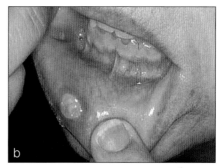

Fig 11-8 Selected mammalian target of rapamycin (mTOR) inhibitors can cause oral mucosal lesions that clinically resemble recurrent aphthous ulceration and often respond to topical, intra-lesional, or systemic corticosteroid management. *(a)* Lesion on the tongue after a patient received three 21-day cycles (63 days) of ridaforolimus. *(b)* Inner lips of a patient who developed mTOR inhibitor–associated stomatitis within 10 days after initiation of treatment with everolimus (10 mg once daily) in combination with figitumumab. (Courtesy of Dr Nathaniel Treister, Dana-Farber Cancer Institute/Brigham and Women's Hospital, Boston, Massachusetts.)

the National Institutes of Health, who are pursuing the use of tempol for prevention of oral mucositis[15] and gene therapy for treatment of chemoradiation-induced oral mucositis.[16] This and related lines of biologic research are being enhanced by development of novel technologies such as in vitro tissue engineering models of oral mucosa[17] as well as prediction of the mucositis trajectory in patients via genetic[6,18–23] and imaging-based[24] approaches. High-throughput deep sequencing of the oral microbiome[25] is permitting delineation of putative pathogens that are not typically cultivable by conventional methods. Systems biology technology is increasingly being utilized to integrate the complex and extensive data sets into cohesive models of pathobiology that translate to the clinical trajectory.[2,26–28] New international conferences, such as the June 2013 first-in-kind Gordon Research Conference,[29] titled "Mucosal Health & Disease," provide further opportunities to create new research models to investigate oral mucositis.

Of further importance are the recent observations of unique oral mucosal lesions caused by selected targeted cancer therapies, such as the mammalian target of rapamycin[30] inhibitors (Fig 11-8). These lesions mimic recurrent aphthous ulcerations in clinical appearance[31,32] and in selected patients respond well to topical, intra-lesional, and/or systemic corticosteroid therapy. These lesions are thus quite different from oral mucositis caused by conventional chemotherapy or head and neck radiation with regard to mucosal distribution, clinical appearance, and response to steroid management. Further research on the molecular pathobiology of these lesions is needed to enhance understanding of their causation as well as the potential for prediction of incidence and severity on a patient-by-patient basis.

Thus, basic, translational, and clinical research has successfully shifted the historic paradigm of "inevitable consequence" to a contemporary model for which prediction of incidence and severity of oral mucositis as well as response to therapeutics is likely to emerge over the next few years. These advances will likely in turn provide an evidence base on which comprehensive clinical guidelines for mucositis management can position the clinician to develop a personalized, customized approach to prevention and treatment of oral mucositis for each individual oncology patient.

| Box 11-3 | Oral complications of hematopoietic stem cell transplantation* |

Phase I: Preconditioning
- Oral infections: dental caries, endodontic infections, periodontal disease (gingivitis or periodontitis), and mucosal infections (ie, viral, fungal, or bacterial)
- Gingival leukemic infiltrates
- Metastatic cancer
- Oral bleeding
- Oral ulceration: aphthous ulcers and erythema multiforme
- Temporomandibular dysfunction

Phase II: Conditioning neutropenic phase
- Oropharyngeal mucositis
- Oral infections: mucosal infections (ie, viral, fungal, or bacterial) and periodontal infections
- Hemorrhage
- Xerostomia
- Taste dysfunction
- Neurotoxicity: dental pain and muscle tremor (eg, jaws or tongue)
- Temporomandibular dysfunction: jaw pain, headache, and joint pain

Phase III: Engraftment hematopoietic recovery
- Oral infections: mucosal infections (ie, viral, fungal, or bacterial)
- Acute graft-versus-host disease (GVHD)
- Xerostomia
- Hemorrhage
- Neurotoxicity: dental pain and muscle tremor (eg, jaws or tongue)
- Temporomandibular dysfunction: jaw pain, headache, and joint pain
- Granulomas/papillomas

Phase IV: Immune reconstitution late posttransplant
- Oral infections: mucosal infections (ie, viral, fungal, or bacterial)
- Chronic GVHD
- Dental and skeletal growth and development alterations (pediatric patients)
- Xerostomia
- Relapse-related oral lesions
- Second malignancies

Phase V: Long-term survival
- Relapse or second malignancies
- Dental and skeletal growth and development alterations

*Adapted from the National Cancer Institute.[36]

Pain management

The complex proinflammatory and neurotransmitter cascade associated with oral mucositis can result in moderate to severe oral pain that can compromise delivery of cancer treatment regimens.[33] The pain can escalate mood changes such as anxiety and depression, which in turn can further contribute to the patient's pain experience.

It is essential that an aggressive and systematic pain assessment and intervention strategy be incorporated. The paradigm begins with education of the patient and caregiver regarding oral mucositis and its consequences prior to initiation of cancer therapy.[34] Systematic oral tissue and pain assessments are then needed throughout the period of cancer treatment. A staged approach to pain relief, ranging from topical anesthetics, doxepin, and fentanyl through nonopioid and opioid systemic analgesics, can be implemented as needed. It is also essential to monitor side effects of the pain therapeutics, particularly with the opioid classes of drugs.

Acute and chronic graft-versus-host disease

The HSCT patient represents a unique cohort among immunocompromised patients, with a broad scope of acute and chronic oral toxicities that may develop[35,36] (Box 11-3). This uniqueness is characterized by a conceptual framework that includes stem cell rescue of bone marrow injury that is caused by a conditioning regimen of high-dose chemotherapy and/or radiotherapy for treatment of the malignancy. This rescue is achieved by postconditioning infusion of hematopoietic cells that are harvested in advance from one of the following donor sources:

- *Autologous:* Patient's own hematopoietic stem cells (human leukocyte antigen [HLA] identical).
- *Syngeneic:* Patient's identical twin or triplet's hematopoietic cells (HLA identical).
- *Allogeneic:* Typically a sibling or donor relative who is genetically similar based on matching at the HLA locus. In some instances, the donor can be unrelated to the patient (HLA identical, haploidentical, or mismatched).

Patients who undergo allogeneic HSCT may develop moderate to severe oral mucositis caused by the conditioning regimen.[37]

In addition, at least 50% of patients develop chronic graft-versus-host disease (GVHD) within about 1 year of the transplant procedure.[35] Risk for development of this condition is directly influenced by the extent to which there is genetic disparity at the HLA locus with either a related or unrelated donor. The reaction is in part mediated via alloreactive donor lymphocytes that recognize and bind to antigens associated with salivary gland and oral mucosa. The resultant cytotoxicity can lead to irreversible oral tissue injury. The oral mucosal lesions associated with chronic GVHD are typically lichenoid in appearance, with an erosive or ulcerative component in selected cases.[38] As such, they mimic naturally occurring mucosal diseases, such as ulcerative lichen planus, pemphigus, and pemphigoid. Oral chronic GVHD is considered a risk factor for development of potentially malignant and malignant oral mucosal neoplasms over time. Clinically significant salivary hypofunction and xerostomia can develop as a result of chronic GVHD as well, with potentially highly adverse impact on the dentition, periodontium, and mucosa.[35]

Considerations for topical management of the mucosal lesions include steroids, immunosuppressants such as azathioprine, and/or oral psoralen and ultraviolet A therapy. Systemic immunosuppression is usually warranted in severe cases, particularly if multiorgan involvement is present.[35,38]

Infection

The dentition, periodontium, and periradicular sites represent potential sources of acute local and systemic infection during myelosuppression.[1] The following preexisting oral lesions can represent clinically significant risk to the patient during the subsequent period of myelosuppression:

- Advanced and/or symptomatic dental caries
- Periapical pathoses symptomatic within the past 90 days
- Severe periodontal disease for which prognosis of the dentition is poor
- Mucosal lesions secondary to trauma from prosthetic or orthodontic appliances

Many of these acute infectious flare-ups can be prevented by stabilization of the oral cavity prior to initiation of the chemotherapy. Unfortunately, there is no definitive prechemotherapy oral care protocol that clearly delineates risk for infectious flare-ups in relation to degree and duration of myelosuppression. Clinicians must therefore incorporate clinical judgment in their prechemotherapy decision making. The history of symptoms within the previous 90 days can serve as a useful guide in this regard.

The oral assessment should occur as early as feasible in relation to the upcoming chemotherapy. Clear communication of the oral findings among the oncology team is essential, with a focus on the extent of preexisting oral disease in relation to likelihood of acute infectious flare-up during myelosuppression.

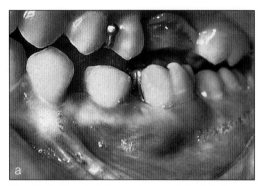
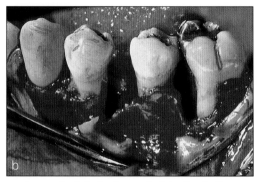

Fig 11-9 Chronic inflammatory periodontal disease represents a potential site for acute infection in the myelosuppressed chemotherapy patient. *(a)* Patient who does not have cancer presenting for periodontal surgical management of severe chronic periodontal disease. *(b)* Intraoperative clinical photograph of the patient in *(a)*. The extensive ulceration provides a direct portal for systemic dissemination of colonizing microflora. In the chemotherapy patient with profound neutropenia (eg, neutrophil count of less than $100/mm^3$), this systemic dissemination can result in morbid or fatal infections.

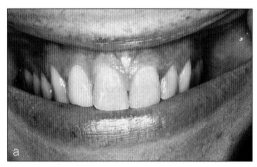
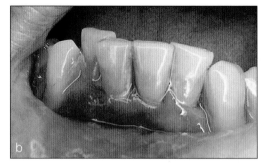

Fig 11-10 *(a)* Acute periodontal infection in a neutropenic cancer patient with a neutrophil count of less than $500/mm^3$. Classic inflammatory signs, including erythema and purulence, are not clinically prominent because the number and function of neutrophils are suppressed. *(b)* Acute periodontal infection in a chemotherapy patient with a neutrophil count of less than $1,000/mm^3$. Classic signs of inflammation are more evident because the neutrophil response is more robust.

Acute periodontal infections

Chronic periodontal disease can undergo acute infectious exacerbation during neutropenia (Figs 11-9 and 11-10). Acute flare-ups are infrequent despite the widespread occurrence of the predisposing chronic inflammatory condition. The microbiologic flora has been historically reported as comprising both periodontopathic organisms as well as acquired pathogens associated with morbidity and mortality in the neutropenic cancer patient.[39] When it does occur, the classic signs of inflammation may be diminished because of the myelosuppressed condition of the patient. Culturing of the attached gingiva, as opposed to direct, subgingival culturing, may not produce microbial specimens reflective of the causative microflora.

Treatment typically consists of oral rinses with 0.12% chlorhexidine digluconate, irrigation of the periodontal pocket with 3% hydrogen peroxide, gentle and supervised dental brushing and flossing, and use of systemic broad-spectrum antibiotics if indicated medically.

Herpes simplex viral infection

The mucosa can also become primarily or secondarily infected during this myelosuppression. Examples of clinical infection with herpes simplex virus (HSV) and *Candida* are discussed, using the HSCT setting as the prototype. Addi-

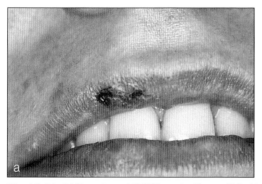 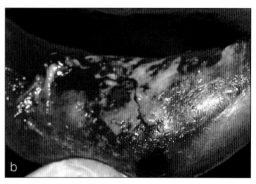

Fig 11-11 *(a)* Reactivated HSV is typically a self-limiting clinical infection in the immunocompetent patient. This patient's lesion has been present for 8 days and is now in the stages of resolution. *(b)* Reactivated HSV can be extensive and fatal in a patient who is immunocompromised following hematopoietic cell transplant. The compromised mucosal and circulating immune defenses result in a rapidly progressing, painful, and sometimes fatal systemic viral infection. (Fig 11-11b courtesy of Dr Mark M. Schubert, Fred Hutchinson Cancer Research Center, Seattle, Washington.)

tional detailed guidelines for prevention of infectious complications among these patients have been provided by Tomblyn et al.[40]

The immunocompromised cancer patient is at risk for either reactivation of latent viruses or activation of newly acquired viruses.[35,41] Latent HSV, varicella-zoster virus, and Epstein-Barr virus can be reactivated, while cytomegalovirus infection can result from either reactivation of latent virus or newly acquired virus.

Unlike the self-limiting recurrent HSV infections in otherwise immunocompetent individuals, reactivation of latent HSV in immunocompromised patients such as those undergoing HSCT can be life-threatening (Fig 11-11). Fortunately, antiviral prophylaxis or treatment with thymidine kinase inhibitors such as acyclovir or its derivatives is highly efficacious. Drug-resistant herpes simplex is an infrequent occurrence. The infection can codevelop in the setting of oral mucositis and/or acute GVHD[35]; this not only confounds the diagnostic process but also intensifies the severity of the mucosal injury.

As with all infections in this population, early diagnosis is key to instituting prompt measures directed to cure. Viral culturing remains the gold standard, while other testing such as direct immunofluorescence, immunoassay, and shell vial testing may be useful in generating more rapid results.

The development of antiviral medications such as acyclovir, valacyclovir, and their derivatives means that the infections in prechemotherapy and pre-HSCT patients who are seropositive for HSV and varicella-zoster virus can essentially be prevented. Breakthrough infections, should they occur, are typically highly responsive to increased doses of the antiviral medications, because viral resistance is rare. Persistent clinical infection is less likely to be due to viral resistance than to less than optimal dosing and/or impaired gastrointestinal absorption of orally administered agents such as acyclovir.

Other, nonherpes viral infections such as human papillomavirus can occur in the immunocompromised HSCT patient as well. As with herpetiform infections, the risk and severity of the human papillomavirus lesion are influenced by the duration and depth of the immunocompromised state. While laser removal or cryotherapy may be implemented, the lesions often regress on immune recovery.

Candidal infection

Opportunistic infections such as candidiasis are common in the immunocompromised HSCT patient[41,42] (Fig 11-12). In addition to the patient's impaired immune response, additional risk factors include oral mucositis as well as pharmacologic- and/or GVHD-induced

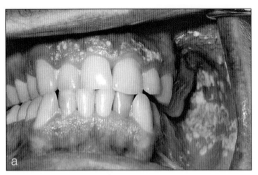
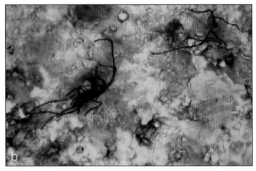

Fig 11-12 Pseudomembranous candidiasis can occur in oncology patients secondary to myelosuppression and/ or compromised salivary defense mechanisms. *(a)* Clinically documented pseudomembranous candidiasis in an allogeneic hematopoietic cell transplant patient with chronic GVHD involving the major salivary glands. *(b)* Cytologic smear demonstrating the dimorphic candidal organism and hyphae.

Box 11-4	Characteristics of candidiasis

Risk factors
- Myelosuppression
- Mucosal injury
- Salivary compromise
- Antibiotics
- Steroids
- Increased length of hospital stay

Diagnosis
- History
- Assessment of risk factors
- Examination
- Culture as needed

Treatment
- Nonmedicated oral rinse
- Topical antifungal (systemic therapy if indicated)
- Removal of dentures

salivary gland hypofunction (Box 11-4). The resultant compromised salivary flow and composition (eg, lactoferrin, salivary immunoglobulin A, transferrin, and mucins) can lead to pseudomembranous candidiasis and other opportunistic infections.

Diagnosis of candidiasis is typically based on history and clinical examination. Smear testing or culturing can be performed if clinically warranted.

Topical oral antifungal therapy with nystatin and clotrimazole can be instituted, although the yeast infection will likely recur on cessation of the medication unless the underlying risk factors are successfully addressed as well. The following regimen of topical therapy (7 to 14 days' treatment) was recommended by Lerman et al[43]:

- Clotrimazole troche (10 mg), 4 to 5 times per day
- Nystatin oral suspension (100,000 U/mL), 5 mL, 4 times per day
- Nystatin pastilles (200,000 U), 4 to 5 times per day
- Fluconazole solution (eg, 10 mg), swished and expectorated, 3 times per day
- Amphotericin B, oral suspension (100 mg/ mL), 1 mL, 4 times per day

Systemic antifungal management with agents such as fluconazole is typically indicated for treatment of persistent oral infection as well as patients with profound immunosuppression.

In addition to candidal infection, other types of fungal infection can occur, including lesions caused by *Aspergillus*, *Mucormycosis*, and *Rhizopus* species. Culturing is essential for diagnosis, because these lesions may mimic the clinical appearance of nonyeast toxicities in HSCT patients.

Conclusion

Oral complications can adversely affect the quality of life of myelosuppressed cancer patients. This impact can range from mild and easily tolerated to severe and debilitating. In some cases, the toxicities can decrease the cancer patient's chances of survival. Treatment of the conditions can be expensive, including the cost of prolonged hospital stays and supportive care interventions such as infection management and nutritional support.

Fortunately, substantial and innovative research in recent years has provided new insights into molecular-based causation. These discoveries are setting the stage for development of novel preventive and therapeutic technologies for future use in the clinical setting. Researchers and clinicians from dental medicine are taking the lead role in these scientific advances for the prevention and management of some toxicities, such as mucositis. In recent years, interdisciplinary collaborations promoted via national and international organizations of health professionals have contributed to the translation of clinically applicable outcomes into high-quality, evidence-based guidelines for oncology practice.

Presentation of this oncology paradigm has been designed to highlight these issues in the context of dental medicine research and clinical care. Insights and lessons learned from this modeling may well be applicable to other patient cohorts in whom disease and/or its treatment has led to immunocompromise.

References

1. National Cancer Institute. Oral complications of chemotherapy and head/neck radiation (PDQ). http://www.cancer.gov/cancertopics/pdq/supportivecare/oralcomplications/HealthProfessional. Accessed 26 Sept 2013.
2. Peterson DE, Srivastava R, Lalla RV. Oral mucosal injury in oncology patients: Perspectives on maturation of a field [epub ahead of print 19 July 2013]. Oral Dis doi:10.1111/odi.12167.
3. Sonis ST, Elting LS, Keefe D, et al. Perspectives on cancer therapy-induced mucosal injury: Pathogenesis, measurement, epidemiology, and consequences for patients. Cancer 2004;100(9 suppl):1995–2025.
4. Peterson DE, Keefe DM, Sonis ST. New frontiers in mucositis. In: Govindan R (ed). 2012 ASCO Educational Book. Alexandria, VA: American Society of Clinical Oncology, 2012:545–551.
5. Sonis ST. Pathobiology of oral mucositis: Novel insights and opportunities. J Support Oncol 2007;5(9 suppl 4):3–11.
6. Al-Dasooqi N, Sonis ST, Bowen JM, et al. Emerging evidence on the pathobiology of mucositis. J Support Care Cancer 2013;21:2075–2083.
7. Brennan MT, Lalla RV, Schubert MM, Peterson DE. Oral toxicity. In: Perry MC, Doll DC, Freter CE (eds). Perry's The Chemotherapy Source Book, ed 5. Philadelphia: Lippincott Williams & Wilkins, 2012:112–138.
8. Carlotto A, Hogsett VL, Maiorini EM, Razulis JG, Sonis ST. The economic burden of toxicities associated with cancer treatment: Review of the literature and analysis of nausea and vomiting, diarrhoea, oral mucositis and fatigue. Pharmacoeconomics 2013;31:753–766.
9. Sonis ST, Oster G, Fuchs H, Bellm L, et al. Oral mucositis and the clinical and economic outcomes of hematopoietic stem-cell transplantation. J Clin Oncol 2001;19:2201–2205.
10. Sonis ST. New thoughts on the initiation of mucositis. Oral Dis 2010;16:597–600.
11. Triantafyllou K, Dervenoulas J, Tsirigotis P, Ladas SD. The nature of small intestinal mucositis: A video-capsule endoscopy study. Support Care Cancer 2008;16:1173–1178.
12. Yasuda M, Kato S, Yamanaka N, et al. 5-HT3 receptor antagonists ameliorate 5-fluorouracil-induced intestinal mucositis by suppression of apoptosis in murine intestinal crypt cells. Br J Pharmacol 2013;168:1388–1400.
13. Sonis ST. Efficacy of palifermin (keratinocyte growth factor-1) in the amelioration of oral mucositis. Core Evid 2010;4:199–205.
14. Niscola P, Tendis A, Cupelli L, et al. The prevention of oral mucositis in patients with blood cancers: Current concepts and emerging landscapes. Cardiovasc Hematol Agents Med Chem 2012;10:362–375.

15. Cotrim AP, Yoshikawa M, Sunshine AN, et al. Pharmacological protection from radiation ± cisplatin-induced oral mucositis. Int J Radiat Oncol Biol Phys 2012;83:1284–1290.

16. Zheng C, Cotrim AP, Sunshine AN, et al. Prevention of radiation-induced oral mucositis after adenoviral vector-mediated transfer of the keratinocyte growth factor cDNA to mouse submandibular glands. Clin Cancer Res 2009;15:4641–4648.

17. Colley HE, Eves PC, Pinnock A, Thornhill MH, Murdoch C. Tissue-engineered oral mucosa to study radiotherapy-induced oral mucositis [epub ahead of print 26 June 2013]. Int J Radiat Biol doi: 10.3109/09553002.2013.809171.

18. Garg MB, Lincz LF, Adler K, Scorgie FE, Ackland SP, Sakoff JA. Predicting 5-fluorouracil toxicity in colorectal cancer patients from peripheral blood cell telomere length: A multivariate analysis. Br J Cancer 2012;107:1525–1533.

19. Sonis S, Haddad R, Posner M, et al. Gene expression changes in peripheral blood cells provide insight into the biological mechanisms associated with regimen-related toxicities in patients being treated for head and neck cancers. Oral Oncol 2007;43:289–300.

20. Al-Dasooqi N, Bowen JM, Gibson RJ, Logan RM, Stringer AM, Keefe DM. Selection of housekeeping genes for gene expression studies in a rat model of irinotecan-induced mucositis. Chemotherapy 2011;57:43–53.

21. Hahn T, Zhelnova E, Suchestion L, et al. A deletion polymorphism in glutathione-S-transferase mu (GSTM1) and/or theta (GSTT1) is associated with an increased risk of toxicity after autologous blood and marrow transplantation. Biol Blood Marrow Transplant 2010;16:801–808.

22. Mougeot JL, Bahrani-Mougeot FK, Lockhart PB, Brennan MT. Microarray analyses of oral punch biopsies from acute myeloid leukemia (AML) patients treated with chemotherapy. Oral Surg Oral Med Oral Pathol Oral Radiol Endod 2011;112:446–452.

23. Mougeot JL, Mougeot FK, Peterson DE, Padilla RJ, Brennan MT, Lockhart PB. Use of archived biopsy specimens to study gene expression in oral mucosa from chemotherapy-treated cancer patients. Oral Surg Oral Med Oral Pathol Oral Radiol 2013;115:630–637.

24. Calantog A, Hallajian L, Nabelsi T, et al. A prospective study to assess in vivo optical coherence tomography imaging for early detection of chemotherapy-induced oral mucositis. Laser Surg Med 2013;45:22–27.

25. Diaz PI, Dupuy AK, Abusleme L, et al. Using high throughput sequencing to explore the biodiversity in oral bacterial communities. Mol Oral Microbiol 2012;27:182–201.

26. Michelson S, Sehgal A, Friedrich C. In silico prediction of clinical efficacy. Curr Opin Biotech 2006;17:666–670.

27. Molina F, Dehmer M, Perco P, et al. Systems biology: Opening new avenues in clinical research. Nephrol Dial Transplant 2010;25:1015–1018.

28. Sonis ST, Antin J, Tedaldi MW, Alterovitz G. SNP-based Bayesian networks can predict oral mucositis risk in autologous stem cell transplant recipients. Oral Dis 2013;19:721–727.

29. Gordon Research Conference. Mucosal Health & Disease. 9–14 June 2013. http://www.grc.org/programs.aspx?year=2013&program=mucosal. Accessed 26 Sept 2013.

30. Pilotte AP, Hohos MB, Polson KM, Huftalen TM, Treister N. Managing stomatitis in patients treated with mammalian target of rapamycin inhibitors. Clin J Oncol Nurs 2011;15(5):E83–E89.

31. Sonis S, Treister N, Chawla S, Demetri G, Haluska F. Preliminary characterization of oral lesions associated with inhibitors of mammalian target of rapamycin in cancer patients. Cancer 2010;116:210–215.

32. Elting LS, Chang YC, Parelkar P, et al. Risk of oral and gastrointestinal mucosal injury among patients receiving selected targeted agents: A meta-analysis. Support Care 2013;21:3243–3254.

33. National Cancer Institute. Oral mucositis. Oral complications of chemotherapy and head/neck radiation (PDQ). http://www.cancer.gov/cancertopics/pdq/supportivecare/oralcomplications/HealthProfessional/page5. Accessed 26 Sept 2013.

34. McGuire DB, Fulton JS, Park J, et al. Systematic review of basic oral care for the management of oral mucositis in cancer patients. Support Care Cancer 2013;21:3165–3177.

35. Schubert MM, Correa MCM, Peterson DE. Oral complications of hematopoietic cell transplantation. In: Appelbaum FR, Negrin RS, Antin JH, Forman SJ (eds). Thomas' Hematopoietic Cell Transplantation, ed 5. London: Blackwell Scientific (in press).

36. National Cancer Institute. Oral and dental management before cancer therapy. Oral complications of chemotherapy and head/neck radiation (PDQ). http://www.cancer.gov/cancertopics/pdq/supportivecare/oralcomplications/HealthProfessional/page3. Accessed 1 Nov 2013.

37. Ringdén O, Erkers T, Aschan J, et al. A prospective randomized toxicity study to compare reduced-intensity and myeloablative conditioning in patients with myeloid leukaemia undergoing allogeneic haematopoietic stem cell transplantation. J Intern Med 2013;274:153–162.

38. National Cancer Institute. Graft-versus-host disease. Oral complications of chemotherapy and head/neck radiation (PDQ). http://www.cancer.gov/cancertopics/pdq/supportivecare/oralcomplications/HealthProfessional/page10. Accessed 26 Sept 2013.

39. Peterson DE, Minah GE, Overholser CD, et al. Microbiology of acute periodontal infection in myelosuppressed cancer patients. J Clin Oncol 1987;5:1461–1468.

40. Tomblyn M, Chiller T, Einsele H, et al. Guidelines for preventing infectious complications among hematopoietic cell transplantation recipients: A global perspective. Biol Blood Marrow Transplant 2009; 15:1143–1238.

41. National Cancer Institute. Infection. Oral complications of chemotherapy and head/neck radiation (PDQ). http://www.cancer.gov/cancertopics/pdq /supportivecare/oralcomplications/Health Professional/page7. Accessed 26 Sept 2013.

42. Muzyka BC, Epifanio RN. Update on oral fungal infections. Dent Clin North Am 2013;57:561–581.

43. Lerman MA, Laudenbach J, Marty FM, Baden LR, Treister NS. Management of oral infections in cancer patients. Dent Clin North Am 2008;52:129–153.

Clinical Considerations:
What You Can Take Back to Your Practice

What is the effect of osteoporosis on oral health?

Despite physicians' well-meaning attempts to prevent and treat osteoporosis and the drug companies' denials, drug-induced osteonecrosis of the jaws, mostly caused by bisphosphonate therapy prescribed for the treatment of osteoporosis, is a real entity and represents one of the most direct examples of an oral-systemic connection.

Are the drugs used to treat osteoporosis independent risk factors for the development of osteonecrosis of the jaws?

Because only those drugs that impair or kill osteoclasts or represent potent antiangiogenic effects have produced osteonecrosis of the jaws, they prove a singular and independent risk factor for patients, relegating other concomitant drugs and medical conditions to be viewed as contributing comorbidities.

What is the biologic plausibility of the association between the drugs used to treat osteoporosis and osteonecrosis of the jaws?

Because these drugs that cause osteonecrosis of the jaws affect bone that continuously remodels (the alveolar bone is the target bone), dental inflammatory disease, traumatic occlusion, and tooth extractions, all of which require accelerated bone remodeling, remain the most significant initiating events.

Does the delivery of oral health care to patients with osteoporosis contribute to reduced incidence of osteonecrosis of the jaws?

For dental practitioners, preventive measures and maintaining oral health should be primary goals. Improving oral health and preventive dentistry can result in as much as a 75% reduction in the incidence of drug-induced osteonecrosis of the jaws.

Is it safe to provide dental care to patients being treated for osteoporosis?

In the patient taking an oral bisphosphonate or intravenous bisphosphonates for osteoporosis, noninvasive dental restorative procedures are safe at all times. For those requiring invasive surgical procedures, the judicial use of drug holidays with the consent of the prescribing physician and/or the morning fasting serum C-terminal telopeptide test can allow these procedures to be accomplished with predictable outcomes and proven safety.

What is the appropriate message to give to the public about the association between the drugs used to treat osteoporosis and osteonecrosis of the jaws?

The public needs to be aware that the mouth is as much a part of the body as the hip and leg bones and that diseases, aging, and medications that affect the hip bone or other bones also affect the jaw bone. Patients would be best served by asking their physicians about the short-term and long-term safety of any drugs they may be required to take. Above all, clinicians should seek out the current FDA recommendations concerning bisphosphonate therapy, which requires retesting after 3 years of treatment, and discourage treatment continued for more than 5 years.

12 Osteoporosis: Its Controversies, Treatment, and Complications

Robert E. Marx, DDS

Osteoporosis literally means "porous bone." However, the disease has a biologic definition and a clinical working definition. The biologic definition is the weakening of bone caused by thinning of the bone cortex and the trabecular struts between the cortices. This is an age-related phenomenon more than an actual disease and is similar to the loss of muscle mass and the thinning of scalp hair that are experienced with age.

The clinical definition was established by the World Health Organization (WHO),[1] which defines osteoporosis via a bone mineral density (BMD) measurement obtained through a dual-energy x-ray absorption (DEXA) scan. The scan gives a value expressed in milligrams or grams per deciliter, similar to the Hounsfield units more familiar to dental practitioners. A diagnosis of osteoporosis is made when the BMD value is 2.5 standard deviations less than the arbitrary norm, which has been set as the mean BMD of a 22-year-old white woman. If the BMD value is only 1.0 to 2.4 standard deviations less than this arbitrary norm, a diagnosis of osteopenia is made. Osteopenia is not considered a disease by the WHO.

The standard deviations of the BMD are referred to as a *T-score*. Because T-scores related to osteopenia and osteoporosis are always lower than the arbitrary norm, they are usually negative values (–2.0, –2.5, –3.4, etc). The WHO[1] defines normal as a T-score greater than –1.0 (–0.5, +1.0, +1.5, etc) and osteopenia as a T-score between –1.0 and –2.5. A T-score of less than –2.5 is considered osteoporosis, and an individual with a history of a "fragility fracture" (nontraumatic fracture) and a T-score of less than –2.5 is considered to have severe osteoporosis (Fig 12-1).

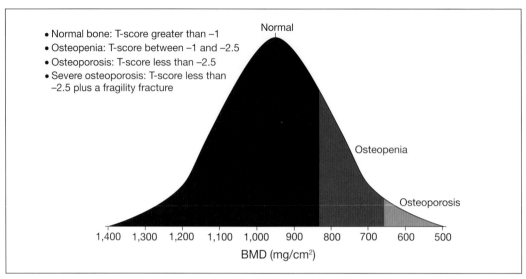

- Normal bone: T-score greater than –1
- Osteopenia: T-score between –1 and –2.5
- Osteoporosis: T-score less than –2.5
- Severe osteoporosis: T-score less than –2.5 plus a fragility fracture

Normal

Osteopenia

Osteoporosis

1,400   1,300   1,200   1,100   1,000   900   800   700   600   500

BMD (mg/cm²)

Fig 12-1 WHO's bell curve defining normal bone mineral density, osteopenia, osteoporosis, and T-scores. (Reprinted from Marx[2] with permission.)

Mechanism of Osteoporosis

Bone remodeling is actually bone renewal. Once an osteoblast becomes entrapped in its own mineral matrix to become an osteocyte, it lives for about 180 days.[3] During that life span, it prevents resorption of its mineral matrix by secreting osteoprotegerin (OPG), which inhibits the signaling mechanism for osteoclasts to resorb bone.[4] The osteoclast signaling mechanism is a protein called *receptor activator of nuclear factor κB ligand* (RANKL).[5] RANKL is secreted by the osteoclast itself and sometimes even by osteoblasts. Young osteocytes secrete sufficient amounts of OPG to inhibit the resorptive signaling effects of RANKL. However, as osteocytes age toward the end of their 180-day life span, their ability to secret OPG declines, and RANKL stimulation tips the scale toward bone resorption[6] (Fig 12-2). In a similar mechanism, necrotic bone, which secretes no OPG, is either resorbed or sequestered, depending on the amount of necrotic bone present.

New bone formation results directly from this resorption. As the osteoclast resorbs the mineral matrix of bone, it releases the bone morphogenetic protein and insulinlike growth factors 1 and 2 originally embedded into it by the osteoblast that formed the bone[7] (Fig 12-3). These growth and differentiating factors act on the local resident and some circulating stem cells as well as adjacent osteoblasts to lay down replacement bone. Osteoporosis develops because, after the age of 22 years, this replacement is not in a 1:1 ratio with resorption.

Epidemiologic Factors

Why is osteoporosis more common in postmenopausal women? The effect of the less than 1:1 ratio of new bone formation to resorption is small but equal between men and women prior to menopause. During and mostly after menopause, women exhibit a much greater rate of BMD decline than do men because estrogen production decreases in menopausal women, and estrogen is required for osteoblastic differentiation.[8] In the absence of estrogen, mesenchymal stem cells and osteoprogenitor cells undergo more lipoblastic differentiation. This

Fig 12-2 *(a and b)* When concentrations of RANKL are greater than concentrations of OPG, osteoclasts are stimulated to resorb bone *(arrow in a)*. Several osteoclasts that recognize decreased OPG secretion from old bone initiate bone resorption *(arrow in a)* but are unable to resorb younger adjacent bone *(double arrows in a)* because of its higher level of OPG secretion. BMP, bone morphogenetic protein; ILG, insulin-like growth factor. (Reprinted from Marx[2] with permission.)

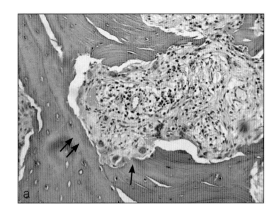

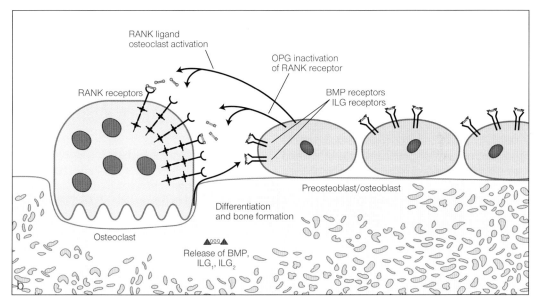

Fig 12-3 Resorption of the bone mineral matrix releases growth and differentiation factors to regenerate bone. BMP, bone morphogenetic protein; ILG, insulinlike growth factor. (Reprinted from Marx[2] with permission.)

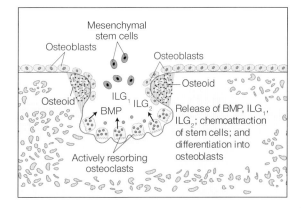

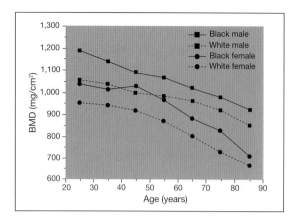

Fig 12-4 WHO graph of declining bone mineral densities related to age, sex, and race. (Reprinted from Marx[2] with permission.)

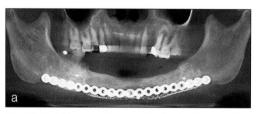 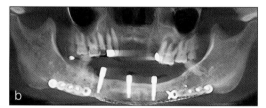

Fig 12-5 (a) Less mature graft prior to functional loading of the dental implants. (b) Graft density indicative of maturity has increased after implants have been loaded with an overdenture.

phenomenon has been graphically observed as fatty marrow in various jaw surgeries and ilium bone harvests for jaw reconstruction.

Although menopause is the most significant factor leading to osteoporosis, genetics, age, activity (functional bone loading), and nutrition also play a role. Most dental practitioners and orthopedic surgeons who perform surgeries on bone know that some individuals possess denser bone than do others. The WHO also recognized this difference related to racial characteristics and sex.[1] That is, black individuals are noted to have higher BMD and T-scores than their age-matched white counterparts, and men of any race or culture have higher BMD values than do women of the same age and race or culture (Fig 12-4).

BMD declines with age in both men and women of any race. However, the rate of decline is nearly equal among races and the sexes until menopause, after which the rate of BMD decline is much greater in women of all races

(see Fig 12-4). Clinical experience suggests that osteoporosis is clinically more common and more significant in white women and Asian women, although this latter group has not been as thoroughly studied.

Because bone is primarily type I collagen into which calcium hydroxyapatite crystals are placed, along with trace amounts of the aforementioned growth factors, the nutrition that supports bone renewal, and therefore resists osteoporosis, centers around protein, calcium, and 25-hydroxyvitamin D. Therefore, adequate dietary protein must be included in the diet, and supplements of calcium and hydroxyvitamin D are often recommended. However, osteoporosis is more a problem of bone turnover than mineral content, which underscores the limited value of the BMD value and of dietary calcium and vitamin D intake.

There is little doubt that activity also plays a key role in BMD, because functionally stimulated bone will tend to respond by thickening the

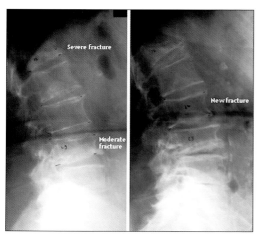

Fig 12-6 Compression fractures of the vertebral bodies, called *spinal fractures*, are attributable to osteoporosis. (Reprinted from Marx[2] with permission.)

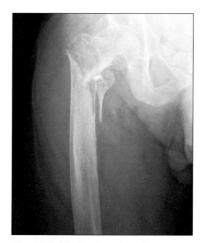

Fig 12-7 Hip fracture from trauma occurs at the trochanteric level. Many individuals are thought to be predisposed to such fractures because of osteoporosis.

cortex and the marrow trabecular network. This is graphically illustrated by astronauts, who lose up to 30% of their bone mass after a prolonged stay in a zero-gravity environment but regain almost all of it with their return to Earth's gravity. Dental practitioners also witness this correlation after functional loading of dental implants. In such cases, the trabecular bone density increases once the implants are restored; this increase is especially evident when the implants are placed in a bone graft (Fig 12-5).

Treatment Strategies and Drugs

The fundamental goal in treating osteoporosis is prevention of fractures. The two skeletal locations of interest related to osteoporosis-linked fractures are the "spine," which is actually the vertebral bodies, and the "hip," which is actually the neck of the femur around the greater and lesser trochanters (Figs 12-6 and 12-7).

Bisphosphonates

The treatment strategy of bisphosphonates is antiresorption, which sounds positive on superficial inspection. That is, preventing resorption in theory should prevent the bone from becoming porous. However, this strategy ignores the known resorption-renewal cycle of bone. Bisphosphonates therefore actually reduce new bone formation and leave old bone in place. Over time and with long-term bisphosphonate use, this old bone becomes brittle and actually more prone to fracture. This phenomenon has become apparent to the dental community as bisphosphonate-induced osteonecrosis of the jaws[9–12] (BIONJ; Figs 12-8 and 12-9) and to orthopedic surgeons as nontraumatic subtrochanteric fractures of the femur[13–17] (Fig 12-10).

A compilation of the studies sponsored by Merck (manufacturer of Fosamax) and independent studies confirmed a bone-strengthening effect for 3 years, after which the therapeutic effect of oral bisphosphonates ceases.[18] Recognizing this, the US Food and Drug Adminis-

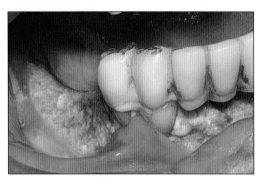

Fig 12-8 Bisphosphonate-induced osteonecrosis of the mandible.

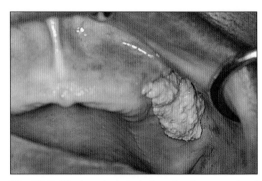

Fig 12-9 Bisphosphonate-induced osteonecrosis of the maxilla.

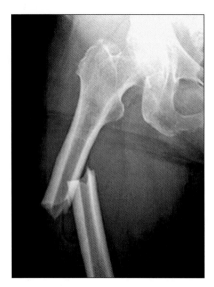

Fig 12-10 Fracture of the midshaft of the femur (subtrochanteric fracture) caused by alendronate. (Reprinted from Marx[2] with permission.)

tration (FDA), as of September 2011, recommended stronger warnings in the product label as well as a limitation on the duration of therapy to the manufacturers of oral bisphosphonates.[18] Specifically, the FDA recommended that physicians treating osteoporosis patients reevaluate them at 3 years and consider withdrawing the drug at or before 5 years.

The jaws are the target for exposed bone osteonecrosis because of the fundamental ac-

tion of bisphosphonates, which is to achieve antiresorption by impairing and mostly killing osteoclasts and their precursors in bone marrow.[19] Because the alveolar bone remodels more and faster than any other bone in the adult skeleton as a result of dental occlusion and the wearing of dentures, BIONJ always begins in the alveolar bone or the surface of a torus, which is another rapidly remodeling bony structure.[20] The midshaft of the femur is another area of significant bone remodeling in the adult skeleton because it is the point of the bending moment during walking. Therefore, bisphosphonate-caused fractures of the femur are always located in this unique area, which does not normally experience fractures from trauma; those occur mostly at the trochanteric level[14,15] (see Fig 12-7).

The oral bisphosphonate drugs used to treat osteoporosis are residronate (Actonel, Warner Chilcott; Atelvia, Warner Chilcott), 35 mg/wk; ibandronate (Boniva, Genentech), 150 mg/mo, which averages out to be 35 mg/wk; and alendronate (Fosamax, Merck), 70 mg/wk. Alendronate is also now available as a generic. Each of these is a nitrogen-containing bisphosphonate that has sufficient potency to treat osteoporosis and to cause BIONJ.

Each pill is irritating to the esophagus and has a high incidence of esophagitis.[21] This is why individuals are instructed to take the pill with two full glasses of water and to remain upright for 1 hour after taking the medication. It is also why the initial daily doses of Actonel and Fosamax created such significant noncompliance that each manufacturer switched to a weekly dose and Boniva was introduced as a monthly dose. This was later followed by the introduction of zoledronic acid (Reclast, Novartis) as an annual intravenous (IV) dose.

The IV form of zoledronic acid, Reclast, is the same as the commercial drug Zometa (Novartis), which is administered as a monthly IV 4-mg dose to limit bony resorption from metastatic cancer deposits in bone and reduce the hypercalcemia of malignancy.[22] As Reclast, zoledronic acid is also administered intravenously, as a once-yearly 5-mg dose, to prevent the development of esophagitis and avoid the resultant noncompliance.[23] Reclast was introduced in 2008 and has already caused cases of BIONJ. Its optimal dose over time and length of therapy have not been stated by the manufacturer.

Denosumab

Denosumab (Prolia, Amgen) has the same strategy as bisphosphonates, that is, prevention of fractures by an antiresorptive mechanism. Like bisphosphonates, denosumab targets the osteoclast and prevents its ability to resorb bone, thereby also preventing new bone formation. Therefore, denosumab has the same disadvantage as the bisphosphonates of retaining old bone, which is initially stronger but with time becomes brittle. This phenomenon is likely to lead to exposed jawbone and possibly to femur fractures.[14,15]

Denosumab is administered as a subcutaneous injection of 60 mg once every 6 months. Prolia was introduced in June 2010. The optimal length of therapy is not known or stated by the manufacturer, but cases of osteonecrosis of the jaws caused by Prolia have already been reported.[24]

Prolia's mechanism of antiresorption, and therefore anti–bone renewal, is somewhat different than that of the bisphosphonates. Whereas bisphosphonates are an internal metabolic poison, Prolia is a monoclonal antibody that inhibits RANKL and thereby impairs the ability of the osteoclast to resorb bone.

Raloxifene

Raloxifene (Evista, Lilly) is a selective estrogen receptor modulator.[25] It is not a bisphosphonate, and therefore no esophagitis or other complications are associated with swallowing the pill. Evista comes as a 60-mg oral capsule to be taken once daily without the precautions required of a bisphosphonate. It has not been known to cause osteonecrosis of the jaws or femur fractures. Because it acts on estrogen receptors in bone in a stimulatory manner, like estrogen itself it promotes osteoblastic differentiation and therefore maintains bone in postmenopausal women in a manner similar to that achieved by the natural estrogen of premenopausal women.[26]

Additionally, raloxifene acts on the estrogen receptors in breast tissue in an inhibitory manner, thus providing some protective measure against invasive breast cancer. This breast cancer–preventive aspect has been related as equivalent to that of the chemotherapy drug docetaxel (Taxotere, Sanofi), and raloxifene has gained FDA clearance for this benefit as well.[27]

Recombinant human parathyroid hormone 1-34

Recombinant human parathyroid hormone 1-34 (rhPTH 1-34, also known as *teriparatide*; Forteo, Lilly) is a recombinant protein that represents the active amino acid sequence of human para-thyroid hormone. Although naturally secreted human parathyroid hormone is known to stimu-late osteoclast-mediated bone resorption, daily microdoses of 20 μg paradoxically stimulate osteoblasts to secrete new osteoid instead. Therefore, rhPTH 1-34 is vastly different in its osteoporosis strategy than bisphosphonates and denosumab. While bisphosphonates and deno-sumab essentially retain old bone, rhPTH 1-34 produces new bone. Therefore, it actually in-creases bone mass, not just BMD.[28]

Forteo is administered as a subcutaneous in-jection of 20 μg daily. It has been cleared by the FDA for three cycles of 28 days each for maxi-mum effect. Its specific FDA-cleared indication is for severe osteoporosis; therefore, it is usually not prescribed for osteopenia or prevention of osteoporosis.

rhPTH 1-34 has not been associated with osteonecrosis of the jaws. However, in some animal models, high doses and long-term use have been associated with cancer development.[29] Although such cancer development has not oc-curred above background rates in humans, its treatment sequences are limited to three 28-day cycles.

Salmon calcitonin

Salmon calcitonin (Miacalcin, Novartis; Forti-cal, Upsher-Smith) comes as a nasal spray and a subcutaneous injection, each delivering 200 IU of synthetic calcitonin for once-daily use. A synthetic of the salmon calcitonin molecule, it is more potent and has a much longer duration of action than mammalian calcitonin.[30]

As do native human calcitonin, the bisphos-phonates, and the denosumab drugs, salmon calcitonin exerts an antiresorptive effect on bone by depressing osteoclast function and reducing their numbers. Therefore, its overall effect is the retention of existing bone at the expense of bone renewal. Salmon calcitonin differs from the bisphosphonates in one critical area: It does not have the long 11-year half-life in bone as do all bisphosphonates.[31] Instead, it is readily metab-olized and therefore does not accumulate in bone.

Most important is a relatively new warning concerning salmon calcitonin by the FDA. As recently as April 15, 2013, the FDA published their review of all the safety data related to salmon calcitonin and identified a small but significant overall increased cancer risk from a background rate of 0.7% to 2.4% (a 3.4-fold increase) with long-term use.[32] The FDA recom-mended limiting administration of salmon cal-citonin to no more than 3 months and stated that the benefits of salmon calcitonin did not outweigh the risk of its use in treatment of os-teoporosis.

Vitamin D and calcium

Calcium supplements and 25-hydroxyvitamin D (the activated form of vitamin D) together are the mainstay of supplements to treat osteope-nia and in some cases osteoporosis. It is usually recommended that they be taken as a supple-ment with all the other osteoporosis medica-tions as well. They are the inorganic building blocks of bone but do not by themselves pro-mote the synthesis of type I collagen, which is the organic building block of bone. Therefore, dietary protein intake is as important as vitamin D and calcium.

Dietary calcium intake is usually adequate or close to adequate. The daily requirement of cal-cium is 1,000 mg. The daily requirement of vita-min D is 800 IU. The daily recommended intake of protein is 4 g in women and 5 g in men.

Discussion

From a bone science perspective, it must be accepted that an age-related reduction in bone mass does occur in most everyone. However, in most people—children, young adults, men, and women, including postmenopausal women—

this reduction does not reach a critical level that causes a fracture without an episode of significant trauma. No doubt many people, especially postmenopausal women, may benefit from osteoporosis treatment. However, the BMD value generated by a DEXA scan is only a surrogate test that does not even correlate to fracture risk and measures the wrong thing. Therefore, the decisions as to who will actually benefit from osteoporosis treatment and what treatment is best are largely left to individual prescribers and the many influences placed on them.

Additionally, bisphosphonates and denosumab represent poor long-term strategies to prevent osteoporosis-related fractures, and alendronate (Fosamax) in particular has actually caused femur fractures and jaw fractures. Raloxifene and rhPTH 1-34 represent an improved strategy to treat osteoporosis via drug therapy. However, raloxifene is less popular than the bisphosphonates and has not been studied or cleared to prevent hip fractures. Forteo is limited at this time to treatment of individuals with severe osteoporosis, leaving bisphosphonates as the mainstay drug therapy for osteoporosis prevention and treatment with exercise, vitamin D, calcium, and an adequate protein diet as the main alternative.

Suffice it to say that fewer individuals actually require drug treatment than are currently receiving it. At this time, the current FDA recommendation of limiting drug therapy to 3 years, after which continued treatment is indicated only if retesting shows that the osteoporosis has worsened, is a reasonable approach until more definitive data or better long-term treatments become available.

Osteoporosis: Clinical Disease or Aging Process?

As a disease entity, osteoporosis today is mired in confusion, controversy, and competition. There seem to be two camps significantly divided as to whether osteoporosis represents a true dis-ease or an aging process and whether drug treatment or exercise and nutrition are the best means of preventing fractures. Those in the camp advocating drug therapy produce a large number of statistical extrapolations as facts that, if taken as accurate, recommend that osteoporosis begins and occurs in children and develops in men as well as in premenopausal women.[33,34] Those groups are not traditionally known to suffer from signs or symptoms of osteoporosis, yet strong proponents of drug therapy suggest drug treatments for this population as well and therefore for nearly everyone.

Those in the nutrition camp counter by relating that low bone density is an aging process, not a disease; they use the analogy of skin laxity and a reduction in muscle mass seen in every human as he or she ages. They also contend that low bone density does not equate to an increase in fracture risk but that poor bone quality does, which undermines many of the drug therapies currently in place.[35]

Both camps are fueled by the large revenues tied to each industry. Osteoporosis drugs represent a US$17 billion per year market, and the exercise, nutritional supplement, and diet control market generates an equal amount.

Caught in the middle of this argument are the public, many of the physicians who are not committed to either camp, and, of course, the dental profession, which must prevent and treat the continually growing number of cases of what is now referred to by the American Medical Association as *drug-induced osteonecrosis of the jaws* (DIONJ).[36]

The case for primary drug therapy

In advocating for the advantages of drug therapy for osteoporosis, bone and mineral organizations, osteoporosis organizations, physicians, and other interests have cited the following statistics[37,38]:

1. Some 50% of women older than 50 years will suffer an osteoporosis-related fracture in their lifetime.

2. Osteoporosis causes 1.5 million fractures every year in the United States.
3. Among women aged 50 to 59 years, 58% have low bone mass, and this percentage increases each year.
4. In women older than 45 years, osteoporosis accounts for more days spent in the hospital than many other diseases, including diabetes, myocardial infarction, and breast cancer.
5. The national direct expenditures for osteoporosis-related fractures are US$14 billion each year.
6. Osteoporosis has been called a "pediatric disease with geriatric consequences."
7. More than 80% of all fractures in people older than 50 years are caused by osteoporosis.
8. Approximately 28% of women and 37% of men who suffer a hip fracture will die within the following year.
9. In the United States today, 10 million individuals have osteoporosis, and 34 million more have low bone mass, placing them at risk for this disease.
10. More than 2 million American men suffer from osteoporosis, and millions more are at risk. Each year, 80,000 men have a hip fracture, and one-third of these die within 1 year.

The case for nutritional and diet therapy

Those in favor of nutritional and diet therapy for management of bone density loss point out the flaws in the aforementioned statistics and make the case that treating an arbitrary standard of bone mineral density is the wrong strategy[39,40]:

1. The United States Surgeon General reports that only 17% of women older than 50 years of age will develop a hip fracture and that the 50% claim comes from incidental radiographic findings of reduced vertebral size unassociated with symptoms but recorded as a fracture.
2. Advocates of nutritional and diet therapy further claim that so-called osteoporosis-caused fractures are actually caused by

falls and other injuries and that a causal effect of osteoporosis has not been proven. This claim is supported by a multicenter European study published in the *British Medical Journal*.[41]
3. "Low bone mass" is not low bone mass at all but low BMD as measured by the DEXA scan, which was developed by Merck, the originator and manufacturer of alendronate (Fosamax), who set the mark of a −2.5 T-score as the firm diagnosis of osteoporosis.[42] The low bone mass as measured by the DEXA scan has been studied by the WHO, which found that women's maximum bone mass occurs around the age of 22 years and set this value as normal. However, nearly everyone over the age of 30 years will naturally have a lower bone mass than at age 22 years and certainly most women over the age 50 years will as well. Furthermore, the BMD does not measure bone quality and does not take into consideration vitamin D levels, steroid history, vitamin K levels, muscle strength, activity level, urine pH, and acidifying drinks and diet.
4. Osteoporosis by itself does not require hospitalization, only the fractures do. If falls and other injuries actually cause these fractures, the actual hospital stays cannot be attributed to osteoporosis. Even the length of hospital stays are found to be related to the many comorbid diseases in this age group and not osteoporosis.
5. While the cost of treating fractures is US$14 billion each year, the expenditures on osteoporosis drugs are US$17 billion, and yet patients taking these drugs still experience fractures. This argument is once again predicated on the fact that osteoporosis causes the fractures, not falls or other injuries that would fracture a bone regardless of drug therapy. The author would be in agreement with this point, as he has followed 104 patients with DIONJ caused by oral bisphosphonates, 14 (13.5%) of whom fractured a bone or the jaw in a fall even though they had been taking an oral bisphosphonate.
6. All diseases can be said to begin in childhood and adolescence. Heart disease and hypertension in particular have been shown

Box 12-1	Measures to reduce the probability of falls in individuals older than 50 years

- Adopt exercise training.
- Build muscle strength.
- Improve home lighting.
- Reduce the use of sleep medications, antidepressants, and other medications that produce drowsiness.
- Firmly secure carpets and throw rugs.
- Add grab bars to shower and bathtub areas and increase the surface texture of floors to prevent slipping.

to follow this epidemiology. This should not be an indication to start drug therapy.

7. Attributing 80% of fractures in people older than 50 years to osteoporosis is an estimate and assumes once again that the osteoporosis is the cause of rather than a coincidence in the fracture. This statistic is also refuted by another multicenter randomized prospective unsponsored study from Europe.[43]

8. The high rate of death each year after a hip fracture in both men and women is not related to osteoporosis but rather to the comorbidities of the diseases of aging, such as heart disease, diabetes, and arthritis, that caused them to fall in the first place.

9. The large numbers of individuals carrying a diagnosis of osteoporosis and/or low bone mass is due to the low threshold values of the BMD set by the proprietary drug company and later adopted by the WHO. The BMD does not consider bone quality, which is protein related.

10. If 80,000 men develop hip fractures caused by osteoporosis and one-third die each year, that would mean that more than 26,000 men die each year of osteoporosis, that is, 3 times more than die of oral pharyngeal cancer and greater than 3 times more than die of leukemia and kidney, thyroid, and esophageal cancers, among others. This is highly unlikely.

Proponents of nutrition- and exercise-based treatment of osteoporosis instead recommend daily exercise; administration of calcium, vitamin D, and vitamin K supplements; and a normal to high-protein diet. They discourage ingestion of alcohol and highly acidic drinks, particularly phosphoric acid–containing soft drinks. They embrace the European studies[41,43] that recommend a number of measures to reduce the probability of falls in those older than 50 years of age (Box 12-1).

Osteopenia/Osteoporosis and the Dental Profession

The dental profession is indirectly and directly affected by the osteoporosis controversy. While treatment is mostly a matter between these groups with divergent opinions and even data, members of the dental profession need to understand the process of bone aging and osteoporosis and the varying treatments that patients may take. Dentists also need to be able to understand the medical language concerning osteoporosis and know how to communicate with physicians who are treating osteoporosis.

More directly, osteoporosis and its treatment affect the type of bone in which dentists place dental implants today and may cause DIONJ.

Related to bone type, almost all dentists who place dental implants know that the maxilla in general and the posterior mandible have less trabecular bone density. That is, these areas consist mostly of type III or type IV bone and indeed worsen with age. These sites and advanced age of the patient are associated with a slightly reduced primary stability and a slightly greater implant failure rate.

Overcoming this reduced trabecular bone density and even combating periodontal bone loss with the use of bisphosphonates were once of great research interest among periodontal researchers.[44] However, with the identification of the bisphosphonates found to be the cause of DIONJ as well as a decrease in manufacturers' sponsorship of such research, few applications have emerged. Instead, postmenopausal women must accept the possibility of a slightly higher failure rate if dental implants are placed or undergo a site improvement or site preparation procedure. Today, this may take the form of socket grafting, ridge splitting procedures with grafting, segmental distraction, sinus augmentation, or horizontal or vertical ridge augmentation using the provider's preferred grafting material.

Drug-Induced Osteo-necrosis of the Jaws

Today, most every dental professional is aware of jaw osteonecrosis caused by IV and oral bisphosphonates, and more are becoming aware of cases caused by denosumab. DIONJ was first introduced to the dental and medical profession by Marx and Stern in 2002.[45] The first publications in the scientific literature occurred in September 2003,[46] and two more followed by the end of that year.[47,48] A decade later, two textbooks and more than 1,400 publications have appeared, relating more than 15,000 cases of DIONJ, attesting to the epidemic proportions predicted in the first publication.[46] Today, dental professionals must be keenly aware of the mechanism of DIONJ, the factors that initiate it, and preventive and treatment measures for patients treated for osteopenia or osteoporosis.

The current drugs that place osteopenia and osteoporosis patients at risk for DIONJ are the following:

- Orally administered bisphosphonates: alendronate (Fosamax and generic equivalents), residronate (Actonel and Atelvia), and ibandronate (Boniva)
- Intravenously administered bisphosphonate: zoledronate (Reclast)
- Subcutaneously injected denosumab (Prolia)

All of these drugs impair osteoclastic bone resorption and therefore bone renewal, thereby leading to the retention of old bone and a reduction in bone turnover. Because the alveolar bone turns over faster and to a greater degree than any other bone in the adult skeleton,[49] it is the focal point for the osteonecrosis caused by these drugs.

Among the oral bisphosphonates, alendronate is the drug linked to 96% of cases of DIONJ; in contrast, residronate and ibandronate are linked to 3% and 1% of cases, respectively.[2] This is mostly due to the fact that alendronate is prescribed at twice the dose of all other bisphosphonates (70 mg/wk) while having the same absorption, distribution, and potency of the others.

Although zoledronate in the form of Reclast is new and is administered in a dose of 5 mg IV only once yearly for osteoporosis, it has already caused several cases of DIONJ in this author's experience. This is because the half-life in bone of 11 years is the same for all the bisphosphonates,[31] and the IV infusion loads the bone 140 times more than any oral bisphosphonate.[2] Therefore, dental professionals must realize that although some cases of DIONJ may occur sooner, the significant risk of DIONJ begins after about 3 years of weekly dosing with an oral bisphosphonate and at about the fourth yearly dose with IV Reclast. Those patients whose medication was changed to Reclast after taking an oral bisphosphonate are at risk for DIONJ before the fourth dose.

Denosumab (Prolia), a RANKL inhibitor, does not seem to bind to bone or to accumulate in bone as do bisphosphonates. Therefore, discontinuation as a "drug holiday" becomes a useful tool for the clinician with this drug as it does with oral bisphosphonates. Drug holidays are useful in patients taking oral bisphosphonates because only 0.64% of any oral bisphosphonate is absorbed through the intestines into the circulation.[21,22,50] This amounts to a slower accumulation in bone and a gradual toxic death to osteoclasts. Therefore, during a drug holiday, the bone marrow is able to replace lost osteoclasts to some degree and repopulate the osteoclast population.

Prevention

When given to adults, these antiosteoclastic drugs do not become bound to tooth structure. Therefore, caries removal, direct restorations, placement of crown and bridge restorations, nonsurgical root canal therapy, dental prophylaxis, and fabrication of removable partial and complete dentures are safe to perform at any time. In fact, it is advisable to accomplish these more preventive dental procedures in these patients to prevent the need for alveolar bone surgeries in the future. The dental practitioner must not defer or neglect needed dental care because of the fear of DIONJ.

For patients requiring surgery within the alveolar bone (tooth extraction, alveoloplasty, dental implants, osseous periodontal surgery, and apical resective root canal therapy) and who have taken an oral bisphosphonate or Prolia for less than 3 years, it is reasonable to assess the bone turnover suppression by requesting a morning fasting serum C-terminal telopeptide (CTX) test. Several studies have shown that a value of 150 pg/mL or greater is consistent with alveolar bone healing.[51–53] If the value shown by the CTX test is greater that 150 pg/mL, the planned alveolar bone surgery can be performed. The prescribing physician should be asked to approve a 3-month drug holiday to cover the healing period.

If the CTX value is less than 150 pg/mL, it is advisable to ask the prescribing physician to approve a drug holiday before the planned alveolar bone surgery is performed. The length of the drug holiday will depend on the drug dose and the length of time the patient took the drug.

Most patients taking these drugs for less than 3 years will either return a CTX value greater than 150 pg/mL initially or require a short drug holiday of 3 months or less to gain a value greater than 150 pg/mL.

For patients who have taken an oral bisphosphonate or Prolia for more than 3 years, the initial CTX value is usually less than 150 pg/mL. For such patients, a longer drug holiday is usually necessary; many are required to be as long as 9 months. If the practitioner has no access to obtain a CTX serum test or the patient declines to take one, the author has found that an arbitrary 9-month to 1-year drug holiday will allow alveolar bone healing after a surgical procedure in most cases.

For urgent surgeries in the alveolar bone, such as painful abscesses, bone fractures, or vertical root fractures, it is better to accomplish the needed surgery and request a drug holiday for the following 3 months than to allow the problem to further damage bone, because such damage may very well initiate osteonecrosis in these patients. Of course, it is advisable for the practitioner to obtain informed consent from the patient after outlining the patient's greater risk for developing DIONJ due to the urgent need for alveolar bone surgery in the face of bone healing that has been compromised by the drug in question.

Despite three peer-reviewed studies documenting the clinical utility of a properly performed CTX test[51–53] as well as the use of the CTX or N-terminal telopeptide (NTX) test in almost all of the research studies sponsored by oral bisphosphonate drug companies,[54,55] the value of this test for oral surgical procedures remains controversial. It is curiously missing from the position papers of the American Association of Oral and Maxillofacial Surgeons,[56] the American Dental Association,[57] and the American Society for Bone and Mineral Research.[58] This is likely due to several misapplications of the CTX test and misunderstandings of what is actually tested and what can interfere with its accuracy.

The CTX test measures an eight–amino acid sequence derived from collagen when the osteoclast resorbs bone. Its name comes from the fact that this amino acid sequence is derived from the carboxy terminal end of collagen.

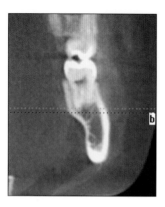

Fig 12-11 The axial loading from molar occlusion on the mandible is directed toward the lingual cortex, resulting in a site of predilection for drug-induced osteonecrosis in the osteoporotic patient. (Reprinted from Marx[2] with permission.)

A less-consistent serum test from the amino terminal end of collagen, the NTX, is a less frequently used alternative test.

Some of the misapplications arise from the fact that cancers split off collagen fragments that cross-react with this test, resulting in abnormally high values. Therefore, use of the CTX is inappropriate in cases of IV bisphosphonate–induced osteonecrosis of the jaw where the bisphosphonate was prescribed to treat metastatic cancer deposits in bone or hypercalcemia of malignancy; such misuse detracts from valid use of the CTX test in noncancerous patients. Additionally, patients who have received methotrexate, which inhibits bone marrow stem cells, and/or steroids, which inhibit collagen synthesis, will have falsely low CTX values because of the reduction of collagen in their bone. Therefore, the CTX test is not to be relied on in such patients.

One other phenomenon may also be noted: Patients beginning a drug holiday after 7 years or more of an oral bisphosphonate will begin with very low CTX values; this will be followed by a rise in values as the drug holiday progresses. However, a paradoxical decrease in the CTX value may occur as the drug holiday progresses further. This decrease results from a recovery of the bone marrow osteoclast precursors, which produce osteoclasts that begin resorbing bone. As they do, they die off and rupture, releasing unmetabolized bisphosphonate with its high affinity for bone. The released bisphosphonate then is taken up by the bone again, suppressing the CTX value. However, a 9-month to 1-year drug holiday will restore alveolar bone healing in these individuals.

Diagnosis and treatment

An updated definition for DIONJ can be derived from the definitions used by most dental associations for bisphosphonate-related, bisphosphonate-induced, or bisphosphonate-associated osteonecrosis of the jaws: *Exposed bone in the maxilla or mandible that fails to heal after 8 weeks in a patient who is receiving a systemic antiresorptive drug and who has not received radiotherapy directly to the jaws.*

About 50% of exposures occur spontaneously; the remainder result after a trauma to the jaws, usually tooth removal or other alveolar bone surgery. About 50% will also occur in the lingual cortex in the molar region of the mandible. This has been attributed to the axial loading forces that are directed at this cortex and to the increased forces on molar teeth during occlusion (Fig 12-11).

Staging of DIONJ

Previous staging systems for osteonecrosis of the jaws have incorrectly included pain as a

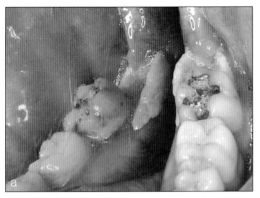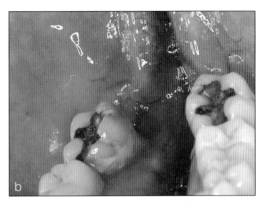

Fig 12-12 *(a)* Exposed bone has resulted from 5.5 years of alendronate therapy for osteopenia. *(b)* Resolution of exposed bone correlated to a 9-month drug holiday and rising CTX values. (Reprinted from Marx[2] with permission.)

major contributor to staging. Because pain associated with DIONJ is the result of secondary infection, the pain changes with antibiotic therapy, the patient's pain tolerance, and the day-to-day activity of the secondary infection. Because any staging system should indicate the severity and extent of the disease regardless of subjective pain, the following staging system is the most appropriate:

- Stage I: Exposed bone limited to one quadrant
- Stage II: Exposed bone involving two quadrants
- Stage III: Exposed bone in three or four quadrants *or* osteolysis to the inferior border *or* a pathologic fracture of the mandible *or* extension into the maxillary sinus

Treatment

The exposed bone represents necrotic bone. If the offending drug is continued, the area of exposed bone is likely to increase, and secondary areas of exposed bone may develop. It is advisable to request a drug holiday from the prescribing physician. The dental practitioner should refrain from instituting the drug holiday directly because osteoporosis therapy is not within the scope of any dental specialty. Studies have shown that a drug holiday of 9 months will result in a spontaneous sequestration and exfoliation of the exposed bone followed by mucosal healing in 50% of cases[2] (Fig 12-12). These cases are usually the smaller areas of exposed bone.

During this drug holiday, clinicians find it useful to prescribe 0.12% chlorhexidine oral rinses three times daily to prevent secondary infection. If a secondary infection does develop, the best antibiotic to prescribe is penicillin VK, 500 mg 4 times daily (or doxycycline, 100 mg once daily, if the patient is allergic to penicillin).

If the exposed bone does not exfoliate after a drug holiday, surgical debridement after a drug holiday of 9 months or after the patient has attained a CTX value greater than 150 pg/mL has been associated with resolution of DIONJ[2] (Fig 12-13). However, such drug holidays and debridement surgeries are not predictable and often are not successful in cancer patients treated with IV bisphosphonates or subcutaneous denosumab (Xgeva, Amgen) because of the 11-year half-life in bone of the bisphosphonates coupled with the 140-times greater bone loading via the IV route and the high dose of denosumab in Xgeva.

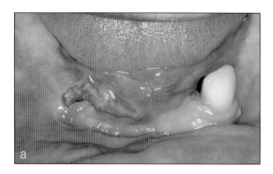
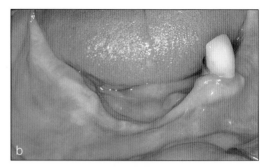
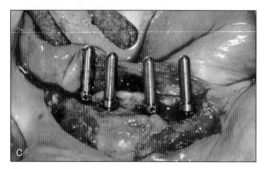
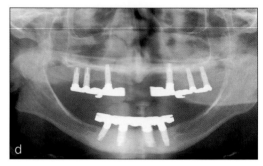

Fig 12-13 Surgical debridement of DIONJ. *(a)* The exposed bone represents bisphosphonate-induced osteonecrosis caused by alendronate. *(b)* A minor office-based debridement that removed the exposed bone after a 9-month drug holiday has resulted in a CTX value greater than 150 pg/mL. *(c)* Implants are placed in the area of previously exposed bone. *(d)* Successful implant placement and long-term outcome (5 years' follow-up) have been achieved because implant placement has followed a 9-month drug holiday and attainment of a CTX value greater than 150 pg/mL. (Parts *b* to *d* reprinted from Marx[2] with permission.)

Long-term use of oral bisphosphonates, especially alendronate, with or without comorbidities (eg, diabetes, cancer, immunosuppression) may result in extensive osteonecrosis (stage III). In the mandible, this destruction of tissue may necessitate a mandibular resection (Fig 12-14). In the anterior maxilla, it may be necessary to perform an alveolar resection (Fig 12-15); in the posterior maxilla, the patient may require an alveolar resection together with a sinus debridement (Fig 12-16). For each of these procedures, a 9-month drug holiday before surgery followed by another 3-month drug holiday during healing has been shown to predictably resolve the DIONJ. If the patient's CTX value rises above 150 pg/mL before the full 9-month drug holiday has ended, the indicated surgery may be accomplished at that time with predictable healing.

It is extremely rare that a prescribing physician will disagree with a drug holiday. If the physician does resist the proposal, the dental team may suggest the use of vitamin D, calcium, and protein or drug therapy with raloxifene or rhPTH 1-34 as an alternative. Additionally, the physi-

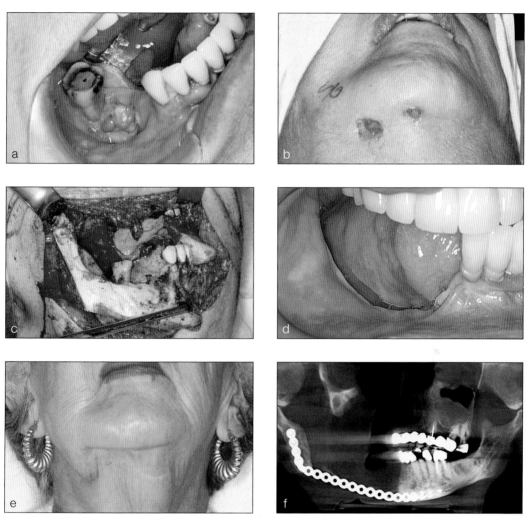

Fig 12-14 Mandibular resection to treat DIONJ. *(a)* Exposed necrotic bone in the mandible represents bisphosphonate-induced osteonecrosis. *(b)* Necrotic bone from bisphosphonate-induced osteonecrosis often becomes secondarily infected. In this case, two cutaneous fistulas have developed. *(c)* A hemimandibulectomy is required to resolve this case of bisphosphonate-induced osteonecrosis. *(d)* The exposed necrotic bone has resolved, and the mucosa has healed after surgery. *(e)* The cutaneous fistulas have also resolved after surgery. *(f)* A long-span titanium plate used to reconstruct the resultant continuity defect has been stable for 4 years.

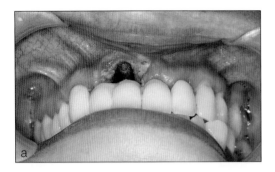
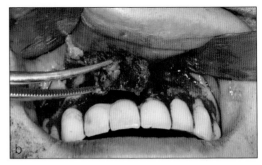
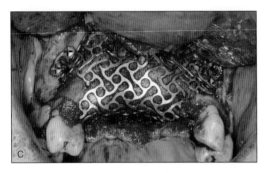
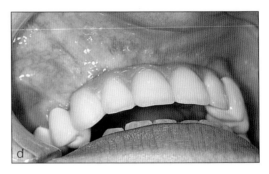
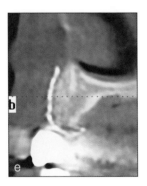

Fig 12-15 Alveolar resection to treat DIONJ. *(a)* Bisphosphonate-induced osteonecrosis of the maxilla is limited to the alveolar bone. *(b)* Necrotic bone is removed after the patient has completed a drug holiday of 9 months and achieved a CTX value greater than 150 pg/mL. *(c)* The resultant alveolar defect is grafted in accordance with in situ tissue engineering principles (platelet-rich plasma, recombinant human bone morphogenetic protein 2, and crushed cancellous freeze-dried allogeneic bone). *(d)* The provisional appliance is made to avoid pressure on the healed graft site. *(e)* The alveolar ridge is fully regenerated after placement of the in situ tissue-engineered graft.

cian can be referred to the article by Black et al.[59] In this multicenter randomized prospective study, discontinuation of a bisphosphonate for 5 years did not result in an extension or worsening of osteoporosis. In addition to the dental utility of drug holidays of 1 year or less to treat or prevent DIONJ, they are well within the limits of proven safety with regard to the course of osteoporosis.[59]

Once DIONJ has been resolved in the patient with osteopenia or osteoporosis, reconstruction of the lost bone is feasible by the usual and individually preferred methods of the practitioner. Where sufficient bone remains to accommodate dental implants, dental implant placements can be accomplished as safely in these patients as in any other patients, provided that the patient does not resume use of one of the drugs known to cause DIONJ (see Fig 12-13).

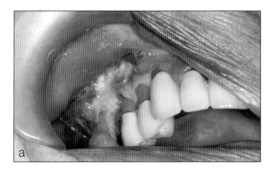
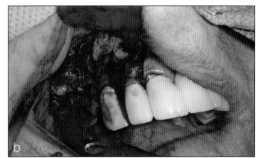
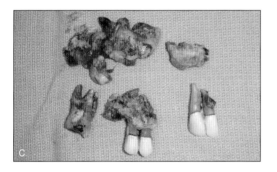
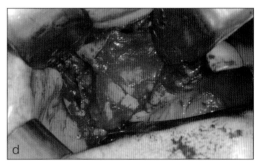
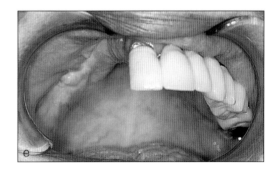

Fig 12-16 Alveolar resection and sinus debridement to treat DIONJ. *(a)* Bisphosphonate-induced osteonecrosis of the maxilla has reached stage III. *(b)* After the patient has completed a 9-month drug holiday and achieved a CTX level greater than 150 pg/mL, bony debridement and aggressive removal of secondarily infected sinus membrane can be accomplished. *(c)* Teeth, necrotic bone, and infected sinus membrane are removed during debridement surgery. *(d)* To assist healing, advancement of the buccal fat pad, with its robust blood supply, is advised before primary mucosal closure is accomplished. *(e)* The surgical site has healed, and the osteonecrosis and sinusitis have resolved.

Conclusion

Opinions conflict as to whether osteoporosis represents a true disease or an aging process. What is known is that an age-related reduction in bone mass occurs in almost everyone and that postmenopausal women are the most severely affected by this loss. Some parties urge the use of drug therapy to prevent fractures that can result from weakened bone, while others suggest that better nutrition and increased physical activity are the best way to improve bone health.

Some drug therapies available for osteoporosis, namely oral and IV bisphosphonates and injectable denosumab, have been found to cause osteonecrosis of the jaws. Dental practitioners must understand osteoporosis and the drugs used to treat it in order to prevent and manage DIONJ. A drug holiday of 9 months will result in spontaneous resolution of DIONJ in about half of cases. For patients in whom invasive treatment such as debridement or resection is needed, a drug holiday of 9 months before and 3 months after the procedure is recommended to aid healing.

References

1. World Health Organization. Assessment of Fracture Risk and Its Application to Screening for Postmenopausal Osteoporosis. Report of a WHO Study Group (WHO Technical Report Series, No. 843). Geneva: World Health Organization, 1994.

2. Marx RE. Oral and Intravenous Bisphosphonate–Induced Osteonecrosis of the Jaws: History, Etiology, Prevention, and Treatment, ed 2. Chicago: Quintessence, 2011.

3. Bringhurst FR, Demay MB, Krane SM, Kronenberg HM. Bone and mineral metabolism in health and disease. In: Jameson JL (ed). Harrison's Endocrinology, ed 3. New York: McGraw-Hill, 2013:384–401.

4. Hofbauer LC, Khosla S, Dunstan CR, Lacey DL, Boyle WJ, Riggs BL. The roles of osteoprotegerin and osteoprotegerin ligand in the paracrine regulation of bone resorption. J Bone Miner Res 2000; 15:2–12.

5. Hofbauer LC, Heufeldes AE. Role of receptor activator of nuclear factor-κB ligand and osteoprotegerin in bone cell biology. J Mol Med (Berl) 2001; 79:243–253.

6. Hofbauer LC, Kühne CA, Viereck V. The OPG/RANKL/RANK system in metabolic bone diseases. J Musculoskelet Neuronal Interact 2004;4:268–275.

7. Wergedal JE, Mohan S, Lundy M, Baylink DJ. Skeletal growth factor and other growth factors known to be present in bone matrix stimulate proliferation and protein synthesis in human bone cells. J Bone Miner Res 1990;5:179–186.

8. Riggs BL. The mechanisms of estrogen regulation of bone resorption. J Clin Investig 2000;106:1203–1204.

9. Ruggiero SL, Mehrotra B, Rosenberg TJ, Engroff SL. Osteonecrosis of the jaws associated with the use of bisphosphonates: A review of 63 cases. J Oral Maxillofac Surg 2004;62:527–534.

10. Marx RE, Sawatari Y, Fortin M, Broumand V. Bisphosphonate-induced exposed bone (osteonecrosis/osteopetrosis) of the jaws: Risk factors, recognition, prevention, and treatment. J Oral Maxillofac Surg 2005;63:1567–1575.

11. Migliorati CA, Schubert MM, Peterson DE, Seneda LM. Bisphosphonate-associated osteonecrosis of mandibular and maxillary bone: An emerging oral complication of supportive cancer therapy. Cancer 2005;104:83–93.

12. Durie BG, Katz M, Crowley J. Osteonecrosis of the jaws and bisphosphonates. N Engl J Med 2005; 353:99–102.

13. Edwards MH, McCrae FC, Young-Min SA. Alendronate-related femoral diaphysis fracture—What should be done to predict and prevent subsequent fracture of the contralateral side? Osteoporos Int 2010;21:701–703.

14. Neviaser AS, Lane JM, Lenart BA, Edobor-Osula F, Lorich DG. Low-energy femoral shaft fractures associated with alendronate use. J Orthop Trauma 2008;22:346–350.

15. Shane E. Evolving data about subtrochanteric fractures and bisphosphonates. N Engl J Med 2010; 362:1825–1827.

16. Park-Wyllie LY, Mamdani MM, Juurlink DN, et al. Bisphosphonate use and the risk of subtrochanteric or femoral shaft fractures in older women. JAMA 2011;305:783–789.

17. Schilcher J, Michaëlsson K, Aspenberg P. Bisphosphonate use and atypical fractures of the femoral shaft. N Engl J Med 2011;364:1728–1737.

18. Food and Drug Administration. Background document for meeting of Advisory Committee for Reproductive Health Drugs and Drug Safety and Risk Management Advisory Committee. 9 Sept 2011. http://www.fda.gov/downloads/Advisory Committees/CommitteesMeetingMaterials/Drugs /DrugSafetyandRiskManagementAdvisory Committee/UCM270958.pdf. Accessed 3 Sept 2013.

19. Eslami B, Zhou S, Van Eekeren I, LeBoff MS, Glowacki J. Reduced osteoclastogenesis and RANKL expression in marrow from women taking alendronate. Calcif Tissue Int 2010;88:272–280.

20. Marx RE. Oral & Intravenous Bisphosphonate–Induced Osteonecrosis of the Jaws: History, Etiology, Prevention, and Treatment. Chicago: Quintessence, 2006.

21. Merck & Co. Fosamax (alendronate sodium) tablets and oral solution. Product information sheet. 2012. http://www.merck.com/product/usa/pi_circulars/f /fosamax/fosamax_pi.pdf. Accessed 18 Nov 2012.

22. Novartis Pharma. Zometa: Zoledronic acid injection. Product Information Sheet. http://www.pharma.us .novartis.com/product/pi/pdf/Zometa.pdf. Accessed 3 Sept 2013.

23. Black DM, Delmas PD, Eastell R, et al. Once-yearly zoledronic acid for treatment of postmenopausal osteoporosis. N Engl J Med 2007;356:1809–1822.

24. Aghaloo TL, Felsenfeld AL, Tetradis S. Osteonecrosis of the jaw in a patient on Denosumab. J Oral Maxillofac Surg 2010;68:959–963.

25. Ozmen B, Kirmaz C, Aydin K, Kafesciler SO, Guclu F, Hekimsoy Z. Influence of the selective oestrogen receptor modulator (raloxifene hydrochloride) on IL-6, TNF-α, TGF-β1 and bone turnover markers in the treatment of postmenopausal osteoporosis. Eur Cytokine Netw 2007;18:148–153.

26. Vogel VG, Costantino JP, Wickerham DL, et al. Effects of tamoxifen vs raloxifene on the risk of developing invasive breast cancer and other disease outcomes: The NSABP Study of Tamoxifen and Raloxifene (STAR) P-2 trial. JAMA 2006;295:2727–2741 [erratum 2007;298:973].

27. Siris ES, Harris ST, Eastell R, et al. Skeletal effects of raloxifene after 8 years: Results from the continuing outcomes relevant to Evista (CORE) study. J Bone Miner Res 2005;20:1514–1524.

28. Neer RM, Arnaud CD, Zanchetta JR, et al. Effect of parathyroid hormone (1-34) on fractures and bone mineral density in postmenopausal women with osteoporosis. N Engl J Med 2001;344:1434–1441.

29. Vahle JL, Sato M, Long GG, et al. Skeletal changes in rats given daily subcutaneous injections of recombinant human parathyroid hormone (1-34) for 2 years and relevance to human safety. Toxicol Pathol 2002;30:312–321.

30. Arnala IO. Salmon calcitonin (Miacalcic NS 200 IU) in prevention of bone loss after hip replacement. Scand J Surg 2012;101:249–254.

31. Lasseter KC, Porras AG, Denker A, Santhanagopal A, Daifotis A. Pharmacokinetic considerations in determining the terminal half lives of bisphosphonates. Clin Drug Investig 2005;25:107–114.

32. In brief: Cancer risk with salmon calcitonin. Med Lett Drugs Ther 2013;55:29.

33. Gafni RI, Baron J. Overdiagnosis of osteoporosis in children due to misinterpretation of dual-energy x-ray absorptiometry (DEXA). J Pediatr 2004;144:253–257.

34. Melton LJ 3rd, Atkinson EJ, O'Connor MK, O'Fallon WM, Riggs BL. Bone density and fracture risk in men. J Bone Miner Res 1998;13:1915–1923.

35. Faulkner KG. Bone matters: Are density increases necessary to reduce fracture risk? J Bone Miner Res 2000;15:183–187.

36. Buck CJ. 2011 ICD-9-CM for Physicians. St Louis: Elsevier/Saunders, 2011:962.

37. International Osteoporosis Foundation: Facts and Statistics. http://www.iofbonehealth.org/facts-statistics. Accessed 28 May 2013.

38. Monson K. eMedTV: Osteoporosis statistics. osteoporosis.emedtv.com/osteoporosis /osteoporosis-statistics.html/. Accessed 3 Sept 2013.

39. Brown SE. Women to Women: Those scary statistics—Banishing fear of fracture with a dose of common sense. www.womentowomen.com /bonehealth/osteoporosis-statistics.aspx. Accessed 3 Sept 2013.

40. Roche JJ, Wenn RT, Sahota O, Moran CG. Effect of comorbidities and postoperative complications on mortality after hip fracture in elderly people: Prospective observational cohort study. BMJ 2005; 331:1374.

41. Järvinen TL, Sievänen H, Khan KM, Heinonen A, Kannus P. Shifting the focus in fracture prevention from osteoporosis to falls. BMJ 2008;336:124–126.

42. Spiegel A. NPR: How a bone disease grew to fit the prescription. http://www.npr.org/templates/story /story.php?storyId=121609815. Accessed 22 Dec 2009.

43. Alonso-Coello P, García-Franco AL, Guyatt C, Moynihan R. Drugs for pre-osteoporosis: Prevention or disease mongering? BMJ 2008;336:126–129.

44. Lane N, Armitage GC, Loomer P, et al. Bisphosphonate therapy improves the outcome of conventional periodontal treatment: Results of a 12-month, randomized, placebo-controlled study. J Periodontol 2005;76:1113–1122.

45. Marx RE, Stern D. Oral and Maxillofacial Pathology: A Rationale for Diagnosis and Treatment. Chicago: Quintessence, 2002.

46. Marx RE. Pamidronate (Aredia) and zoledronate (Zometa) induced avascular necrosis of the jaws: A growing epidemic. J Oral Maxillofac Surg 2003;61: 1115–1117.

47. Migliorati CA. Bisphosphonates and oral cavity avascular bone necrosis. J Clin Oncol 2003;21: 4253–4254.

48. Wang J, Goodger NM, Pogrel MA. Osteonecrosis of the jaws associated with cancer chemotherapy. J Oral Maxillofac Surg 2003;61:1104–1107.

49. Dixon RB, Trickler ND, Garetto LP. Bone turnover in elderly canine mandible and tibia. J Dent Res 1997; 76:2579.

50. Novartis Pharma. Aredia. Pamidronate disodium for injection, for intravenous infusion. Product Information sheet. http://www.pharma.us.novartis.com /product/pi/pdf/aredia.pdf. Accessed 3 Sept 2013.

51. Marx RE, Cillo JE Jr, Ulloa JJ. Oral bisphosphonate-induced osteonecrosis: Risk factors, prediction of risk using serum CTX testing, prevention, and treatment. J Oral Maxillofac Surg 2007;65:2397–2410.

52. Kwon YD, Ohe JY, Kim DY, Chung DJ, Park YD. Retrospective study of two biochemical markers for the risk assessment of oral bisphosphonate-related osteonecrosis of the jaws: Can they be utilized as risk markers? Clin Oral Implants Res 2011;22:100–105.

53. Kunchur R, Need A, Hughes T, Goss A. Clinical investigation of C-terminal cross-linking telopeptide test in prevention and management and management of bisphosphonate-associated osteonecrosis of the jaws. J Oral Maxillofac Surg 2009;67:1167–1173.

54. Bone HG, Hosking D, Devogelaer JP, et al. Ten years' experience with alendronate for osteoporosis in postmenopausal women. N Engl J Med 2004; 350:1189–1199.

55. Black DM, Thompson DE, Bauer DC, et al. Fracture risk reduction with alendronate in women with osteoporosis: The Fracture Intervention Trial. FIT Research Group. J Clin Endocrinol Metab 2000;85: 4118–4124.

56. Ruggiero SL, Dodson TB, Assael LA, et al. American Association of Oral and Maxillofacial Surgeons position paper on bisphosphonate-related osteonecrosis of the jaw—2009 update. J Oral Maxillofac Surg 2009;67(suppl 5):2–12.

57. Migliorati CA, Casiglia J, Epstein J, Jacobsen PL, Siegel MA, Woo SB. Managing the care of patients with bisphosphonate-associated osteonecrosis: An American Academy of Oral Medicine position paper. J Am Dent Assoc 2005;136:1658–1668.

58. Khosla S, Burr D, Cauley J, et al. Bisphosphonate-associated osteonecrosis of the jaw: Report of a task force of the American Society for Bone and Mineral Research. J Bone Miner Res 2007;22:1479–1491.

59. Black DM, Schwartz AV, Ensrud KE, et al. Effects of continuing or stopping alendronate after 5 years of treatment: The Fracture Intervention Trial Long-term Extension (FLEX): A randomized trial. JAMA 2006; 296:2927–2938.

13 Oral Manifestations of Systemic Diseases

Alessandro Villa, DDS, PhD, MPH

Sook-Bin Woo, DMD, MMSc

The general dentist in daily practice encounters a variety of oral mucosal disorders, most of which are straightforward and easy to diagnose. However, even a banal-appearing lesion may be a manifestation of systemic disease or side effect of treatment for systemic disease. Moreover, the oral signs may be the first presentation of a systemic disorder, and the dentist is in a unique position to facilitate an early diagnosis. Early diagnosis and management can often diminish the morbidity associated with a systemic disease, improve well-being, and reduce health care costs.

This chapter presents seven common oral conditions that are encountered in routine general dental practice (Box 13-1). For each condition, the discussion first presents one or two "most likely" diagnoses based on the frequency of occurrence and then offers a detailed description of other conditions that may look similar but represent the oral presentation of a systemic condition or drug effect. The differences in history, clinical findings, and diagnostic tests that may help distinguish between each entity are also presented.

Box 13-1 — Common oral conditions that are encountered in routine general dental practice

Oral ulcers
- Traumatic ulcers
- Recurrent aphthous ulcers/stomatitis
- Aphthous-like ulcers from systemic disease
- Drug-induced oral ulcers
- Viral infections
- Erythema multiforme
- Deep fungal infections
- Vesiculobullous disease

White-red lesions
- Frictional/factitial keratoses
- Leukoplakia and proliferative leukoplakia
- Oral lichen planus and lichenoid lesions
- Candidiasis
- Coated or hairy tongue
- Migratory glossitis

Gingivitis
- Conventional gingivitis
- Desquamative gingivitis and hypersensitivity reactions
- Human immunodeficiency virus/AIDS–associated linear gingivitis and necrotizing ulcerative gingivitis

Diffuse gingival hyperplasia
- Drug-induced gingival hyperplasia
- Acute leukemia

- Hereditary and syndromic gingival hyperplasia
- Destructive membranous periodontal disease (ligneous gingivitis and periodontitis)

Pigmented lesions
- Extrinsic pigmentation
  - Foods and dentifrices
  - Amalgam tattoo
  - Heavy metal pigmentation
  - Other causes
- Intrinsic pigmentation
  - Melanin
  - Blood pigment
- Drug-induced oral pigmentation

Poorly healing or nonhealing extraction sockets and osteonecrosis
- Dry socket
- Infection
- Osteoradionecrosis
- Drug-induced osteonecrosis
- Metastatic tumor to the jaw

Xerostomia and hyposalivation
- Hyposalivation associated with normal glands
- Hyposalivation associated with damaged glands

Oral Ulcers

An ulcer is a loss of epithelium over an area of the mucosa covered by a yellow or whitish-gray fibrin pseudomembrane. Traumatic ulcers are the most common type, followed by aphthous ulcers. Other ulcerative conditions include aphthous-like ulcers seen in systemic diseases, drug-induced ulcers, infections in immunocompromised patients, vesiculobullous diseases, and erythema multiforme.

Traumatic ulcers

Traumatic ulcerations may be caused by sharp or broken teeth, rough restorations, acute biting of the mucosa, and friction from ill-fitting dentures. Traumatic ulcers also occur on protruding lesions (such as fibromas). The side of the tongue, buccal mucosa, and lower lip are the most frequently affected sites, and removal of traumatic factors leads to resolution.[1]

Fig 13-1 Recurrent aphthous stomatitis. Aphthous ulcer with yellow fibrin pseudomembrane and erythematous halo.

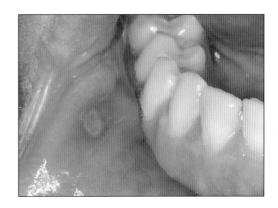

Table 13-1	Classification of recurrent aphthous stomatitis		
	Type of presentation		
Characteristic	**Minor***	**Major**	**Herpetiform**
Size and number	< 1 cm; usually 1 to 5 ulcers	≥ 1 cm; usually 1 ulcer	< 0.5 cm; usually 10 ulcers or more
Duration	7 to 10 d	Months	7 to 10 d
Scarring	No	Yes/No	No

*There is a severe variant of minor RAS in which an affected individual is almost never without ulcers.

Recurrent aphthous ulcers/stomatitis

Recurrent aphthous stomatitis (RAS), popularly known as canker sores, affects 10% to 20% of the population and usually first manifests in childhood or adolescence; the frequency of episodes usually diminishes with age.[2] The etiology is multifactorial, and some factors include trauma, smoking cessation, hormonal changes, stress, genetics, some hypersensitivity reactions, and immunologic factors; many cases are idiopathic.[3]

RAS generally presents as shallow, oval or round ulcers covered by a grayish-white fibrin pseudomembrane with an erythematous halo (Fig 13-1). The ulcers occur on the nonkeratinized mucosa and resolve completely between episodes. Except in patients with major RAS, ulcers rarely occur on the hard palatal mucosa, dorsum of the tongue, or attached gingiva. The frequency of episodes varies from monthly to only a few times a year. A minority of women develop minor RAS just before their menses.

There are four main forms: minor, major, herpetiform, and severe (Table 13-1). Biopsy, usually performed to rule out other conditions, shows an ulcer with nonspecific acute and chronic inflammation. RAS is not caused by a virus or other infectious agent.

Treatment depends on the severity and frequency of the lesions and centers around pain control, definitive treatment of the ulcers, and reducing the number of outbreaks. Patients who experience one or two episodes a year probably just require reassurance and the use of over-the-counter local anesthetics (such as 10% benzocaine) or mucoadhesive agents such as

Table 13-2	**Topical immunosuppressive agents and pain medications for the treatment of oral ulcers**

Medication	Instructions
Topical immunosuppressive agents	
Triamcinolone, 0.1% in methylcellulose paste (for solitary lesions only)	Apply to affected site three to four times a day; methylcellulose is an effective covering agent, although triamcinolone is only of moderate potency.
Clobetasol, 0.05% gel Bethametasone, 0.05% gel Fluocinolone, 0.05% gel Tacrolimus, 0.1% ointment	Dry area and apply to affected site three to four times a day (on gauze if appropriate). Do not consume any food or drink for 20 min after application. *or* Place gel in stent and wear for 15 to 30 min, two to three times a day (for extensive gingival lesions).
Dexamethasone elixir, 0.5 mg/5 mL Tacrolimus solution, 5 mg/mL	Dispense 300 mL. Swish 5 mL for 3 min (timed) and spit out, three to four times a day. Do not consume any food or drink for 20 min after use.
Intralesional steroid injection with triamcinolone	Administer in a dose of 5 to 10 mg of triamcinolone per 1 cm^2 of ulceration.
Topical pain medications	
Benzydamine hydrochloride, 0.15% Dyclonine hydrochloride, 1% Viscous lidocaine, 2%	Swish and spit out 5 to 15 mL, three to four times a day, when in pain. Viscous lidocaine may be mixed in equal volume with diphenhydramine, aluminum/magnesium, and bismuth subsalicylate.
Benzocaine, 10%	Apply to the affected area three to four times a day, when in pain.

methylcellulose paste (Orabase Paste, Colgate-Palmolive) and polyvinylpyrrolidone sodium hyaluronate (Gelclair, Helsinn Healthcare). Amlexanox (OraDisc A, ULURU), a prescription anti-inflammatory agent incorporated in a mucoadhesive, is sometimes effective. More frequent or severe outbreaks may be treated with topical corticosteroids and other immunosuppressive agents, and larger, recalcitrant ulcers or those of major RAS may require intralesional therapy such as injections of triamcinolone at a dosage of 10 mg/cm^2 of ulcer size (Table 13-2). The same topical management strategies are used for ulcers associated with other disorders. Systemic therapy for severe outbreaks is with prednisone (usually at a dosage of 1 mg/kg), pentoxifylline, colchicine, azathioprine, or thalidomide.

Aphthous-like ulcers from systemic disease

Several systemic conditions have been associated with aphthous-like ulcers. Aphthous-like lesions may occur in patients deficient in folic acid, iron, or vitamins B_1, B_2, B_6, or B_{12}; these deficiencies are readily diagnosed with a blood test, and ulcers typically resolve or improve with repletion, although not always.[3]

Inflammatory bowel diseases such as Crohn disease and ulcerative colitis often lead to oral ulcers. Patients experience abdominal pain, diarrhea, fever, fatigue, weight loss, and anemia, and these can be elicited by a careful history, although oral findings may precede systemic symptoms. Crohn disease is a granulomatous inflammatory disorder of unknown etiology, although genetic, immunologic, environmental, microbial, dietary, and vascular factors have been implicated. It affects the ileum and large bowel in more than 90% of patients, although any part of the gastrointestinal tract may be affected.[4]

Crohn disease is strongly associated with aphthous-like ulcers, which generally have a linear appearance if located in the oral vestibule. Other findings include angular cheilitis; swelling of the lips, face, and gingiva (orofacial granulomatosis); and edema of the oral mucosa resulting in fissuring, or a "cobblestone" appearance. In addition to aphtheiform ulcers, patients with ulcerative colitis may present with pustular and ulcerative eruptions in the oral cavity that are known as *pyostomatitis vegetans*. The pustules often coalesce and break down, leaving superficial erosions.

Management of intestinal symptoms involves the use of systemic medications (eg, corticosteroids, salicylates, immunosuppressant agents, and biologic agents such as tumor necrosis factor-α [TNF-α] inhibitors) or surgical resection.

Gluten-sensitive enteropathy (also known as *celiac disease* or *celiac sprue*) is an autoimmune disease of the small intestines caused by a reaction to gliadin, a gluten protein. Almost all patients have the HLA-DQ2 allele and some the HLA-DQ8 allele. Aphthous-like ulcers are observed in 3% to 61% of patients, and dental enamel defects have been reported.[5] If this condition is suspected, blood tests for antigliadin, antiendomysial, and anti–tissue transglutaminase antibodies should be performed. Signs and symptoms are relieved with a gluten-free diet. Because of malabsorption after iliectomy, patients may develop aphthous-like ulcers from vitamin B_{12} deficiency.

Behçet disease is a systemic vasculitis associated with the *HLA-B51* gene. It is characterized by aphthous-like ulcers, genital ulcers, ocular lesions (especially anterior uveitis), and skin lesions (such as erythema nodosum). Cardiovascular, musculoskeletal, gastrointestinal, and neurologic symptoms are variably present. Onset is usually during the third and fourth decade of life, and it is more prevalent in individuals from Turkey, Japan, the Middle East, and other Asian countries.[6,7] MAGIC (mouth and genital ulcers with inflamed cartilage) syndrome combines features of both relapsing polychondritis and Behçet disease with major aphthous ulcers and, rarely, multifocal neurologic abnormalities. Oral ulcers in these patients are treated with the same approach used for RAS. Treatment includes the use of anti–TNF-α biologic agents, such as etanercept and infliximab.

A syndrome with periodic fever, aphthous stomatitis, pharyngitis, and adenitis affects mostly children, and the etiology is unknown.

Cyclic neutropenia is a rare inherited condition caused by mutations in the gene for neutrophil elastase. Patients usually have a circulating neutrophil count that fluctuates and severe neutropenia that occurs about every 3 weeks and lasts for 3 to 5 days. During these periods, patients are susceptible to bacterial infections and may report a history of recurrent fever, lymph node enlargement, malaise, aphthous-like ulcers, and pharyngitis. Other oral findings include gingivitis, gingival ulcers, and periodontitis. Blood tests during these episodes reveal low neutrophil counts. Treatment is usually topical (see Table 13-2) because of its relapsing-remitting nature.

The prevalence of oral complications in patients with human immunodeficiency virus (HIV)/AIDS has decreased since the advent of antiretroviral therapy. Patients affected by HIV/AIDS often present with major aphthous-like oral ulcers that may affect both nonkeratinized and keratinized epithelium. All such ulcers in patients with HIV/AIDS must be biopsied to rule out infectious etiologies before a diagnosis of aphthous-like ulcer can be confirmed. Topical and systemic therapy is often required for resolution.

Drug-induced oral ulcers

Several medications, especially those used in oncology settings, have been associated with ulcers in the oral cavity. Targeted therapies and biologic agents are used increasingly in the treatment of cancers, autoimmune diseases, and even chronic mucosal disease. The dentist should be familiar with the names of these med-

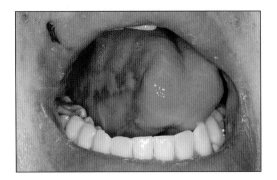

Fig 13-2 Oral mucositis after radiation therapy. Large ulcers of the tongue.

ications. These ulcers do not represent aphthous ulcers but rather are considered aphthous-like ulcers because they resolve when the drug is withdrawn and recur only when the patient is rechallenged with the drug. Therefore, a detailed drug history is extremely important when the clinician is evaluating abrupt-onset oral ulcers.

Oral mucositis, ulcerative or otherwise, still represents a major acute complication of cancer chemotherapy. The most stomatotoxic agents include antimetabolites, such as capecitabine, fluorouracil, or methotrexate; alkylating agents, such as cyclophosphamide or melphalan; antimitotics, such as paclitaxel, vinblastine, or vincristine; and anthracycline antibiotics, such as daunorubicin, doxorubicin, carboplatin, cisplatin, or hydroxyurea. Mucosal soreness and sensitivity generally begin about 3 to 5 days after the first infusion; oral erythema or ulcers develop a few days later, and resolution occurs in approximately 15 days.[8] Lesions involve mostly nonkeratinized sites and tend to be more diffuse than discrete (Fig 13-2). Ulcers that affect the keratinized mucosa of the hard palatal mucosa, gingiva, or dorsal tongue during chemotherapy are likely related to herpes viral infections (discussed later). Topical anesthetics (such as viscous lidocaine or morphine rinses for severe cases) or systemic or narcotic pain medications help relieve symptoms until the ulcers heal.

Methotrexate is an immune-modulating and antimetabolite drug. Methotrexate at low doses is used to control chronic inflammatory disorders such as psoriasis and rheumatoid arthritis. At higher doses, methotrexate acts as a chemotherapeutic agent in the treatment of non-Hodgkin lymphoma, leukemia, and some solid tumors. Oral lesions associated with methotrexate toxicity are typically characterized by dose-dependent erythema and ulceration (broadly termed *mucositis*). Folate supplementation is an effective way to reduce such mucosal damage. These lesions are treated with topical corticosteroids and, if necessary, dose reduction.

Hydroxyurea has been used for the treatment of chronic myeloid leukemia, myeloproliferative disorders, and sickle cell anemia. Painful oral ulcers and atrophic glossitis may occur during treatment in association with skin lesions; these resolve following completion of therapy.

Mammalian target of rapamycin (mTOR) inhibitors are a group of agents prescribed for the management of soft tissue sarcomas (temsirolimus and ridaforolimus), advanced metastatic renal cell carcinoma (everolimus), and immunosuppression following organ transplantation (sirolimus and everolimus). The side effect of mTOR inhibitors of most significance to dentists is that of aphthous-like oral ulcers, clinically distinct from the more diffuse ulcers and erythema of chemotherapy-induced mucositis. This condition has been termed *mTOR inhibitor-associated stomatitis* and occurs within 10 days of start of the drug. The ulcers are managed with topical or intralesional corticosteroids.

Sodium lauryl sulfate (SLS) is the most commonly used detergent in dentifrices. Patients often experience a burning sensation while brushing their teeth with a toothpaste that contains

SLS. The denaturing effect of SLS on the mucin layer overlying the epithelium may result in epithelial inflammation of the oral mucosa, sloughing, and ulcers. SLS has also been shown to be a predisposing factor for recurrent aphthous stomatitis, although this finding is equivocal because it may represent a contact irritation rather than true RAS.[9]

Finally, nonsteroidal anti-inflammatory drugs (NSAIDs) such as piroxicam, indomethacin, or ibuprofen may cause oral ulcers. For SLS- or medication-induced lesions, discontinuation leads to resolution.

Viral infections

Herpes simplex virus 1 (HSV-1), also known as *human herpesvirus 1* (HHV-1), is one of the most common viral infections that produces oral ulcers as part of primary herpetic gingivostomatitis, recrudescent oral disease, mucocutaneous orofacial disease, and ocular disease. Occasionally oral lesions are caused by HSV-2, a virus that historically was considered specific for the anogenital area but is no longer so classified because of changing sexual practices. Primary herpetic gingivostomatitis typically occurs in children and young adults. Most primary HSV infections are asymptomatic or cause only very mild symptoms.

Seroepidemiologic evidence reveals that 50% to 60% of adults in the United States have circulating antibodies to the virus, although few individuals would remember experiencing a primary infection.[10] Following an incubation period of 2 to 20 days, HSV will cause flulike symptoms (such as fever, lethargy, and headache) in some patients 2 or 3 days before the onset of a sore throat and painful oral ulcers. These ulcers resolve within 1 to 2 weeks. The virus then establishes latency within the sensory ganglion. Subsequently, trigger factors such as sunlight, illness, trauma, emotional stress, or menses may reactivate the latent virus in the ganglia, resulting in viral replication and transport via nerves to the skin or mucosal surfaces.

HSV reactivation results in either asymptomatic shedding in bodily fluids or secretions, or the development of recurrent clinical lesions (recrudescent HSV). Asymptomatic shedding remains one of the most important causes of transmission. Differences in presentation are described in Table 13-3, and a typical ulcer is shown in Fig 13-3. Hydration, nutritional support, topical and systemic pain control, and use of antipyretics are important management strategies. Antiviral therapy reduces contagiousness (Table 13-4).[11]

Primary varicella-zoster virus (VZV) infection usually occurs in childhood and begins with flulike symptoms and a pruritic papular rash followed by vesicle formation. These lesions eventually become crusted and fall off in 1 to 3 weeks. In the oral cavity, primary VZV infection presents as small (0.1- to 0.5-cm), painful ulcers that heal in approximately 2 weeks. Reactivation of VZV infection leads to oral shingles. These lesions may resemble recrudescent HSV except they are almost always unilateral. A culture differentiates between the two. Treatment of primary VZV is described in Table 13-4.

Infection with cytomegalovirus (CMV), or *human herpesvirus 5*, remains one of the major complications after solid organ transplantation and may result in severe pulmonary, gastrointestinal, or neurologic disease. Seroepidemiologic studies show that 60% to 65% of the adult population in the United States has antibodies to CMV.[12] Primary CMV infection may be asymptomatic or present with infectious mononucleosis-like or mild flulike symptoms. Recrudescent CMV in the oral cavity occurs mostly in immunocompromised patients and manifests as large (usually larger than 1-cm), painful ulcers on the oral mucosa.

Because CMV, unlike HSV, infects cells deep in the connective tissue, a swab culture may not be diagnostic. A biopsy is the most useful tool for the diagnosis of CMV, and the presence of virus can be detected by immunohistochemistry and in situ hybridization techniques. CMV can also be detected in blood by testing for CMV antigen on white blood cells or polymerase chain reaction studies to detect CMV DNA. Management is directed toward pain control, and definitive therapy is with ganciclovir, cidofovir, or valganciclovir.

Table 13-3 **Clinical presentation of herpesvirus infections**

Virus	Type	Clinical presentation	Location of ulcers in the oral cavity
HHV-1 (HSV-1)	Primary herpetic gingivo-stomatitis	Painful clusters of 1- to 5-mm ulcers; flulike symptoms	Keratinized and nonkera-tinized mucosa
	Recrudescent herpetic infection in healthy indi-viduals	Lip prodrome of tingling, followed by a nodule, blister, clustered vesicles, and ulcer, scabbing, and resolution on lip vermilion; oral ulcers	Junction of lip vermilion and skin (most common); intraoral keratinized mu-cosa (less common)
	Recrudescent herpetic infection in immunocom-promised individuals	Clustered vesicles, coalescent ulcers, or single aphthous-like ulcers	Keratinized and nonkera-tinized mucosa
HHV-2 (HSV-2)		Same as HSV-1 in all three categories	Usually found on skin and mucosa below the waist; may also be found in the mouth
HHV-3 (VZV)	Primary varicella-zoster virus (chicken pox)	Flulike symptoms and pruritic papu-lar skin rash followed by vesicle formation; oral form (uncommon): 0.1- to 0.5-cm painful oral ulcers	Skin; intraoral (uncommon)
	Shingles (herpes zoster infection)	Skin shingles; oral lesions are clus-tered vesicles or coalescent ulcers; usually unilateral	Facial or oral shingles along distribution of tri-geminal nerve
HHV-4 (EBV)	Primary EBV infection	Infectious mononucleosis	
	Recrudescent EBV infec-tion	Asymptomatic white plaques with vertical lines (hairy leukoplakia) often secondarily infected with *Candida* species	Lateral or dorsal tongue (most common sites)
HHV-5 (CMV)	Primary CMV infection	Asymptomatic or infectious mononucleosis-like symptoms or mild flulike symptoms	
	Recrudescent CMV infec-tion	Mostly in immunocompromised patients; large (usually > 1 cm), painful, penetrating ulcers	Oral mucosa

VZV, varicella-zoster virus; EBV, Epstein-Barr virus; CMV, cytomegalovirus.

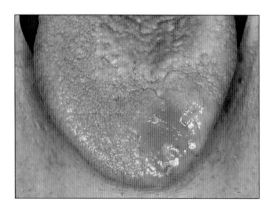

Fig 13-3 Recurrent herpes simplex virus infection in a cancer patient. Large ulcer on the dorsum of the tongue. Note coated tongue due to poor oral intake and poor hydration.

Table 13-4	Antiviral agents for the treatment of oral viral infections
Medication	**Dosage and instructions**
Topical agents	
Acyclovir, 5% ointment or cream Penciclovir, 1% cream Docosanol, 10% cream	Apply to lesions every 2 h for 7 d
Systemic agents	
Acyclovir, 400- or 800-mg tablet	*Primary HSV infection:* 400 mg, three times a day for 7 to 10 d 800 mg, two to five times a day for 7 to 10 d
	Recurrent HSV infection: 400 mg, three times a day for 5 d 800 mg, two times a day for 5 d
Valacyclovir, 500- or 1,000-mg caplet	*Primary HSV infection:* 1 g, two times a day for 7 to 10 d
	Recurrent HSV infection: 500 mg, two times a day for 3 d
	Labial HSV infection: 2 g at first sign of recurrence; then 2 g 12 hours later
	Prophylaxis (when precipitating event is known): 2 g, two times on the day of the dental procedure or event; then 1 g, two times the next day (up to 1 to 3 d after the event or procedure)
	Immunosuppressed individuals: 1 g daily
	VZV infection: 1 g, three times a day for 7 to 14 d
Famciclovir, 125- or 250-mg tablet	*Primary HSV infection:* 250 mg, three times a day for 7 to 10 d
	Recurrent HSV infection: 125 mg, two times a day for 5 d
	VZV infection: 500 mg, three times a day for 7 to 14 d

VZV, varicella-zoster virus.

Coxsackievirus (a group of enteroviruses) infection is associated with two diseases most commonly seen in children: hand, foot, and mouth disease and herpangina. The incubation period is 3 to 7 days and is followed by flulike symptoms in some patients. Herpangina is characterized by multiple small, coalescent ulcers on the tonsillar pillars and the soft palate. Hand, foot, and mouth disease has a similar oral manifestation along with cutaneous vesicles of the hands and feet. Both diseases occur as seasonal outbreaks among young schoolchildren. The infection is typically self-limiting, resolving within 7 to 10 days. Coxsackievirus is also implicated in lymphonodular pharyngitis that causes a sore throat. Treatment includes pain management, hydration, and soft diet until signs and symptoms have resolved.

Erythema multiforme

Erythema multiforme (EM) is a self-limiting mu-cocutaneous hypersensitivity reaction, usually to an infectious agent, with an acute onset; how-ever, some cases may be recurrent. From a dermatologic point of view, EM can be divided into minor and major forms. EM minor is mainly cutaneous (less than 10% skin involvement), with minimal or no mucosal involvement. EM major involves either the skin and at least one mucosal site or a single mucosal site with ex-tensive involvement. However, some cases may involve only the oral cavity. Approximately 70% of cases of EM represent a hypersensitivity re-action to a recent HSV infection or to asymp-tomatic HSV reactivation; less commonly, EM is a reaction to the use of certain medications.[13,14] The most common disease-precipitating medi-cations include NSAIDs, sulfonamides, and anti-convulsants.

Patients with EM may report fever, headache, malaise, and sore throat a few days or 1 to 2 weeks prior to the onset of lesions. Oral lesions present as painful ulcers that typically affect the nonkeratinized mucosa with crusting of the lips. Skin lesions are symmetric, erythematous and edematous papules with a target or bull's eye appearance and typically affect the extremities (especially the palms). The ocular and genital areas can also be affected.

EM is self-limiting, lasting from 2 to 4 weeks, and lesions heal without scarring. The history and the clinical presentation are usually suf-ficient for a diagnosis, and a biopsy is confir-matory. Cultures for HSV and a biopsy should be obtained when the clinical presentation is atypical. EM may also arise from *Mycoplasma pneumoniae* infection, and when this infection is suspected, the evaluation includes a chest radiograph, polymerase chain reaction testing of throat swabs, and serologic tests. Therapy for EM includes topical and systemic admin-istration of analgesics, skin wound care, and hospital-based supportive care.[15]

Stevens-Johnson syndrome is a separate entity from EM and considered an epidermal necrolytic disease. The more severe form is toxic epidermal necrolysis, usually associated with the use of medications such as allopurinol, imidazole antifungals, anticonvulsants, sulfon-amides, or NSAIDs. EM major, Stevens-Johnson syndrome, and toxic epidermal necrolysis mani-fest with similar extensive mucosal ulcers, ero-sions, and hemorrhagic crusts on the lips. Skin blistering is always present. Treatment includes thalidomide, intravenous immunoglobulin, and supportive care. The mortality rate is 6% to 20%.[16]

Deep fungal infections

Deep fungal infections are invasive and often lead to necrotic ulcers of the oral cavity; sys-temic dissemination is common.[17] These include mucormycosis and aspergillosis in patients with cancer and diabetes mellitus; coccidioidomycosis and histoplasmosis, which are endemic in the southwestern United States and Ohio-Mississippi valleys, respectively; and blastomycosis, which is endemic in many areas of Central and South America.

Mucormycoses appear as black, necrotic, and/or fungating lesions that resemble malig-nancy; patients with diabetes mellitus (espe-cially if ketoacidotic), neutropenia, or malignan-cy and individuals who have undergone organ transplantation may develop rhinocerebral mu-cormycosis, and the mortality rate is 60% to 90%.[18,19] Aspergillosis (caused by *Aspergillus fumigatum* or *Aspergillus flavus*) is a fungal infection characterized by noninvasive and in-vasive forms. Noninvasive aspergillosis affects a normal host and may present as a "fungus ball" (mycetoma) within the maxillary sinus or a hypersensitivity to the fungus, leading to aller-gic fungal sinusitis. Invasive infections tend to affect immunocompromised patients such as those with leukemia, and the clinical presenta-tion is similar to that of mucormycosis. Vascular involvement leads to necrosis.

The primary infection of histoplasmosis is usually mild and presents as a self-limiting pulmonary disease. Immunosuppressed indi-viduals may develop a disseminated form with multiorgan involvement (lung, liver, spleen, me-ninges, and adrenal glands). Oral lesions are usually present in patients with disseminated

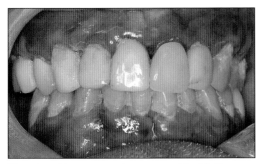

Fig 13-4 Mucous membrane pemphigoid. Desquamative gingivitis with erythematous attached gingiva.

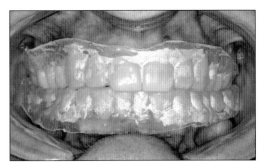

Fig 13-5 Custom tray to hold topical immunosuppressive agent covering the involved gingiva in a patient with mucous membrane pemphigoid presenting as desquamative gingivitis.

histoplasmosis and begin with an erythematous area that eventually forms a papule and then an ulcer.

Blastomycosis is characterized by a pulmonary infection with mild symptoms. If untreated, the symptoms worsen, and the microorganism spreads to the mucosa, skin, and bone, forming indurated ulcers. Oral lesions include verrucous ulcers and radiolucent jawbone lesions.

Diagnosis is made after biopsy and histopathologic examination, as well as culture and serologic and polymerase chain reaction studies. Imaging studies are recommended to assess the extent of systemic involvement. Treatment requires surgical debridement and aggressive systemic antifungal therapy for all such infections.[17]

Vesiculobullous disease

Similar to the vesicles of HSV, the blisters of autoimmune vesiculobullous disease rupture, creating shallow erosions that over time become covered by fibrin, forming an ulcer. Necrotic, whitish, ragged epithelial tags from the ruptured blister roof may be piled up at the edges of such erosions and ulcers.

Mucous membrane pemphigoid (MMP) is an autoimmune vesiculobullous disease associated with increased frequency of the HLA-DQB1*0301 allele. It is characterized by autoreactive antibodies, usually immunoglobulin G (IgG) and sometimes IgA, that target antigens in the epithelium-attachment complex, resulting

in subepithelial blistering and mucosal fragility.[20] MMP may involve the larynx, nose, eyes, and genital mucosa. One of the major complications is conjunctival scarring that can lead to blindness (hence the older term, *cicatricial pemphigoid*). Scarring may also involve the larynx and esophagus but is uncommon in the oral mucosa.

The oral mucosal lesions almost always affect the gingiva, leading to bright red or desquamative gingivitis (Fig 13-4). This develops when epithelium peels off the gingiva, leaving only exposed connective tissue, which is the basis for a positive Nikolsky sign (slight rubbing leads to dislodgment of the epithelium). Ulcers may develop on the gingiva and elsewhere in the mouth, such as the palatal, buccal, and tongue mucosa. These ulcers differ from RAS because they are more diffuse and tend not to heal completely. Biopsy of a perilesional area for histopathologic examination and direct immunofluorescence studies are essential to a definitive diagnosis; direct immunofluorescence shows deposition of IgG, C3, and sometimes IgA at the basement membrane zone.

Management of desquamative gingivitis includes topical treatment with corticosteroids or tacrolimus delivered in a custom tray that covers the involved gingiva (Fig 13-5). This technique also may be used for management of other diffuse gingival inflammatory conditions. Systemic agents such as prednisone, dapsone, azathioprine, tetracycline, nicotinamide, and cyclophosphamide may be required for management of oral MMP refractory to topical ther-

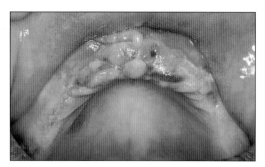

Fig 13-6 Pemphigus vulgaris. Shallow erosions and ulcers of the maxillary ridge mucosa in an edentulous patient, likely from denture trauma.

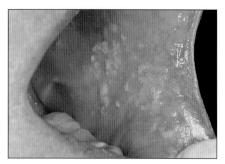

Fig 13-7 Frictional/factitial keratosis. White, irregular papules and plaques resulting from a parafunctional habit.

apy. When the skin is involved, the diagnosis is usually bullous pemphigoid.

Pemphigus vulgaris (PV) is an uncommon autoimmune vesiculobullous disorder that affects mainly older adults and was fatal in the presteroid era. PV has a predilection for people of Ashkenazi Jewish descent (who exhibit a high frequency of the HLA-B38 or HLA-B35 serotype), people of Arab ethnicity, and other individuals from the Mediterranean region. Different HLA subtypes are implicated in PV in non-Jewish persons and Asians. Autoantibodies, mostly IgG, are directed toward the interepithelial cementing substance, leading to intraepithelial blistering.[21]

Oral ulcers, present in 95% of patients, are often the first sign of PV; skin lesions often develop later. Oral lesions are characterized by painful, irregular, erythematous, depressed erosions with whitish tissue tags at the edges; yellow ulcerations may also be present (Fig 13-6). The most commonly affected oral sites are the hard and soft palatal mucosa (likely because of physiologic trauma from swallowing), gingiva (also presenting as desquamative gingivitis), buccal mucosa, and tongue. Diagnosis is established through a perilesional tissue biopsy specimen subjected to histopathologic evaluation and direct immunofluorescence, which shows intercellular deposition of IgG.

Topical corticosteroid therapy and topical tacrolimus are the mainstays of therapy (see Table 13-2). More severe or refractory cases require administration of systemic agents such as prednisone, mycophenolate mofetil, azathioprine, and cyclosporine. For severe cases and if the skin is involved, specialist referral is indicated; in such cases, treatment generally involves prednisone, rituximab (a monoclonal antibody), intravenous immunoglobulin, or extracorporeal photopheresis.

White-Red Lesions

White papules (less than 5 mm) and plaques (greater than 5 mm) are extremely common in the mouth, and often they have a red or erythematous component. Only the most common lesions are discussed in this section.

Frictional/factitial keratoses

Because the mouth is a trauma-intense environment, white or keratotic lesions resulting from friction of the mucosa against the teeth are common, especially if the individual has a parafunctional habit. The linea alba of the buccal mucosa is considered an anatomical variant and is an area of mild reactive frictional keratosis. More extensive frictional keratoses are characterized by poorly demarcated white, rough or shaggy papules and plaques that may be associated with areas of erythema and ulceration, if the parafunctional chewing habit is severe (Fig 13-7). Benign alveolar ridge kerato-

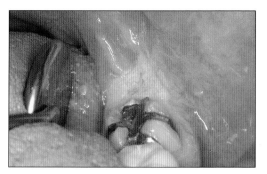

Fig 13-8 Benign alveolar ridge keratosis. Poorly demarcated white plaque of the keratinized mucosa on the retromolar pad.

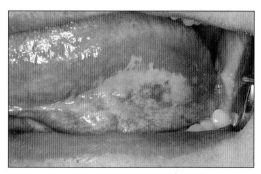

Fig 13-9 Leukoplakia (homogenous form). Uniform white plaque, partially well-demarcated, affecting the left ventral surface of the tongue.

sis is another form of frictional keratosis. It is caused by crushing of food against the alveolar mucosa or the gingiva and is characterized by poorly demarcated white plaques of the keratinized mucosa on the retromolar pad, edentulous ridge, and palatal mucosa (Fig 13-8). Biopsy may be needed to reassure the patient, but no other treatment is necessary.

Leukoplakia and proliferative leukoplakia

Leukoplakia is defined as "a white plaque of questionable risk having excluded (other) known diseases or disorders that carry no increased risk for cancer."[22] Leukoplakia is therefore a clinical diagnosis used when other specific clinical and histopathologic entities are excluded (eg, frictional keratoses). Dysplasia or invasive cancer is present at initial biopsies of leukoplakias in 20% to 40% of patients,[23] and the ventral tongue, floor of the mouth, and soft palate are considered high-risk sites for such dysplasia and cancer.

Leukoplakia presents in different forms. Localized leukoplakia is more frequent in men, is associated with smoking, and may be homogenous or nonhomogenous. The homogenous form presents as a uniform, well-demarcated, white plaque with or without fissuring (Fig 13-9). Nonhomogenous leukoplakia may have red areas (erythroleukoplakia) or nodular or verrucous areas. All forms of leukoplakia, especially nonhomogenous types, are associated with a high-

er frequency of dysplasia and development of cancer. Risk factors for localized leukoplakia are tobacco smoking, excessive alcohol consumption, areca nut habit, age, history of prolonged immunosuppression, history of cancer and cancer therapy, and family history of cancer.[23] Leukoplakia is also observed in patients affected by dyskeratosis congenita, a very rare inherited condition of progressive bone marrow failure with skin hyperpigmentation and dystrophic nail changes.

A second form of leukoplakia is proliferative verrucous leukoplakia (PVL), although not all cases are verrucous. PVL is usually slowly progressive over 10 to 20 years and usually multifocal. It may affect contiguous sites and often affects the gingiva. PVL is more common in women and is not usually associated with smoking. It is mostly characterized by verrucous nodular or erythroleukoplakic lesions, and transformation to cancer occurs in 60% to 100% of patients.[24]

All leukoplakia or PVL must be biopsied to rule out dysplasia or carcinoma; multiple biopsy specimens should be obtained from large lesions. Dysplastic lesions must be removed if this can be achieved without excessive morbidity, because these have the highest association with development of cancer, although management strategies vary from one center to another.[25] Otherwise, monitoring and periodic biopsies are essential, especially for patients with PVL. Other treatments include photodynamic therapy.

Oral lichen planus and lichenoid lesions

Oral lichen planus (OLP) is a fairly common, chronic, immune-mediated inflammatory mucocutaneous condition that occurs in 1% to 2% of adults.[26] Middle-aged women are twice as likely to be affected as men. OLP can affect any mucosal surface. Approximately 70% of individuals with cutaneous disease develop concomitant OLP, while only 10% to 15% of patients with OLP have concomitant cutaneous lesions.[27]

OLP may be idiopathic or associated with a variety of local and systemic conditions. Amalgam and composite resin restorations may cause localized contact lichenoid hypersensitivity reactions, possibly to mercury and formaldehyde. Some cases are caused by a hypersensitivity to medications such as thiazide diuretics, angiotensin-converting enzyme inhibitors, beta blockers, gold salts, sulfasalazine, sulfonylureas, and penicillamine. New biologic agents, such as TNF-α inhibitors, may also cause lichen planus–like eruptions.

Patients with hypothyroidism, including Hashimoto thyroiditis, also develop OLP, but it is unclear whether it is thyroid disease that predisposes the individual to OLP or the medications used to treat hypothyroidism, such as levothyroxine. Hepatitis C virus infection has also been associated with the development of OLP in individuals living in areas of southern Europe, particularly Italy, Portugal, and Spain, and there may be a genetic or ethnic predilection.[26]

OLP most commonly affects the buccal mucosa and tongue bilaterally and can present with three distinct forms: reticular/keratotic (classic), erosive/erythematous, and ulcerative. The reticular/keratotic form, characterized by Wickham striae, is the most common form and is often asymptomatic; white papules may be present. Occasionally patients report discomfort and describe the buccal mucosa as "rough," "thick," or "tight" (Fig 13-10). The erosive/erythematous form typically presents as desquamative gingivitis. Patients may complain of discomfort while eating acidic, spicy, or crunchy foods. The ulcerative form is the most severe and presents as shallow ulcers that have a yellow fibrin membrane on the surface. Often, patients exhibit a combination of the three forms at different sites or at different times.

Most patients exhibit characteristic bilateral and usually symmetric distribution of lesions, typically involving the buccal mucosa, dorsum and ventral surfaces of the tongue, and/or gingiva. A biopsy specimen should be obtained for histopathologic examination when the presentation is not typical (such as unilateral presentation or lack of reticulations). Histopathologic examination usually reveals degeneration or loss of the basal cell layer and a lymphocytic band of variable thickness at the interface.

Treatment is aimed at relieving pain and resolving or reducing erythema and ulcerations. The primary therapies include topical corticosteroids and topical tacrolimus (see Table 13-2). Occasionally systemic corticosteroids and other immunosuppressive agents (such as the antimalarial drug hydroxychloroquin) may be necessary. Malignant transformation to squamous cell carcinoma may occur in approximately 0.1% to 0.2% of cases of OLP, and patients should be followed on a regular basis.[28]

Two other conditions may present with oral lesions similar to OLP: lupus erythematosus and chronic graft-versus-host disease (GVHD). Lupus erythematosus is an autoimmune connective tissue disorder with many subtypes characterized by distinct clinical features, serologic findings, and patterns of humoral and cellular autoimmunity. Women are 9 times more commonly affected than men, and the onset is in young adulthood. Two common presentations often associated with oral findings are systemic lupus erythematosus (SLE) and discoid lupus erythematosus (DLE).

Common signs and symptoms of SLE include weight loss, arthritis, fever, fatigue, and general malaise. Clinically, 30% to 60% of patients may present with an erythematous "butterfly" rash over the malar area. The kidneys, heart, skin, nervous system, and joints are commonly involved. Often, patients affected by SLE develop secondary Sjögren syndrome, resulting in dry mouth. Oral lesions develop in up to 44% of patients, and these may be red with white reticulations (lichenoid) or ulcerative. A biopsy obtained from normal-appearing mucosa

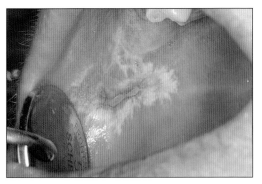

Fig 13-10 Oral lichen planus. Typical white, lacy reticulations with an ulcer surrounded by an erythematous halo.

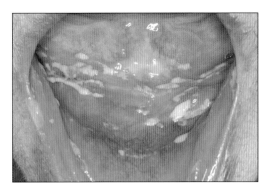

Fig 13-11 Pseudomembranous candidiasis. White, curdy papules and plaques with mild erythema.

for direct immunofluorescence shows a positive result for a lupus band (linear deposition of IgG at the basement membrane zone). Serology is positive for antinuclear antibodies (in more than 95% of patients), anti–double-strand DNA antibodies, anti-Smith antibodies, and antiribonucleoprotein.[29]

DLE is characterized by scaly, atrophic, and red plaques on the skin. Oral lesions develop in up to 20% of patients and are similar to those seen in SLE.[30] A biopsy obtained from lesional tissue exhibits a positive lupus band test in 90% of active lesions. Because there is no systemic involvement, serologic studies are not helpful.

For both SLE and DLE, topical and systemic therapy for oral involvement depends on the severity of the lesions (see Table 13-2). Systemic treatment includes immunosuppressive or immunomodulatory therapy.

Chronic GVHD remains a significant complication of allogeneic hematopoietic cell (bone marrow) transplantation and continues to be the leading cause of nonrelapse mortality. The oral cavity is affected in around 80% of cases, and mucosal lesions resemble those of OLP and are characterized by erythema, reticulation, and ulceration.[31] Topical therapy is similar to that for OLP (see Table 13-2).

Candidiasis

Oral candidiasis is the most common fungal infection encountered in dental patients. *Candida*

albicans is a commensal organism of the oral cavity in approximately 20% to 30% of individuals.[32] It is an opportunistic organism, and candidiasis develops when the normal flora is altered, in hyposalivation, or when there is an immune dysfunction; it also commonly overlies dysplastic lesions.[33] Local factors include use of topical immunosuppressive agents, hyposalivation, wearing of dentures, and smoking. Contributing systemic factors include diabetes mellitus, anemia, immunosuppression (eg, HIV or AIDS), antibiotic use, infancy, advanced age, and endocrine dysfunction.

Candidal infections present in three main forms: pseudomembranous, erythematous, and hyperplastic. Pseudomembranous candidiasis (thrush) is characterized by thick, white, cheesy papules and plaques that can be rubbed off, leaving, in some cases, a bleeding area (Fig 13-11). The erythematous form of candidiasis is mainly encountered on the palatal mucosa under dentures, presenting as diffuse erythema demarcated by the shape of the denture base. Tongue lesions show atrophy of the filiform papilla, erythema, and a smooth tongue surface. Hyperplastic candidiasis is an uncommon chronic variant that presents as white plaques that do not rub off, suggestive of leukoplakia.

Oral candidiasis is treated with topical and systemic antifungal agents. The most commonly used topical agents include clotrimazole troches (10 mg), which are dissolved in the mouth 4 times a day for 7 to 10 days, and nystatin suspension (100,000 U/mL), which is swished

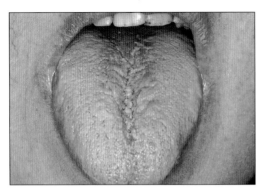

Fig 13-12 Hairy/coated tongue. Hyperplastic filiform papillae forming a matted area.

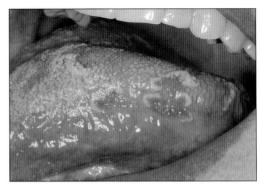

Fig 13-13 Migratory glossitis. White, arcuate lines enclosing erythematous mucosa.

around the mouth in a dose of 5 mL 4 times a day. Systemic therapy with fluconazole, 100 to 200 mg daily for 7 to 10 days, is extremely effective because patients usually exhibit good compliance. Dentures should be soaked overnight in an antibacterial solution such as 0.12% to 2% chlorhexidine digluconate or 3% sodium hypochlorite diluted in water (1:10 solution); they should not be worn overnight.

Candidal infection also causes angular cheilitis, which manifests as bilateral, bright red erythematous fissures at the corners of the mouth. Angular cheilitis is managed with topical nystatin/triamcinolone cream or ointment. Aggravating factors include poor support of the perioral musculature from lack of vertical dimension and hematinic deficiencies.

Coated or hairy tongue

Coated or hairy tongue is a benign, painless condition characterized by hyperplastic filiform papillae and accumulation of keratin on the dorsum (Fig 13-12). It is often mistaken for candidiasis, although treatment with antifungal agents is invariably unsuccessful. In the absence of symptoms, a positive culture for *Candida* (normally present in 20% to 30% of the population[32]) is indicative of carriage rather than candidal infection. The two common etiologic mechanisms are increased retention and reduced exfoliation of keratin of the filiform papillae, which become elongated and "hairy." Increased retention is related to dehydration

and hyposalivation so that there is less watery saliva and proportionally more mucinous, sticky saliva. Precipitating factors include a recent history of illness and antibiotic therapy, radiation therapy, smoking, and use of alcoholic mouthrinses. Poor diets in which meals are composed primarily of soft rather than coarse foods (such as fresh fruits and vegetables) also lead to reduced keratin exfoliation, and therefore coated tongue is common in patients convalescing from illness.

The tongue has a white, coated, matted, or hairy appearance and may become pigmented from food and intrinsic bacteria. Patients may complain of a pasty, stale taste in the mouth and even gagging because the coating tends to localize to the posterior region of the tongue near the circumvallate papillae; however, most do not experience symptoms. Management is directed toward hydration, stopping alcoholic or dehydrating mouthrinses, smoking cessation, improving the diet, and/or gentle brushing or scraping of the tongue 2 or 3 times a day.

Migratory glossitis

Migratory glossitis (also known as *geographic tongue, migratory stomatitis*, and *erythema areata migrans*) is a chronic resolving-relapsing condition that occurs in 1% to 2% of the population,[34] mainly adults (Fig 13-13). It presents as well-demarcated, patchy erythematous depapillation of the dorsum of the tongue with a raised, linear or ringlike, white peripheral rim.

Migratory glossitis is associated with fissured tongue in 25% of cases as well as with atopy (history of asthma, eczema, hay fever, or food intolerance) and psoriasis.[35] Some cases are associated with the HLA-Cw6 allele. Management includes pain control with viscous lidocaine and diphenhydramine as a mouthrinse preparation. Topical corticosteroid treatment is usually necessary because of the chronic, relapsing-resolving nature of the disorder.

Gingivitis

Conventional gingivitis

The most common gingival pathology in dentistry is plaque-induced gingivitis. Plaque-induced gingivitis is a common inflammatory disease of the gingiva resulting from production of inflammatory cytokines in response to bacterial lipopolysaccharides in plaque located in the gingival sulcus and on teeth. Gingivitis is common in adolescents and pregnant women because of hormonal changes. Progesterone associated with pregnancy seems to increase the permeability of gingival blood vessels and render the area more sensitive to physical, bacterial, and chemical irritants. Conventional gingivitis is characterized by erythema, edema, bleeding on provocation, tenderness, and sensitivity of the gingiva. Patients who are mouthbreathers have a unique pattern of gingivitis, with red and swollen anterior facial gingiva.

Good oral hygiene and mechanical plaque removal reduce or eliminate the inflammation, thereby allowing gingival tissue to heal.[36] Some patients may require antibiotic therapy with low-dose doxycycline or metronidazole, especially if there is underlying periodontitis.

Desquamative gingivitis and hypersensitivity reactions

Desquamative gingivitis is a common chronic condition of adults with a female predilection, most often representing OLP, MMP (discussed earlier), plasma cell gingivitis, and other hyper-

sensitivity reactions.[37] Other immunobullous disorders such as PV (discussed earlier), linear IgA disease, and epidermolysis bullosa aquisita are less common conditions that may also present in this fashion, although the last two do not present in the oral cavity without concomitant skin findings.

Desquamative gingivitis is characterized by fiery red, denuded attached gingiva, sometimes ulcerated (with a yellow fibrin pseudomembrane), primarily on the buccal or facial aspect. The gingiva is painful, and oral hygiene procedures may be challenging. Plaque accumulation secondary to poor oral hygiene further aggravates the pain, erythema, and propensity for gingival bleeding. The patient's diet may also be limited because of pain. Patients with desquamative gingivitis respond well to topical corticosteroid treatment applied within custom trays.

Plasma cell gingivitis is a contact hypersensitivity reaction to contactants such as flavoring agents (eg, cinnamic aldehyde) in toothpaste, chewing gum, or candies and presents as desquamative gingivitis. Plasma cell gingivitis may be accompanied by glossitis and cheilitis; sometimes the term *plasma cell orificial mucositis* is used because lesions may involve the upper airway. Examination of a biopsy specimen reveals sheets of plasma cells that raise the suspicion for a plasma cell malignancy, but in situ hybridization studies for light chain restriction show the cells to be polyclonal, typical for an inflammatory process.

Plasma cell gingivitis is reversible and resolves completely with avoidance of the allergen. However, treatment with topical immunosuppressive agents speeds the healing process. A patch test may help to identify the causative agent. However, some hypersensitivity reactions may be of a nonspecific nature, and a biopsy specimen may not exhibit sheets of plasma cells.

HIV/AIDS–associated linear gingivitis and necrotizing ulcerative gingivitis

HIV/AIDS-associated linear gingivitis is characterized by a 2- to 3-mm linear band of marked

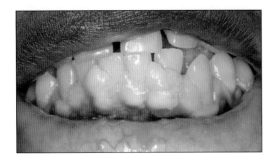

Fig 13-14 Drug-induced gingival hyperplasia. Diffuse dense, fibrotic gingival hyperplasia secondary to use of nifedipine and cyclosporine. (Courtesy of Dr Hani Mawardi, Harvard School of Dental Medicine, Boston, Massachusetts.)

erythema along the gingival margin that does not respond to conventional oral hygiene procedures and represents a form of erythematous candidiasis. Treatment involves antifungal medications together with mechanical debridement.

Immunocompromised individuals are also at higher risk of developing necrotizing ulcerative gingivitis.[38] This condition presents as ulcerated and necrotic, edematous and hemorrhagic interdental papillae and marginal gingiva and is a result of a polymicrobial infection by spirochetes, *Fusobacterium* sp, *Treponema* sp, and *Prevotella intermedia*. These patients may also report pain and halitosis. Treatment includes use of antibiotics, daily rinses with chlorhexidine gluconate, and debridement under local anesthesia.

Diffuse Gingival Hyperplasia

Diffuse gingival hyperplasia has been associated with multiple factors, including poor oral hygiene, as a long-term sequelae to conventional gingivitis, hormonal changes (such as pregnancy and puberty), adverse drug effects, and hereditary conditions. Gingival hyperplasia is caused by a proliferation of fibroblasts and accumulation of connective tissue fibers and extracellular matrix. Bacterial plaque and hormones, such as progesterone, may exacerbate this process. Clinically, the gingiva is overgrown either diffusely or multifocally throughout the mouth. When the cause is hereditary or syndromic, the tissue tends to be densely fibrotic, while hyperplastic gingiva caused by other conditions tends to be edematous and tender and bleeds easily. Good oral hygiene practices may resolve this condition if it is mild, but once there is significant fibrosis, surgery is usually required to remove the excess tissue.

Drug-induced gingival hyperplasia

Gingival hyperplasia is commonly induced by three main classes of drugs: anticonvulsants (phenytoin and less commonly sodium valproate, primidone, vigabatrin, and phenobarbital), calcium channel blockers (such as amlodipine, bepridil, diltiazem, felodipine, nicardipine, nifedipine, nimodipine, nitrendipine, and verapamil) and immunosuppressants (such as cyclosporine and rarely tacrolimus).[39] Drug-induced gingival enlargement associated with long-term phenytoin use occurs in approximately 15% to 50% of cases (Fig 13-14). For calcium channel blockers the prevalence ranges from 10% to 20%, and for cyclosporine the prevalence is approximately 27%. Patients who have received renal transplants are particularly susceptible because they are on both calcium channel blockers and cyclosporine. There are rare cases associated with trimethoprim sulfamethoxazole and erythromycin. These medications cause a reduction in metalloproteinases (leading to accumulation of matrix) and/or an increase in fibroblastic activity.

Not all patients taking these medications develop gingival hyperplasia, and it is more common in patients with poor oral hygiene.[40] There may be a genetic predisposition, perhaps related to drug metabolism.

Unlike plaque-induced gingival hyperplasia, the drug-induced form tends to be less erythematous, more fibrotic, and less inflamed, although inflammation often results if pseudopockets form. The gingival enlargement may resolve on discontinuation of the medication if the condition is mild. For more severe cases, excision of the hyperplastic tissue is required together with maintenance of good oral hygiene and daily use of chlorhexidine rinses. A low dose of doxycycline may reduce the risk of recurrence.

Acute leukemia

Acute monocytic leukemia is the most serious systemic condition associated with diffuse gingival enlargement. The leukemic cells infiltrate the tissues, resulting in gingival enlargement. Bone marrow involvement by leukemia reduces the body's ability to form the normal components of the blood, such as platelets, resulting in petechiae and ecchymosis of the mucosa and gingiva and spontaneous bleeding. Lack of red blood cells leads to anemia, fatigue, and pallor of the mucosa, and poorly functioning cancerous white cells lead to recurrent infections in the mouth that may exacerbate periodontal disease. Teeth may become mobile, and suppuration may be noted around the gingiva. In addition, systemic symptoms such as night sweats, recurrent infections, or lethargy may be present.

Dentists play an important role in the diagnosis of leukemia by taking a careful history, performing a biopsy of the gingiva or referring the patient for a biopsy, and obtaining a complete blood count to establish a preliminary diagnosis. Gingival hyperplasia typically resolves with effective chemotherapy.

Hereditary and syndromic gingival hyperplasia

Fibromatosis gingivae is a diffuse gingival fibrous overgrowth that occurs either in combination with rare syndromes or as an isolated disease caused by spontaneous mutation. Some associated syndromes are Cowden syndrome (associated with trichilemmomas, oral mucosal papillomatosis, acral and palmoplantar keratoses, and increased risk for breast and thyroid carcinoma), Zimmerman-Laband syndrome (ear, nose, bone, and nail defects), Murray-Puretic-Drescher syndrome (juvenile hyaline fibromatosis with nodular/papular skin lesions), Rutherford syndrome (corneal dystrophy), and Cross syndrome (microphthalmia, hypopigmentation, mental retardation, and athetosis).

Hereditary gingival fibromatosis is a rare hereditary gingival condition that usually develops during childhood and is transmitted through both autosomal-dominant and autosomal-recessive modes. This disease is characterized by firm, pink gingival enlargement that is nonhemorrhagic and asymptomatic. The growth is multifocal, diffuse, and nodular or smooth surfaced. The enlargement is slow growing and becomes more prominent during the eruption of both primary and permanent teeth. The gingival enlargement often leads to impaction and displacement of teeth, diastemas, and malocclusion. Patients may also experience difficulty speaking and painful mastication. Treatment for both hereditary and syndromic gingival hyperplasia includes surgical removal of excess gingival tissue and recontouring.

Destructive membranous periodontal disease (ligneous gingivitis and periodontitis)

Ligneous gingivitis, or destructive membranous periodontal disease, is a rare condition characterized by generalized nodular gingival enlargement with or without ulceration. It is associated with plasminogen deficiency that leads to the formation of fibrin deposits that accumulate in the connective tissue. Ligneous gingivitis is found in approximately one of three patients with severe homozygous plasminogen deficiency and is often accompanied by ligneous conjunctivitis. Additional clinical manifestations include involvement of the mucosa of the female genital tract, nasopharynx, and tracheo-bronchial tree. Some patients may benefit from use of topical and systemic corticosteroids or systemic warfarin.

Pigmented Lesions

Pigmentations of the teeth and oral mucosa result from pigments of either extrinsic or intrinsic origin.

Extrinsic pigmentation

Foods and dentifrices

Extensive use of tobacco products, tea, or coffee often results in yellow, brown, or black stains of teeth. Prolonged use of chlorhexidine mouthwash may cause a brown stain along the cervical areas of teeth. These pigmentations can be removed by simple dental prophylaxis.

Black hairy tongue is a pigmented form of coated/hairy tongue (see Fig 13-12). The tongue has a thick matte on the dorsum, varying in color from black-brown to green or even to yellow-orange, depending on food pigment and/or pigments produced by chromogenic bacteria that reside on the tongue. Management considerations are the same as those already described for coated/hairy tongue.

Amalgam tattoo

Amalgam tattoo is the most common extrinsic intramucosal pigmentation. Amalgam tattoos appear as localized or diffuse (less common), asymptomatic slate-blue, gray, or black macules of the oral mucosa. Most patients are unaware of the presence of the pigmentation until it is brought to their attention by a dentist or hygienist.

Patients may become concerned regarding the possibility of melanoma. The diagnosis is straightforward when the tattoos are located on the gingiva near an amalgam restoration or crown or near an apicoectomy scar. However,

some pigmentations caused by traumatic implantation are located on the ventral surface of the tongue, the floor of the mouth, or buccal mucosa, and these are often biopsied (Fig 13-15). The silver of amalgam stains connective tissue fibers, and this is readily identified on histopathologic examination.

Heavy metal pigmentation

Poisoning with heavy metals such as lead, mercury, silver, platinum, arsenic, or bismuth presents as a dark or black band along the gingival margin, likely caused by deposition of sulfides of heavy metals within the gingiva. These pigmentations are mostly of historical interest, and it is extremely rare to see oral manifestations of such heavy metal toxicity now. However, blackening of the tongue may be seen in patients who chronically use bismuth subsalicylate (Pepto-Bismol, Procter & Gamble).

Other causes

Graphite (pencil lead) presents as a dark gray or black pigmentation that is explained by a history of traumatic implantation, usually during childhood. Other extrinsic pigmentations include those from foreign substances intentionally introduced for cosmetic reasons (eg, in some African countries) or from cigarette ash (eg, some prison tattoos).

Intrinsic pigmentation

The two most common pigmented lesions in the oral cavity caused by intrinsic agents arise from melanin deposition and blood or its breakdown products.

Melanin

Physiologic pigmentation. The most common melanosis is physiologic pigmentation that typically affects the gingiva of dark-skinned individuals. The palatal mucosa, buccal mucosa, and tongue are less commonly affected. Such pigmentation is usually brown-to-black, symmet-

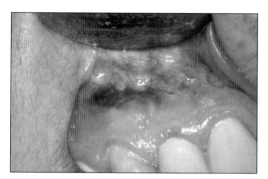

Fig 13-15 Amalgam tattoo. Dark gray to black macule of oral mucosa located at a scar from apical surgery.

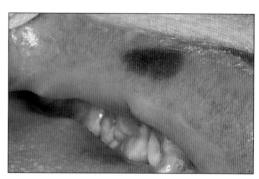

Fig 13-16 Labial melanotic macule. Solitary brown, painless macule.

ric, and macular (flush with the nonpigmented mucosa). The diagnosis is based on the clinical appearance.

Melanotic macules. Melanotic macules are common in the adult population, especially in the fifth decade and beyond. They present as brown or tan, painless macules, evenly pigmented, usually smaller than 1 cm, on the lower vermilion, palatal mucosa, or attached gingiva (Fig 13-16). Some lesions may be so dark as to appear black.[41] Although most melanotic macules are solitary, they may also be multiple. Such macules of sudden onset may lead to concerns about primary adrenocortical insufficiency (discussed later). Lesions are often biopsied to rule out a melanoma, and the specimens show melanin in the basal cells and in the connective tissue. Treatment is not necessary for the condition unless it is of cosmetic concern.

Postinflammatory hypermelanosis. Postinflammatory hypermelanosis is associated with nonspecific or specific inflammatory conditions, such as OLP, oral chronic GVHD, and post-chemotherapy or radiation mucositis. The brown macules appear in the areas involved by the mucosal inflammatory lesion, usually the buccal mucosa and tongue. Lesions tend to occur in dark-skinned individuals, are usually asymptomatic, and fade over time.

Melanoacanthosis is a rare, benign pigmented lesion that is seen most frequently in young black women. It typically presents as a tan to brown macule on the buccal mucosa that may rapidly grow to several centimeters.[42] A biopsy will reveal a benign proliferation of melanocytes within thickened epithelium. Melanoacanthosis may represent a form of postinflammatory hypermelanosis because it resolves over time.

Melanocytic nevi and melanoma. Oral melanocytic nevi occur most frequently on the palatal mucosa. Intramucosal and compound melanocytic nevi are fleshy nodules resembling fibromas that may or may not be pigmented.[43] Junctional nevi (rare) and blue nevi (more common) are macular and brown or blue-black. Melanocytic nevi are evenly pigmented (when pigmented) and usually less than 1 cm in size. A biopsy establishes the diagnosis.

Oral melanoma accounts for 0.2% to 8% of all melanomas.[44] It is more common in black and Japanese individuals and in men in their 50s to 70s and is more frequent in the sinonasal tract than in the oral cavity. The most affected oral sites are the palatal mucosa and gingiva, and they arise within a preexisting dysplastic melanocytic lesion. Unlike skin melanomas, which are caused by sun damage, the etiopathogenesis of oral melanoma is unclear.

Clinically, oral melanoma is greater than 1 cm with irregular borders and irregular pigmentation; nodularity and areas of hemorrhage within a pigmented lesion are suspicious signs of melanoma. Treatment includes excision with clear margins. The recurrence rate is 50%, and adjuvant radiotherapy reduces metastases and local relapse.[45] Chemotherapeutic regimens are currently under investigation.

Melanotic macular lesions associated with syndromes. Melanotic macules may be associated with Addison disease and lentiginous syndromes such as neurofibromatosis, Peutz-Jeghers syndrome, McCune-Albright syndrome, Carney complex, and Laugier-Hunziker syndrome.

Addison disease (primary adrenocortical insufficiency) is a rare condition in which the adrenal cortex does not produce enough glucocorticoids, and sometimes mineralocorticoids, leading to compensatory overproduction of adrenocorticotropic hormone (ACTH). Most cases are autoimmune, but it can also be caused by infection or other etiologies. Addison disease is typically diagnosed in middle-aged or young adults. Patients report fatigue, dizziness, hypotension, and abdominal pain. β-melanocyte-stimulating hormone is integral to the ACTH molecule, so whenever levels of ACTH are high, regardless of the etiology, melanosis results. Patients present with generalized bronze coloration of the genitalia and skin (especially flexural areas) and sites of trauma. The oral mucosa may exhibit a sudden onset of melanotic macules. Diagnosis is made by observation of clinical signs and symptoms and confirmation of elevated levels of ACTH.

Neurofibromatosis is a group of genetic disorders with autosomal-dominant inheritance; the most common form is neurofibromatosis type 1 (von Recklinghausen disease of skin). Neurofibromatosis type 1 is characterized by pigmented lesions that are usually present at birth. These lesions appear as freckles and tan to brown café-au-lait macules with smooth edges (resembling the coast of California). Other clinical manifestations include oral and skin neurofibromas and Lisch nodules in the eyes.

Peutz-Jeghers syndrome is a rare autosomal-dominant disorder characterized by intestinal polyposis and multiple mucocutaneous melanocytic macules. Brown macules are generally several millimeters and typically "peppered" on the skin around periorificial sites such as the mouth, nose, and eyes; on the extremities; and in the oral cavity. Peutz-Jeghers syndrome is also associated with short bowel syndrome, small intestine intussusception, and anemia. Management consists of surveillance of intestinal polyps and laparotomies and laparoscopies for both gastrointestinal and extraintestinal problems.

McCune-Albright syndrome is characterized by fibrous dysplasia of bone, irregularly shaped café-au-lait skin macules (resembling the coast of Maine), and precocious puberty. Oral melanotic macules may occur in some individuals, although these lesions are rare.

Carney complex is an autosomal-dominant family of disorders characterized by multiple lentigines of the skin and oral mucosa, cardiac and skin myxomas, and endocrine hyperactivity.

Laugier-Hunziker syndrome is a rare acquired disorder characterized by multiple melanotic macules of the oral mucosa and occasionally the genital mucosa, conjunctiva, esophagus, and acral surfaces as well as brown melanotic bands on the nails (melanonychia). Lesions may be treated with a laser as necessary.

Blood pigment

Pigmentations may result from vascular lesions or from extravasated blood and their breakdown products.

Petechiae and ecchymoses. The most common oral lesions caused by blood pigment are those resulting from trauma, namely petechiae (less than 5 mm, clustered and pinpoint), ecchymoses, and hematomas, which tend to be deeper. These lesions are readily diagnosed if a history of trauma can be elicited from the location of lesions (such as acute bite trauma). These resolve without treatment, although hematomas may require evacuation and antibiotics to prevent secondary infection. The onset of frequent and extensive petechiae and ecchymoses in the mucosa raises the specter of a blood dyscrasia, such as leukemia, where the platelets are reduced in number and/or function.

Vascular lesions. Vascular lesions may lead to pigmented lesions that appear as small red, blue, or purple blebs or nodules on the mucosa; these lesions often blanch on pressure.

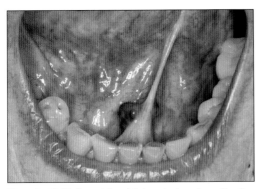

Fig 13-17 Varices. Blue blebs clustered on the lingual frenum.

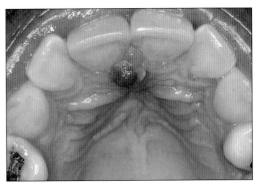

Fig 13-18 Pyogenic granuloma. Red nodule on the incisive papilla.

The most common type of vascular lesion is a varix or venous lake (Fig 13-17). More than one vessel may be involved, leading to a multilobulated or bosselated nodule. These are common on the lips, tongue, or buccal mucosa in older individuals.

Another vascular lesion common on the gingiva, lips, and tongue is the pyogenic granuloma, presenting as red or bluish-purple nodules (Fig 13-18). Pregnant women may develop these lesions (granuloma gravidarum). If small, they usually regress postpartum, but they may also fibrose and require excision.

Vascular lesions may bleed excessively when traumatized and are readily excised or ablated with a laser. Larger lesions represent venous anomalies, and these may involve the muscle, especially of the tongue. True hemangiomas are usually present from birth, are uncommon in the oral cavity, and regress over time.

Sturge-Weber syndrome. Sturge-Weber syndrome (encephalofacial angiomatosis) is a rare congenital neurocutaneous condition characterized by a port-wine stain of the skin, typically along the ophthalmic and maxillary distributions of the trigeminal nerve. Patients may present with bluish-purple plaques on the buccal mucosa and gingiva on the same side as the skin lesions. These plaques represent hamartomatous vascular hyperplasia. Abnormal vessels in the leptomeninges of the brain and choroid are the cause of seizures.

Diagnosis is made through clinical examination, angiography, and imaging. The treatment is symptomatic and includes laser therapy to remove or lighten the skin and mucosal lesions, anticonvulsants for seizure control, symptomatic and prophylactic therapy for headache, and treatments to reduce intraocular pressure.

Hereditary hemochromatosis. Hereditary hemochromatosis results from an inherited autosomal-recessive disorder, while hemosiderosis may follow a history of multiple transfusions. Hereditary hemochromatosis is caused by increased absorption of dietary iron in the gut, leading to iron accumulation in parenchymal organs and end-organ damage. Iron deposition in the form of hemosiderin and ferritin leads to skin bronzing, cirrhosis, hypopituitarism, diabetes mellitus, nephrogenic diabetes insipidus, and cardiomyopathy. Brown to gray diffuse macules of the palatal mucosa and gingiva occur in approximately 15% to 20% of patients.[46] Phlebotomy and chelation therapy are the preferred treatment for these patients.

Drug-induced oral pigmentation

Several medications, including antibiotics of the tetracycline family, antimalarial agents, oral contraceptive agents, antipsychotics (phenothiazines such as chlorpromazine), and chemotherapeutic agents may cause oral pigmentation.[47] While many chemotherapeutic agents have been reported to cause pigmentation, some of these instances may represent postinflammatory hypermelanosis (discussed earlier) at sites where mucositis and ulcers had developed (such as the buccal mucosa, tongue, and lips) and should not be considered true drug-induced pigmentation.

Three mechanisms have been proposed to explain drug-induced pigmentation:

1. Drug metabolites that are pigmented are deposited in the connective tissue, causing pigmentation.
2. The pigmentation is caused by breakdown products of the drug that chelate with melanin or iron.
3. The drug (or drug metabolite) stimulates an increase in melanin production.

Diagnosis of drug-induced pigmentation is typically made from a history of exposure to medications. Oral lesions present as diffuse, painless, symmetric, bluish-gray macular pigmentations of the hard palatal mucosa that may occur concomitantly with skin and nail pigmentation.

Tetracycline is a broad-spectrum antibiotic used to treat bacterial infections. It chelates to bone and teeth and results in brown or gray discoloration, which is revealed as fluorescence under ultraviolet or other light sources. Minocycline is a long-acting compound with powerful anti-inflammatory properties that is widely used to treat dermatologic conditions such as acne as well as systemic infections and periodontal disease. Tetracycline and minocycline pigmentation typically occurs after long-term use and involves the skin, thyroid, nails, conjunctiva, sclera, and oral mucosa. Bone and teeth developing during the time of minocycline administration are discolored similarly to bone and teeth affected by tetracycline. In the oral cavity, the mucosa may darken because the grayish-black color of the underlying bone shows through the mucosa. However, breakdown products of minocycline may be noted within the connective tissue.

Antimalarial agents, such as chloroquine, hydroxychloroquine, quinacrine, and amodiaquine, have anti-inflammatory and immunosuppressive functions. Chloroquine is also widely used as an adjunct in the treatment of autoimmune diseases. Long-term use of chloroquine may cause diffuse grayish-black pigmentation of the palatal mucosa, as does imatinib, a tyrosine kinase inhibitor that is used as a first-line treatment for chronic myelogenous leukemia. Skin and nails may also be affected.

Oral pigmentations induced by minocycline, antimalarial agents, and imatinib have a similar histopathologic appearance. Small, regular spherical particles are noted in the connective tissue chelated to melanin and sometimes iron.

Estrogens, either alone or in combination with progesterone, have also been reported to cause oral pigmentation. Hyperpigmentation is the result of an increase in the activity of melanogenic enzymes. Oral involvement most often involves the palatal mucosa and facial gingiva. On cessation of the medication, the oral and cutaneous lesions (melasma or chloasma) slowly resolve.

Poorly Healing or Nonhealing Extraction Sockets and Osteonecrosis

After dental extractions, a blood clot is formed within 24 to 48 hours. The clot is replaced with granulation tissue, and bone formation is well established by 6 to 8 weeks and completed by 6 months. Intact mucosa is noted within 2 to 3 weeks.

Dry socket

Dry socket (alveolitis sicca dolorosa, postoperative osteitis, alveolar osteitis) is a common postoperative complication that occurs after a dental extraction. It has an onset of 2 to 4 days after surgery. The incidence ranges from 3% to 4% following routine dental extractions to 1% to 45% after the removal of third molars.[48]

The etiology of dry socket is still unclear. Studies suggest that the blood clot that forms after dental extraction is not replaced with granulation

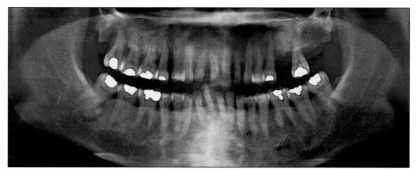

Fig 13-19 Multifocal cemento-osseous dysplasia. Panoramic radiograph showing multiple radiolucencies with opacities of the mandible and maxilla.

tissue but rather early fibrinolysis and clot breakdown occur, leaving the socket empty with exposed bare bone.[48] Risk factors include a previous experience of dry socket; extraction of deeply impacted mandibular third molars, especially those with pericoronitis; poor oral hygiene; active or recent history of acute ulcerative gingivitis; heavy smoking; use of oral contraceptives; and an immunocompromised state.[48]

Patients typically complain of severe pain and halitosis 24 to 72 hours after the extraction. The socket presents with exposed alveolar bone with little tissue in it, hence the term *dry socket*. Healing may not occur without intervention. Pain control is of utmost importance, and this can be accomplished with NSAIDs and/or narcotic analgesics. The surgical site should be irrigated with saline, and gentle debridement and packing with zinc oxide–eugenol paste on iodoform gauze may be useful as well. Patients must be followed at least weekly to ensure that granulation tissue forms in the socket to start the process of bone healing. Preventive strategies include rinsing with chlorhexidine (0.12% or 0.2%) before and after the extraction or placement of chlorhexidine gel (0.2%) in the sockets of extracted teeth.

Infection

Infections of the jawbones lead to pain, swelling, suppuration, and, in the most severe cases, osteomyelitis. This may occur after extractions, other surgical procedures, or trauma (such as fractures). However, some systemic and local factors greatly increase the risk of infection.

Diabetes mellitus

Patients with poorly controlled type 1 diabetes mellitus are at risk for poorly healing sockets because these patients are prone to infections and more severe periodontal disease, which in itself may impair glycemic control. Conversely, treatment for severe periodontitis has been shown to improve glycemic control. Studies in diabetic animals have shown that the formation of the collagenous framework in the tooth extraction socket is inhibited and that aberrant endothelial activation and impaired angiogenic response result in delayed socket healing and the development of dry socket.[49]

Primary bone diseases

Cemento-osseous dysplasia is a fairly common disorder of the jaws that occurs in focal, periapical, and florid (or multifocal) forms and is of unknown etiology.[50] Black women in particular develop the periapical form that involves the apices of the anterior mandibular teeth, as well as the multiquadrant florid form. The associated teeth are vital, and this disorder is usually first noticed on routine radiographic examination. Early lesions are generally radiolucent; over time, the centers of the radiolucencies exhibit radiopacities that may become extremely dense and sclerotic (Fig 13-19). As a result, dental extractions may lead to necrosis of the bone because of poor perfusion, infection, and osteomyelitis.

Paget disease of bone (osteitis deformans) is a disease of unknown etiology characterized by hyperactivity of osteoclasts and increased bone remodeling that lead to the formation of disorganized bone. Paget disease usually occurs after the age of 55 years and typically affects the axial skeleton, especially the pelvis. The skull is involved in about 40% of patients, and involved bones enlarge over time.[51]

The most common symptom of Paget disease is bone pain and neurologic signs related to pressure on the cranial nerves when their ostia become progressively narrowed from bone deposition. Enlargement of the maxilla and mandible may result in development of diastemas and malocclusion. Early lesions are radiolucent with coarsening of the trabecular pattern. Later, cortical thickening develops and radiopacities form, resulting in a cotton wool–like appearance. Patients with Paget disease are at higher risk of developing osteosarcoma (less than 1% of cases).[52]

The diagnosis is made on the basis of serology (greatly increased bone-specific alkaline phosphatase and other bone-turnover markers), histopathology, and radiographic appearance. Histopathologic studies reveal haphazard bone formation.

Dentists should recognize the symptoms and signs of Paget disease and be aware that a dental extraction may be associated with postextraction bleeding and secondary osteomyelitis. Mild cases of Paget disease do not require treatment, but patients with pain and severe involvement are treated with antiresorptive therapy.

Osteopetrosis is a genetic heterogenous group of heritable diseases of the bone characterized by osteoclastic dysfunction that results in osteosclerosis. Infection, osteonecrosis, and osteomyelitis may ensue after extractions because of the reduced blood supply.

Osteoradionecrosis

Osteoradionecrosis is a severe complication of radiation therapy of the head and neck re-

gion with a prevalence of 4%.[53] Radiation of the bone (50 Gy or more) causes damage to the microvasculature system and osteocytes, which can lead to poor wound healing, infection, and bone necrosis.

The majority of cases of osteoradionecrosis occur after trauma or dental extraction in patients who have undergone radiation therapy. Signs and symptoms include pain, swelling, tooth mobility, mucosal breakdown, fistula formation, exposed necrotic bone, and pathologic fracture.[54] Radiographs show a poorly defined radiolucency with areas of radiopacity consistent with sequestra.

Initial treatment is directed at controlling infection through surgical debridement, removal of sequestra, and gentle tissue irrigation. Hyperbaric oxygen may be used to improve wound healing through increased oxygen tension, stimulation of vascular proliferation, and direct bacteriostatic effects on certain microorganisms.

To reduce the incidence of osteoradionecrosis, patients should complete a comprehensive dental evaluation by a dentist or an oral medicine specialist prior to starting radiation. All carious teeth should be restored, and nonvital teeth should be endodontically treated (if they are without significant periapical pathosis) or extracted. Any nonrestorable tooth with a poor prognosis (3+ mobility) should be extracted 2 to 3 weeks prior to radiation treatment to allow sufficient time for healing. Teeth that are symptomatic after endodontic therapy or exhibit sinus tracts may require retreatment, apicoectomy, or extraction. Areas with periodontal pocketing of more than 4 to 5 mm should receive deep scaling and curettage.

If the patient has already received radiation therapy and requires extraction, the patient may need hyperbaric oxygen therapy prior to the extraction, although more recent studies suggest that extraction under prophylactic antibiotic therapy may be sufficient.[54] Much may depend on the state of the teeth to be extracted, that is, whether the teeth are firmly encased in bone or whether they are severely periodontally involved and merely surrounded by granulation tissue.

Table 13-5   **Staging of bisphosphonate-induced osteonecrosis of the jaw***

Stage	Description
Stage 0	*Stage 0, suspicious asymptomatic:* Asymptomatic, persistent sinus tracts or localized deep periodontal pockets and typical radiographic findings for BIONJ (thickening or loss of the lamina dura, osteosclerosis, mottled radiolucency and/or radiopacity, persistent extraction sockets)
	Stage 0, suspicious symptomatic: Symptomatic with same findings as stage 0, suspicious asymptomatic
Stage 1	Exposed necrotic bone with absence of pain and infection
Stage 2	Exposed necrotic bone with pain, suppuration, or intraoral sinus tract all suggesting ongoing infection
Stage 3	Same as stage 2 plus one of the following: extraoral fistula, osteolysis extending to the inferior border, exposed necrotic bone extending beyond the region of the alveolar bone, pathologic fracture, or oroantral and oronasal communication

*According to the American Association of Oral and Maxillofacial Surgeons[58] and Mawardi et al.[59]

Drug-induced osteonecrosis

Drug-induced osteonecrosis of the jaw (DIONJ) is a sequela of the use of antiresorptive agents, such as bisphosphonates and denosumab, as well as antiangiogenic agents. Bisphosphonates are potent inhibitors of osteoclast-mediated bone resorption and have been used in the management of multiple myeloma, bone metastases, osteoporosis, and Paget disease of bone. The most common adverse effects associated with the use of bisphosphonates include acute-phase reactions, gastrointestinal upset, renal toxicity, and bisphosphonate-induced osteonecrosis of the jaw (BIONJ). Acute-phase reaction (a nonspecific physiologic reaction associated with fever, flulike symptoms, and increased levels of inflammatory cytokines) and impaired renal function occur primarily with use of intravenous bisphosphonates. Oral bisphosphonates can also cause esophagitis; patients are therefore instructed to remain upright for 30 to 60 minutes after ingestion.

The use of bisphosphonates is associated with BIONJ in treatment of both osteoporosis (frequency of 0.02%)[55] and cancer (frequency of 3% to 8%).[56] The single most important risk for BIONJ is cumulative dose, which is related to duration of therapy.[57] Patients with osteoporosis who are prescribed intravenous bisphosphonates generally receive a single annual 5-mg infusion of zoledronic acid, compared with patients with myeloma or metastatic cancer to the bones, who receive a 4-mg infusion monthly, usually for 24 months. Other risk factors include dental extractions, other dentoalveolar surgery, physiologic trauma, and oral infections, although some cases of BIONJ are idiopathic.

The American Academy of Oral and Maxillofacial Surgeons defines BIONJ on the basis of three criteria: prior or current exposure of the patient to bisphosphonates, presence of a necrotic bone lesion for at least 8 weeks, and no history of irradiation of the involved bone; stage 0 disease without exposed bone also exists. Staging and clinical and radiographic findings are described in Table 13-5.[58,59]

Patients present with painful or painless areas of exposed bone, often located on the mylohyoid ridge or tori, or nonhealing extraction sockets with exposed bone. Some patients may develop ulcers on the tongue from trauma caused by sharp bone edges. Sinus tracts are often seen around the exposed bone and are a particularly important finding in stage 0 disease.

Treatment is aimed at pain and infection control. At every visit, the dental practitioner should attempt to gently dislodge the bone fragment (nonsurgical sequestrectomy) (Fig 13-20). Stag-

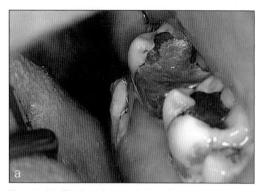
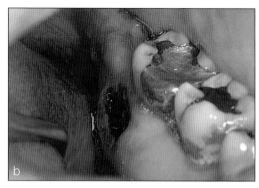

Fig 13-20 Bisphosphonate-induced osteonecrosis of the jaw. *(a)* Nonviable sequestrum on the mylohyoid ridge. *(b)* Bed of hemorrhagic granulation tissue after dislodgment (nonsurgical sequestrectomy).

es 2 and 3 are treated with antibiotics (amoxicillin with or without clavulanic acid, clindamycin, or metronidazole) for a 2- to 4-week or 1- to 2-month course of therapy. Chlorhexidine or other antimicrobial oral rinses should be prescribed for all patients at any stage.

If the patient has had substantial exposure to bisphosphonate therapy, endodontic therapy is preferable to extraction for nonmobile teeth that have good bone support; nonrestorable teeth can be decoronated. However, there is no absolute contraindication to extraction. Extraction may be the most appropriate treatment for teeth that are located within obvious areas of BIONJ that are extremely mobile and at risk for aspiration, if the patient has continued to have pain and infection in spite of multiple courses of antibiotic therapy. Contrary to earlier findings, more recent data show that surgical resection may lead to durable remission of disease.[60] Prevention of BIONJ, especially in cancer patients, involves a protocol similar to that for patients who are scheduled for head and neck radiation.

Denosumab (Prolia, Amgen; Xgeva, Amgen) is a monoclonal antibody with bone antiresorptive properties that has been cleared by the US Food and Drug Administration for use in patients with osteoporosis and metastatic cancer to the bone, as an alternative medication to bisphosphonates. Denosumab binds to a molecule on the osteoclast, inhibiting its activity and thereby causing inhibition of bone resorption. As such,

use of denosumab has also been associated with the development of DIONJ in patients with cancer at a frequency of 2% to 3%, similar to that associated with bisphosphonates.[61]

Prolia is used for treatment of osteoporosis and is administered at a dose of 60 mg subcutaneously once every 6 months, while Xgeva is indicated for bone metastases from solid tumors in adult patients and is administered at a dose of 120 mg subcutaneously every 4 weeks. Prevention and treatment strategies for denosumab-associated DIONJ are the same as for BIONJ.[62]

Antiangiogenic agents (such as bevacizumab and sunitinib) are prescribed for the management of metastatic cancers and are also associated with an increased risk of DIONJ, especially when used together with bisphosphonates that themselves have antiangiogenic properties. Both agents act against blood vessel growth factors essential for normal jawbone remodeling and wound repair and can lead to BIONJ. Management principles for DIONJ are the same as for BIONJ.

Metastatic tumor to the jaw

Metastases to the oral cavity are rare and represent approximately 1% of all oral malignancies. Two-thirds of metastatic tumors to the oral cavity occur to the jawbones, and nearly 80%

involve the mandible; one-third occur in the soft tissues, usually involving the gingiva and sometimes the tongue.[63] Cancers of the breast, lung, prostate, kidney, and colon/rectum are the most common primary sites.

Patients with metastasis to the jaw may complain of pain, paresthesia, or anesthesia of the skin or mucosa, tooth mobility, and gingival or jaw swelling. Radiographically, the lesions present as poorly defined radiolucencies. When such involved mobile teeth are extracted, a common scenario is that the socket fails to heal but is instead filled with fleshy soft tissue.[63]

Xerostomia and Hyposalivation

Saliva plays a critical role in lubrication, buffering, mastication, swallowing, speech, taste, tooth remineralization, and prevention of oral infection. Therefore, patients with hyposalivation are at risk of developing erythematous areas from friction; experience difficulty with eating, swallowing, taste, and speech; and are at greater risk of caries and candidiasis.[64]

Xerostomia is a common subjective complaint of dryness in the mouth. It is only a symptom and may or may not be associated with a reduced quantity of saliva in the mouth. *Salivary gland hypofunction* and *hyposalivation* are the terms used for objective and measurable reductions in the amount of saliva in the mouth. The measurable reduction occurs because saliva production and flow are reduced either in normally functioning glands or in damaged glands.

A simple subjective test for dryness from hyposalivation that correlates well with saliva collection studies involves asking the following four questions[65]:

1. Do you feel you have less saliva than normal?
2. Does your mouth feel dry when eating a meal?
3. Do you have difficulty swallowing?
4. Do you need to drink water to swallow dry foods?

A positive answer to all four is strongly associated with hyposalivation. A modified Schirmer test (normally used in the eyes) also identifies patients with marked hyposalivation.[66]

Besides feeling that the mouth is dry, patients may report that they experience sensitivity on eating foods that are spicy, acidic, or crunchy or have symptoms of burning. Food may not taste the way it used to, and patients may report a metallic or salty taste. In less severe cases, the saliva is frothy, ropey, or thick. In more severe cases, the mucosa looks dry and erythematous (especially the tongue) and there is little to no pooling of saliva in the floor of the mouth.

Hyposalivation associated with normal glands

Hyposalivation associated with normal glands is by far the most common type of hyposalivation. Causative factors include dehydration (eg, from poor oral intake of fluids, overconsumption of caffeinated beverages, and/or smoking), the use of drugs with anticholinergic activity, the use of multiple medications (polypharmacy), and chronic anxiety. Strongly xerogenic medications include antidepressants, antipsychotics, diuretics, anticholinergics, antihypertensives, anxiolytics, sedatives, NSAIDs, antihistamines, and opioid analgesic agents.

Hyposalivation associated with damaged glands

Radiation therapy of the head and neck region, especially for head and neck cancer, and Sjögren syndrome occur less commonly but result in severe hyposalivation because of destruction of salivary glands. Parotid glands exposed to doses of greater than 60 Gy sustain permanent damage with no recovery in salivary hypofunction over time.

Sjögren syndrome is a systemic autoimmune disorder that mainly affects middle-aged women. Affected individuals produce autoantibodies that attack and destroy the salivary and other exocrine glands.[67] The primary form involves mostly the exocrine glands (especially the salivary and lacrimal glands), while the secondary form is associated with other autoimmune diseases such as lupus erythematosus and rheumatoid arthritis. Patients typically report a dry mouth, dry eyes (keratoconjunctivitis sicca), and dry nasal passages. Patients with Sjögren syndrome are at higher risk for lymphoma and should be followed regularly.

To establish a diagnosis of Sjögren syndrome, individuals with symptoms and signs suggestive of Sjögren syndrome need to have at least two of the following three objective features: (1) positive serum anti–SSA/Ro and/or anti–SSB/La or positive rheumatoid factor and antinuclear antibody titer ≥ 1:320; (2) labial salivary gland biopsy exhibiting focal lymphocytic sialadenitis with a focus score of ≥ 1 focus/4 mm²; (3) keratoconjunctivitis sicca with an ocular staining score of 3 (assuming that individual is not currently using daily eye drops for glaucoma and has not had corneal surgery or cosmetic eyelid surgery in the last 5 years).

Other possible conditions that may contribute to hyposalivation are IgG4-related disease, which results in salivary gland enlargement and hyposalivation similar to Sjögren syndrome, chronic GVHD, poorly controlled diabetes, and malnutrition.

Treatment of xerostomia aims to relieve symptoms and, in cases of true salivary gland hypofunction, increase salivary flow. Therapeutic strategies include improved hydration and avoidance of harsh and dehydrating dentifrices; avoidance of crunchy hard foods; use of saliva substitutes, mucosal lubricants, and saliva stimulants such as sugar-free candy or gum; and daily fluoride treatment for caries prevention. Nonalcoholic oral care products such as Biotene products (GlaxoSmithKline) and children's toothpaste are good options. Medications include pilocarpine (5 mg, 3 times a day for at least 3 months) and cevimeline (30 mg, 3 times a day for at least 3 months). Saline nasal sprays help in lubrication and sometimes improve flavor discernment in food.

Damage to the salivary glands with radiation can be somewhat mitigated with the use of intensity-modified radiation therapy, where the radiation is better targeted; with the use of amifostine (a free radical scavenger that protects the glands); and with the use of pilocarpine during radiation.

Conclusion

Seven common findings in the oral mucosa that may also indicate systemic disease have been discussed. Many patients go to their dentist on a regular basis for scaling and prophylaxis, and the dental hygienist and dentist are therefore in a unique position to notice subtle changes in the mucosa or bone that may be the first indication of a systemic disease, be it as common as iron-deficiency anemia or as life-threatening as leukemia.

References

1. Budtz-Jorgensen E. Oral mucosal lesions associated with the wearing of removable dentures. J Oral Pathol 1981;10:65–80.
2. Scully C. Clinical practice. Aphthous ulceration. N Engl J Med 2006;355:165–172.
3. Baccaglini L, Lalla RV, Bruce AJ, et al. Urban legends: Recurrent aphthous stomatitis. Oral Dis 2011; 17:755–770.
4. Baumgart DC, Sandborn WJ. Crohn's disease. Lancet 2012;380:1590–1605.
5. Scully C, Hodgson T. Recurrent oral ulceration: Aphthous-like ulcers in periodic syndromes. Oral Surg Oral Med Oral Pathol Oral Radiol Endod 2008;106:845–852.
6. Dalvi SR, Yildirim R, Yazici Y. Behcet's syndrome. Drugs 2012;72:2223–2241.
7. Mendes D, Correia M, Barbedo M, et al. Behcet's disease—A contemporary review. J Autoimmun 2009;32:178–188.
8. Sonis ST. Oral mucositis. Anticancer Drugs 2011; 22:607–612.
9. Shim YJ, Choi JH, Ahn HJ, Kwon JS. Effect of sodium lauryl sulfate on recurrent aphthous stomatitis: A randomized controlled clinical trial. Oral Dis 2012;18:655–660.
10. Xu F, Schillinger JA, Sternberg MR, et al. Seroprevalence and coinfection with herpes simplex virus type 1 and type 2 in the United States, 1988–1994. J Infect Dis 2002;185:1019–1024.

11. Woo SB, Challacombe SJ. Management of recurrent oral herpes simplex infections. Oral Surg Oral Med Oral Pathol Oral Radiol Endod 2007;103(suppl):S12e1–S12e18.

12. Griffiths PD. Burden of disease associated with human cytomegalovirus and prospects for elimination by universal immunisation. Lancet Infect Dis 2012;12:790–798.

13. Williams PM, Conklin RJ. Erythema multiforme: A review and contrast from Stevens-Johnson syndrome/toxic epidermal necrolysis. Dent Clin North Am 2005;49:67–76.

14. Leaute-Labreze C, Lamireau T, Chawki D, Maleville J, Taieb A. Diagnosis, classification, and management of erythema multiforme and Stevens-Johnson syndrome. Arch Dis Child 2000;83:347–352.

15. Ayangco L, Rogers RS 3rd. Oral manifestations of erythema multiforme. Dermatol Clin 2003;21:195–205.

16. Bastuji-Garin S, Fouchard N, Bertocchi M, Roujeau JC, Revuz J, Wolkenstein P. SCORTEN: A severity-of-illness score for toxic epidermal necrolysis. J Invest Dermatol 2000;115:149–153.

17. Lerman MA, Laudenbach J, Marty FM, Baden LR, Treister NS. Management of oral infections in cancer patients. Dent Clin North Am 2008;52:129–153.

18. Lee FY, Mossad SB, Adal KA. Pulmonary mucormycosis: The last 30 years. Arch Intern Med 1999;159:1301–1309.

19. Spellberg B, Edwards J Jr, Ibrahim A. Novel perspectives on mucormycosis: Pathophysiology, presentation, and management. Clin Microbiol Rev 2005;18:556–569.

20. Chan LS, Ahmed AR, Anhalt GJ, et al. The first international consensus on mucous membrane pemphigoid: Definition, diagnostic criteria, pathogenic factors, medical treatment, and prognostic indicators. Arch Dermatol 2002;138:370–379.

21. Scully C, Mignogna M. Oral mucosal disease: Pemphigus. Br J Oral Maxillofac Surg 2008;46:272–277.

22. Warnakulasuriya S, Johnson NW, van der Waal I. Nomenclature and classification of potentially malignant disorders of the oral mucosa. J Oral Pathol Med 2007;36:575–580.

23. Napier SS, Speight PM. Natural history of potentially malignant oral lesions and conditions: An overview of the literature. J Oral Pathol Med 2008;37:1–10.

24. Bagan J, Scully C, Jimenez Y, Martorell M. Proliferative verrucous leukoplakia: A concise update. Oral Dis 2010;16:328–332.

25. Brennan M, Migliorati CA, Lockhart PB, et al. Management of oral epithelial dysplasia: A review. Oral Surg Oral Med Oral Pathol Oral Radiol Endod 2007;103(suppl):S19e1–S19e12.

26. Al-Hashimi I, Schifter M, Lockhart PB, et al. Oral lichen planus and oral lichenoid lesions: Diagnostic and therapeutic considerations. Oral Surg Oral Med Oral Pathol Oral Radiol Endod 2007;103(suppl):S25e1–S25e12.

27. Schlosser BJ. Lichen planus and lichenoid reactions of the oral mucosa. Dermatol Ther 2010;23:251–267.

28. Au J, Patel D, Campbell JH. Oral lichen planus. Oral Maxillofac Surg Clin North Am 2013;25:93–100.

29. Habash-Bseiso DE, Yale SH, Glurich I, Goldberg JW. Serologic testing in connective tissue diseases. Clin Med Res 2005;3:190–193.

30. Brennan MT, Valerin MA, Napenas JJ, Lockhart PB. Oral manifestations of patients with lupus erythematosus. Dent Clin North Am 2005;49:127–141.

31. Schubert MM, Correa ME. Oral graft-versus-host disease. Dent Clin North Am 2008;52:79–109.

32. Lalla RV, Patton LL, Dongari-Bagtzoglou A. Oral candidiasis: Pathogenesis, clinical presentation, diagnosis and treatment strategies. J Calif Dent Assoc 2013;41:263–268.

33. Akpan A, Morgan R. Oral candidiasis. Postgrad Med J 2002;78:455–459.

34. Assimakopoulos D, Patrikakos G, Fotika C, Elisaf M. Benign migratory glossitis or geographic tongue: An enigmatic oral lesion. Am J Med 2002;113:751–755.

35. Woo SB. A Comprehensive Atlas and Text. Philadelphia: Saunders, 2012:58.

36. Armitage GC. Diagnosis of periodontal diseases. J Periodontol 2003;74:1237–1247.

37. Casiglia J, Woo SB, Ahmed AR. Oral involvement in autoimmune blistering diseases. Clin Dermatol 2001;19:737–741.

38. Holmstrup P, Westergaard J. Necrotizing periodontal disease. In: Lindhe J, Lang NP, Karring T (eds). Clinical Periodontology and Implant Dentistry, ed 5. Ames, Iowa: Blackwell Munksgaard, 2008:459–476.

39. Kataoka M, Kido J, Shinohara Y, Nagata T. Drug-induced gingival overgrowth—A review. Biol Pharm Bull 2005;28:1817–1821.

40. Seymour RA, Ellis JS, Thomason JM. Risk factors for drug-induced gingival overgrowth. J Clin Periodontol 2000;27:217–223.

41. Kaugars GE, Heise AP, Riley WT, Abbey LM, Svirsky JA. Oral melanotic macules. A review of 353 cases. Oral Surg Oral Med Oral Pathol 1993;76:59–61.

42. Carlos-Bregni R, Contreras E, Netto AC, et al. Oral melanoacanthoma and oral melanotic macule: A report of 8 cases, review of the literature, and immunohistochemical analysis. Med Oral Patol Oral Cir Bucal 2007;12:E374–E379.

43. Buchner A, Leider AS, Merrell PW, Carpenter WM. Melanocytic nevi of the oral mucosa: A clinicopathologic study of 130 cases from northern California. J Oral Pathol Med 1990;19:197–201.

44. Hicks MJ, Flaitz CM. Oral mucosal melanoma: Epidemiology and pathobiology. Oral Oncol 2000;36:152–169.

45. Mendenhall WM, Amdur RJ, Hinerman RW, Werning JW, Villaret DB, Mendenhall NP. Head and neck mucosal melanoma. Am J Clin Oncol 2005;28:626–630.

46. Sanchez-Pablo MA, Gonzalez-Garcia V, del Castillo-Rueda A. Study of total stimulated saliva flow and hyperpigmentation in the oral mucosa of patients diagnosed with hereditary hemochromatosis. Series of 25 cases. Med Oral Patol Oral Cir Bucal 2012;17:e45–e49.

47. Li CC, Malik SM, Blaeser BF, et al. Mucosal pigmentation caused by imatinib: Report of three cases. Head Neck Pathol 2012;6:290–295.

48. Cardoso CL, Rodrigues MT, Ferreira Junior O, Garlet GP, de Carvalho PS. Clinical concepts of dry socket. J Oral Maxillofac Surg 2010;68:1922–1932.

49. McKenna SJ. Dental management of patients with diabetes. Dent Clin North Am 2006;50:591–606.

50. Eversole R, Su L, ElMofty S. Benign fibro-osseous lesions of the craniofacial complex. A review. Head Neck Pathol 2008;2:177–202.

51. Colina M, La Corte R, De Leonardis F, Trotta F. Paget's disease of bone: A review. Rheumatol Int 2008; 28:1069–1075.

52. Hansen MF, Seton M, Merchant A. Osteosarcoma in Paget's disease of bone. J Bone Miner Res 2006; 21(suppl 2):P58–P63.

53. Peterson DE, Doerr W, Hovan A, et al. Osteoradionecrosis in cancer patients: The evidence base for treatment-dependent frequency, current management strategies, and future studies. Support Care Cancer 2010;18:1089–1098.

54. Nabil S, Samman N. Incidence and prevention of osteoradionecrosis after dental extraction in irradiated patients: A systematic review. Int J Oral Maxillofac Surg 2011;40:229–243.

55. Solomon DH, Mercer E, Woo SB, Avorn J, Schneeweiss S, Treister N. Defining the epidemiology of bisphosphonate-associated osteonecrosis of the jaw: Prior work and current challenges. Osteoporos Int 2013;24:237–244.

56. Kuhl S, Walter C, Acham S, Pfeffer R, Lambrecht JT. Bisphosphonate-related osteonecrosis of the jaws—A review. Oral Oncol 2012;48:938–947.

57. Almazrooa SA, Woo SB. Bisphosphonate and non-bisphosphonate-associated osteonecrosis of the jaw: A review. J Am Dent Assoc 2009;140:864–875.

58. Ruggiero SL, Dodson TB, Assael LA, Landesberg R, Marx RE, Mehrotra B. American Association of Oral and Maxillofacial Surgeons position paper on bisphosphonate-related osteonecrosis of the jaws—2009 update. J Oral Maxillofac Surg 2009; 67(5 suppl):2–12.

59. Mawardi H, Treister N, Richardson P, et al. Sinus tracts—An early sign of bisphosphonate-associated osteonecrosis of the jaw? J Oral Maxillofac Surg 2009;67:593–601.

60. Carlson ER, Basile JD. The role of surgical resection in the management of bisphosphonate-related osteonecrosis of the jaws. J Oral Maxillofac Surg 2009;67(5 suppl):85–95.

61. Epstein MS, Ephros HD, Epstein JB. Review of current literature and implications of RANKL inhibitors for oral health care providers [epub ahead of print 15 Aug 2012]. Oral Surg Oral Med Oral Pathol Oral Radiol doi:10.1016/j.oooo.2012.01.046.

62. Diz P, Lopez-Cedrun JL, Arenaz J, Scully C. Denosumab-related osteonecrosis of the jaw. J Am Dent Assoc 2012;143:981–984.

63. Hirshberg A, Shnaiderman-Shapiro A, Kaplan I, Berger R. Metastatic tumours to the oral cavity—Pathogenesis and analysis of 673 cases. Oral Oncol 2008;44:743–752.

64. Gupta A, Epstein JB, Sroussi H. Hyposalivation in elderly patients. J Can Dent Assoc 2006;72:841–846.

65. Fox PC, Busch KA, Baum BJ. Subjective reports of xerostomia and objective measures of salivary gland performance. J Am Dent Assoc 1987;115:581–584.

66. Chen A, Wai Y, Lee L, Lake S, Woo SB. Using the modified Schirmer test to measure mouth dryness: A preliminary study. J Am Dent Assoc 2005;136: 164–170.

67. Shiboski SC, Shiboski CH, Criswell L, et al. American College of Rheumatology classification criteria for Sjögren's syndrome: A data-driven, expert consensus approach in the Sjögren's International Collaborative Clinical Alliance cohort. Arthritis Care Res (Hoboken) 2012;64:475–487.

Index

immunosuppressive agents for, 264t
recurrent aphthous stomatitis, 263f,
    263–264
traumatic, 262
vesiculobullous disease as cause of,
    271f–272f, 271–272
viral infections as cause of, 267–269,
    268t–269t
Oral-systemic connections
description of, 54–57
overview of, 103–104
summary of, 116–117
Oropharyngeal cancers, 92
Osteitis deformans. *See* Paget disease of
    bone.
Osteoblast, 240
Osteoclasts, 241f
Osteocytes, 240
Osteomyelitis, 285
Osteonecrosis of the jaw
bisphosphonate-induced. *See*
    Bisphosphonate-induced
    osteonecrosis of the jaw.
denosumab as cause of, 250–251
drug-induced. *See* Drug-induced
    osteonecrosis of the jaw.
Osteopenia, 249–250, 253f
Osteopetrosis, 286
Osteoporosis
as aging process, 247
bone mineral density criteria for, 239, 240f
clinical definition of, 239
as clinical disease, 247
definition of, 239
dental care considerations, 238
dietary therapy for, 248–249
epidemiologic factors, 240, 242–243
fractures secondary to, 243, 243f–244f,
    247–249
hip fractures secondary to, 243f,
    248–249
incidence of, 248
mechanism of, 240, 241f
nutritional therapy for, 248–249
oral health affected by, 238
in postmenopausal women, 240
treatment of
    bisphosphonates, 243–245, 247
    calcium, 246
    denosumab, 245, 247, 288
    diet, 248–249
    fracture prevention as goal of, 243,
        243f

nutrition, 248–249
pharmacologic, 243–245, 247–248
raloxifene, 245, 247
recombinant human parathyroid
    hormone 1-34, 246–247
salmon calcitonin, 246
vitamin D, 246
Osteoprotegerin, 240, 241f
Osteoradionecrosis, 223t, 286
Outcome variables, 26
Overweight
body mass index criteria for, 158t
definition of, 157
global rates of, 159

P

P value, 46
Paget disease of bone, 286
Pain, oral
in drug-induced osteonecrosis of the
    jaw, 253
management of, 230
topical medications for, 264t
Pancreatic cancer, 96
Parafunctional habits, 272, 272f
Pemphigus vulgaris, 272, 272f
Periodic fever, aphthous stomatitis,
    pharyngitis, and adenitis syndrome,
    265
Periodontal disease. *See also* Gingivitis;
    Periodontitis.
breast cancer and, 91
burden of, 121–122
characteristics of, 108
cigarette smoking and, 166
coronary heart disease and, 14
description of, 107
destructive membranous, 279–280
diabetes mellitus and, 121–125,
    126b–129b
host-parasite interaction, 107
inflammation and, 114
in myelosuppressed patients, 232f
obesity and, 167t, 167–170, 169f
risk factors for, 135
systemic conditions and, 108–114
treatment of, 146–147
weight gain and, 177
Periodontal infections, 232, 232f
Periodontal inflammation
adverse pregnancy outcomes associated
    with, 207f
description of, 107–108, 111

Periodontal pathogenic bacteria, 62–63
Periodontal therapy
atherosclerotic cardiovascular disease
    affected by, 148–150
C-reactive protein concentrations
    affected by, 150t, 170
during pregnancy, 213–214
preterm birth affected by, 212t
Periodontitis. *See also* Periodontal
    disease.
animal studies of, 115t–116t
atherosclerotic cardiovascular disease
    and, 146, 152
atherothrombogenesis and, 143f
cardiovascular disease and, 110–113
C-reactive protein and, 110–111,
    140t–141t, 170
definition of, 144b
description of, 62, 79, 81, 107
diabetes mellitus and, 108–110
etiology of, 108
glycemic control affected by, 124–125,
    125f, 135
metabolic syndrome and, 169–170
obesity and, 167t, 167–170
pregnancy and, 113–114, 210–213
rates of, 122f
risk factors for, 145, 152
systemic diseases and, 144b
Periodontitis and vascular events, 148
Periopathogens, 142
Peritonitis, 115t
Peroxisome proliferator activator receptor
    gamma, 164
Personal standards, 42
Petechiae, 282
Peutz-Jeghers syndrome, 282
Pharyngeal cancer, 92, 93f
Phenytoin-induced gingival hyperplasia,
    278
Physical activity, 162
Pigmented lesions, 280–284
Pilocarpine, 290
Placental growth factor, 209
Plaque, dental
description of, 190
gingival hyperplasia caused by, 279
gingivitis caused by, 277
Plasma cell gingivitis, 277
Platelet aggregation, 142
Plausibility, of causation, 36
Pleiotropy, 30–32, 31f

Pneumonia
aspiration, 189, 191
community-acquired, 187–189
definition of, 187
health care-associated, 189
nosocomial, 189–190
nursing home-associated, 187, 190, 194
subtypes of, 187
ventilator-associated
antiseptics to prevent, 191–194, 192t
oral hygiene guidelines, 194–196
oral interventions to prevent, 191–194
prevalence of, 189
toothbrushing to prevent, 194
Polymorphonuclear leukocytes, 105, 109
Poorly healing extraction sockets, 284–285
Porphyromonas gingivalis, 66, 75, 93, 111, 113, 142, 205
Post hoc fallacy, 39
Postinflammatory hypermelanosis, 281
Prediabetes, 6, 134
Preeclampsia, 202
Pregnancy
adolescent, 214
adverse outcomes, oral infection correlation with
biologic plausibility of, 205–210, 207f
description of, 200–203
indirect pathway of, 209–210
periodontal inflammation, 207f
gestational diabetes, 160–161
gingival inflammation during, 204
granulomas during, 204, 205f
maternal weight gain in, 160
oral infections during, 200
periodontal health during, 200
periodontal therapy during, 213–214
periodontal tissues affected by, 203–205
periodontitis and, 113–114, 210–213
preterm birth, 201–203, 202f, 203b, 206, 210
sex steroids during, 203–204
Pregnancy gingivitis, 204
Preterm birth
C-reactive protein and, 206, 210
description of, 201–203, 202f, 203b
periodontal treatment effects on, 212t
Prevalence, 46

Prevalence-incidence bias, 21
Prevotella, 205
Primary bone diseases, 285–286
Probabilistic cause, 29
Progranulin, 170
Proinflammatory cytokines, 105, 111
Proliferative verrucous leukoplakia, 273
Prophylactic antibiotics
for artificial joints, 88–90
for infective endocarditis, 83–84, 85b–87b, 88t
Proportional hazards model, 45
Prostaglandin E$_2$, 105, 206
Protectin D1, 115t
Proteomics, 52
Pseudomembranous candidiasis, 234f, 234t, 275, 275f
Psoralen and ultraviolet A therapy, 231
Publication bias, 28b
Pulmonary aspiration, 74
Pulmonary diseases
oral cavity as reservoir for, 190–191
oral health effects on, 186
pneumonia. *See* Pneumonia.
Pyogenic granuloma, 204, 283, 283f
Pyostomatitis vegetans, 265

Q

Quackery, 39

R

Radiation therapy
hyposalivation caused by, 289
osteoradionecrosis induced by, 286
salivary gland damage caused by, 290
Raloxifene, 245, 247
Randomization, for controlling for confounding, 32
Randomized controlled trials, 16, 19–20, 215
Recall bias, 27
Receptor activator of NFκB ligand, 105, 240, 241f
Receptor for advanced glycation end products, 124f
Recombinant human parathyroid hormone 1-34, 246–247
Recurrent aphthous stomatitis, 263f, 263–264
Regularity of nature, 15
Relative risk, 19–20, 28–29, 46
Remodeling, of bone, 240
Residual confounding, 37, 46

Resolution, of inflammation, 114
Resolvin D1, 115t
Resolvin D2, 116t
Resolvin E1, 115t–116t
Response variables, 26
Restriction, for controlling for confounding, 32
Rhetorical tactics, 41–42
Rheumatoid arthritis, 163
Ribonucleases, 55
Ribosomal RNA, 62
Risk, 46
Risk factors
for atherosclerotic cardiovascular disease, 145
for bisphosphonate-induced osteonecrosis of the jaw, 287
for coronary heart disease, 5
definition of, 46
for obesity, 177f
for periodontal disease, 135
for periodontitis, 145, 152
Rutherford syndrome, 279

S

Saliva
antibiotics and, 81
biomarkers, 51, 51f, 54
composition of, 49
functions of, 289
hyposalivation, 289–290
proteins in, 49, 52
RNA species in, 49
xerostomia, 130, 224t, 289–290
Salivaomics
definition of, 50
immunomics, 53
metabolomics, 54
methylomics, 52–53
microbiome, 53–54
proteomics, 52
transcriptomics, 51–52
Salivary diagnostics
in current practice, 57
description of, 50–51
future of, 57
mechanism-based, 56, 56f
microvesicles in, 55
Salivary glands
description of, 49, 50f
hypofunction of, 224t
radiation therapy-induced damage to, 290